Computer Systems Experiences of Users with and without Disabilities

An Evaluation Guide for Professionals

REHABILITATION SCIENCE IN PRACTICE SERIES

Series Editors

Marcia J. Scherer, Ph.D.
President
Institute for Matching Person and Technology
Professor
Orthopaedics and Rehabilitation
University of Rochester Medical Center

Dave Muller, Ph.D.
Executive
Suffolk New College
Editor-in-Chief
Disability and Rehabilitation
Founding Editor
Aphasiology

Published Titles

Assistive Technology Assessment Handbook, *edited by Stefano Federici and Marcia J. Scherer*

Assistive Technology for Blindness and Low Vision, *Roberto Manduchi and Sri Kurniawan*

Computer Access for People with Disabilities: A Human Factors Approach, *Richard C. Simpson*

Computer Systems Experiences of Users with and without Disabilities: An Evaluation Guide for Professionals, *Simone Borsci, Maria Laura Mele, Masaaki Kurosu, and Stefano Federici*

Multiple Sclerosis Rehabilitation: From Impairment to Participation, *edited by Marcia Finlayson*

Paediatric Rehabilitation Engineering: From Disability to Possibility, *edited by Tom Chau and Jillian Fairley*

Quality of Life Technology Handbook, *Richard Schultz*

Forthcoming Titles

Ambient Assisted Living, *Nuno M. Garcia, Joel Jose P. C. Rodrigues, Dirk Christian Elias, and Miguel Sales Dias*

Devices for Mobility and Manipulation for People with Reduced Abilities, *Teodiano Bastos-Filho, Dinesh Kumar, and Sridhar Poosapadi Arjunan*

Neuroprosthetics: Principles and Applications, *Justin C. Sanchez*

Rehabilitation Goal Setting: Theory, Practice and Evidence, *Richard Siegert and William Levack*

Computer Systems Experiences of Users with and without Disabilities

An Evaluation Guide for Professionals

Simone Borsci

Masaaki Kurosu

Stefano Federici

Maria Laura Mele

Forewords by
Constantine Stephanidis and
Esteban Levialdi

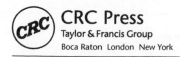

CRC Press
Taylor & Francis Group
Boca Raton London New York

CRC Press is an imprint of the
Taylor & Francis Group, an **informa** business

CRC Press
Taylor & Francis Group
6000 Broken Sound Parkway NW, Suite 300
Boca Raton, FL 33487-2742

First issued in paperback 2017

ISBN-13: 978-1-4665-1113-2 (hbk)
ISBN-13: 978-1-138-07348-7 (pbk)

Library of Congress Cataloging-in-Publication Data

Computer systems experiences of users with and without disabilities : an evaluation guide for professionals / authors, Simone Borsci, Masaaki Kurosu, Stefano Federici, Maria Laura Mele.
    pages cm -- (Rehabilitation science in practice series)
"A CRC title."
Includes bibliographical references and index.
ISBN 978-1-4665-1113-2 (hardcover : alk. paper)
    1. User interfaces (Computer systems)--Evaluation--Handbooks, manuals, etc. 2. Computers and people with disabilities--Handbooks, manuals, etc. I. Borsci, Simone, editor of compilation author.

QA76.9.U83C6594 2014
005.4'37--dc23
    2013018308

Visit the Taylor & Francis Web site at
http://www.taylorandfrancis.com

and the CRC Press Web site at
http://www.crcpress.com

Contents

Chapter 8 Evaluation Techniques, Applications, and Tools 193

8.1   Introduction 195
8.2   Inspection and Simulation Methods of the Expected
       Interaction 196
       8.2.1   Inspection of the Interaction 197
       8.2.2   Heuristic Evaluation 198
       8.2.3   Cognitive Walkthrough Method 200
       8.2.4   Task Analysis 202
       8.2.5   Summary of Inspection and Simulation Methods
                of the Expected Interaction 204
8.3   Qualitative and Subjective Measurements for Interaction
       Analysis 205
       8.3.1   Questionnaires and Psychometric Tools 206
       8.3.2   Interview 211
       8.3.3   Observation 213
       8.3.4   Diary 214
       8.3.5   Eye-Tracking Technologies and Biofeedback 214
                8.3.5.1   Biofeedback Usability and UX Testing ... 215
                8.3.5.2   Eye-Tracking Usability and UX Testing .. 216
       8.3.6   Summary of the Qualitative and Subjective
                Measurements for Interaction Analysis 218
8.4   Usability Testing and Analysis of Real Interaction 219
       8.4.1   Usability Testing 219
       8.4.2   Concurrent Thinking Aloud in Usability Testing ... 221
       8.4.3   Retrospective Thinking Aloud in Usability Testing . 224
       8.4.4   Alternative Verbal Protocols for Parallel Thinking
                and Partial Concurrent Thinking Aloud 225
       8.4.5   Remote Testing 227
       8.4.6   Summary of Usability Testing and the Analysis
                of Real User Interaction 229
8.5   Conclusion 230

References ....
Index ....

Foreword by Constantine Stephanidis

The advent of the information society has brought about a paradigm shift, whereby computers are conceived as everyday tools, available to anyone, anytime, anywhere. This shift has altered both parts of the human–computer interaction equation. On the one hand, computers are no longer just the machinery on our desks; they are also ubiquitous devices that we may use everywhere, i.e., at work, at home, on the go, in private and public spaces, and while engaged in a variety of activities. On the other hand, the user has long ago shifted from the archetypical young computer expert to a much wider population, including, for instance, children, teenagers, older users, technology-naive users, as well as users with disabilities. Therefore, it is now more crucial than ever before to design high-quality systems, ensuring an efficient, effective, and enjoyable interaction.

The myth of designing for the average user has collapsed and has been substituted by the reality of actually involving users in the design process in order to cater to the requirements of the broadest possible user population. To this end, and in the context of an iterative design process, the role of evaluation is central in acquiring the user's point of view and understanding the interaction experience. Recent evaluation approaches take into consideration not only the usability of an interactive system in terms of users' effectiveness, efficiency, and satisfaction, but also the overall user experience, considering how a user thinks and feels about using a system, before, during, and after use. It should be noted that an important factor affecting the usability and overall user experience of a system is its accessibility by diverse user groups with different cultural, educational, training, and employment background, novice and experienced computer users, the very young and the elderly, as well as people with different types of disabilities. As the authors of this book argue, accessibility, usability, and user experience have to be considered as three different perspectives on interaction, and any evaluator should assess these aspects in sequence in order to produce a complete interaction evaluation.

This book is addressed to professionals dealing with the design, implementation, and evaluation of interactive systems and to those who are interested in studying the topic of usability and user experience analysis. The book introduces a new evaluation model, the integrated model of interaction evaluation, aiming to equalize the roles of the design and the evaluation processes by considering them as two opposite and separate points of view toward reaching the same goal: a successful system. In summary, the book consists of eight chapters, providing the reader with all the necessary related literature and background information in order to comprehend the proposed model, discussing the need for an integrated model of interaction evaluation, presenting the model itself, and explaining the evaluation methods and techniques that can be used in the context of the proposed framework.

Besides being an excellent textbook, this highly recommended work makes for pleasant reading and equips usability and UX practitioners with a novel evaluation model that clearly defines the role of evaluators in the design process and drives them through a step-by-step process to assess interaction in any design life cycle. An important aspect of the model is that it takes into account a very much discussed, but unfortunately often partially implemented, component of usability and user experience, namely, accessibility.

Constantine Stephanidis
Professor, Department of Computer Science, University of Crete
Director, Institute of Computer Science—FORTH

Foreword by Esteban Levialdi

This book can be used in two different ways: (1) as a comprehensive description of the main features that identify how an information application can be evaluated, through accessibility, usability, and user experience (UX), and (2) how such features can be evaluated by means of a coordinated view based on an integrated model of intrasystemic evaluation called the integrated model of interaction evaluation (IMIE) by the authors. The nature of human–computer interaction is a complex one, essentially due to the difficulty in modeling user mindset, at least in a large number of cases.

This book starts with a comprehensive review, including an extensive list of references, of what has been achieved in the past (before 1980) in the study of human–computer interaction, a field that in most cases, cannot be anticipated and thus leads to errors that should be avoided. As the authors say, "interaction is gradually learned by doing," and this path should be as natural as possible in a well-designed system.

In order to enable evaluators to perform their tasks, a system should be analyzed through both an expert-based and a model-based approach. An interesting view, as reported in this book, is the idea that systems should be able to be used by any person–i.e., the design for all (DA) approach. This approach seems utopic, since impaired users should also be considered; the aging population, who have hearing problems and are vision impaired, and the number of disabled users are growing, and in order to eliminate the digital divide, such users should also be included.

In short, the designed systems need to be perceivable, operable, understandable, and robust. In this context, the UX must be integrated with accessibility and usability, and a number of international standards should be regularly updated to keep pace with the latest technology and different modes of triggering system functions should be made available.

The contents of this book focus on how accessibility, usability, and UX are defined as ISO international standards, how they can be evaluated, and what difficulties are encountered when analyzing the interaction dialogue between the user and his or her system, mostly through the interface. In fact, for the user, the application *is* the interface, since it is the only controlling component. In other words, accessibility refers to the openness of the system, while usability includes effectiveness (i.e., achieving one's goal), efficiency, satisfaction, freedom from risk (not losing any data), and context coverage (encompassing a wide scope).

From the software point of view, however, the quality depends on its scalability, efficiency, compatibility, usability, reliability, security, maintainability, and portability. As a reader may understand by looking at these two lists of properties (for usability from the user's point of view) and software quality itself, the system's evaluation is awkward. Therefore, standards that are incorporated within UX include users' emotions, beliefs, preferences, perceptions, physical and psychological responses, and behavior before, during, and after use.

The authors of this book introduce the term *psychotechnology* as "any technology that emulates, extends, amplifies, or modifies sensory motor, psychological, or cognitive functions of the user's mind." In short, they indicate the relationship between cognitive ergonomics (perception, attention, memory), the socioenvironmental system (between the technology and the user), and the socialization aspect (generally known as media technologies) of the human–computer interaction complex.

Extending the concept of psychotechnology, the authors refer to *biopsychotechnology,* which includes three different variables: hedonic (technologies that induce positive experiences, like joy of use), eudaimonic (technologies that help reach one's goal and that engage in self-actualizing experiences), and social/interpersonal (technologies that improve connectedness between individuals and groups).

One of the main points stressed in this book is the relationship between the evaluator and the designer, which must drive the intrasystemic dialogue within three nested spaces: the context of use, the shared aim, and the shared perspective (the outermost layer). The suggested interaction model (IMIE) considers a meta-evaluator that matches the problems detected by the evaluator and the user (false, missed, real problems), a user-driven evaluation process, and the intrasystemic dialogue containing subjective and objective dimensions.

As pointed out in the literature, the distance between the designer's and the user's mental model is the main source of difficulties and misunderstandings. In fact, IMIE evaluates the distance between these two models by considering the system evaluation, the subjective evaluation of interaction, and the user evaluation of the interaction quality. In order to perform a comprehensive evaluation, different techniques and methods can be employed for assessing accessibility, usability, and UX in a cascaded sequence. A number of issues must be considered, such as miscommunication (designers versus evaluators), so as to relay feedback to designers to improve their designs. There are also certain criteria for choosing the right users (including disabled ones) to perform controlled experiments, to precisely define the user's goals, and even to employ a time scale (before using, during use, and after having used the system to be evaluated).

In conclusion, this book is a gold mine for understanding accessibility, usability and UX of information systems, both in qualitative and quantitative terms. This is not the only positive feature of the book, since it may also be used to define and design a controlled experiment with a number of methods to evaluate both the system and, particularly, the interaction quality between the user and the system itself.

Esteban Levialdi
IEEE Life Fellow
Head of the Usability and Accessibility Lab
Sapienza University of Rome

Preface

When we interact with a technological system, each of our senses is somehow engaged in a particular kind of communication. This communication forms the basis for a dialogue between person and technology (intrasystemic dialogue), that is to say, a dynamic relationship among three components: (i) the designer's mental model, which generates the conceptual system model of the interface; (ii) the user's mental model; and (iii) the image of the system (Norman, 1983, 1988).

In this book, we investigate the complexity of the intrasystemic dialogue between person and technology by focusing on both the evaluator's and the user's perspectives. We choose to follow this holistic approach to create an integrated model of interaction evaluation (IMIE) that is adequate to distinguish clearly (but that does not separate) the evaluator's role from the designer's, thus providing an evaluation process that is able to consider all the different dimensions of the interaction.

As Steve Krug claims in his most famous work *Don't Make Me Think*, a user has a good interaction experience only when the interface is "self-evident" (2000, p. 11)—that is, when the user does not have to expend effort in perceiving the interface. The implementation of a self-evident interface should be considered one of the most important issues to be solved when it comes to creating a good system, i.e., a good architecture of information. Therefore, Krug's assumption strongly relates only to the designer perspective and can be epitomized as "the better the system works, the better the interaction will be." However, even though a well-designed interface can be achieved only by considering the properties of the object, the evaluation process also needs to take into account other dimensions of the interaction. In particular, since the goal of the evaluation process is to measure the human–computer interaction (HCI), the user's point of view somehow needs to be integrated into the evaluation methodologies.

Our objective differs from Krug's. Krug intends to provide developers with the tools for creating successful systems: he expresses the success of a system using the metaphor of good navigation or of navigation without barriers, and this kind of navigation corresponds, according to his approach, to his motto "don't make me think." With this book, we do not aim to provide tools for system development; instead, we want to provide tools for an evaluation of the interaction that even takes into account "what the user thinks" about the system, because, from our point of view, this constitutes an essential element. From Krug's perspective, the user "should not think" since the developer should already have thought about the possible barriers that could occur during the interaction. Conversely, from our perspective, the simulation carried out by the developers during the design process cannot alone be enough to create a fully accessible and usable system. We claim that the key factors for developing a usable and accessible interface are (i) a well-planned assessment process and (ii) a harmonized and equalized relationship between evaluator and designer during the life cycle. For this reason, this book is not only concerned with the developer's perspective, but it also takes into account all the actors who are involved in the evaluation process according to our integrated model of interaction evaluation: the expert evaluators—who are supposed to detect the barriers that usually prevent the interaction; the users—who can estimate the extent to which a detected barrier actually prevents their navigation; and the coordinator of the evaluation—who is supposed to integrate the results of the expert-based tests with those of the user-based ones by performing an evaluation of the evaluation.

Rather than providing the tools for developing a good system where the user "should not think," in this book we propose an evaluation process that is able to assess the users' satisfaction and experience with a developed system. Given that users should be called to judge the system with which they are interacting, we shall focus on the user, who can be considered as someone who thinks about the system. In particular, we shall describe a user-driven process to observe the user's behavior during his or her actual interaction with the system. Giving back to users their point of view on the system, we let the users' thoughts offer valuable information on the quality of the interaction.

The perspective and the models shown in this book are a new synthesis in the HCI field, and they are able to distinguish and integrate the evaluator's and the designer's perspectives in the evaluation process. Moreover, our work is based on three fundamental pillars: the interaction between designers and evaluators, an integrated evaluation, and the involvement of disabled users in the assessment cohort. The first pillar is built on the fact that to achieve the aims of "design for all and user interfaces for all" (Stephanidis, 1995, 2001), designers and evaluators should work together iteratively using a well-planned and integrated methodology that guarantees a successful dialogue between device and user. The product of this collaboration is a technology with a certain level of functioning and capacity, which facilitates users' interaction: the more the functioning of the technology is perceived and experienced by users to be accessible and usable, the more the technology can be considered to be an intrasystemic solution. We call the outcome of this process of collaboration between designers and evaluators *psychotechnology,* by which we mean a technology that plays an active role in the context of use by emulating, extending, amplifying, and modifying the cognitive functions of the users involved in the interaction (Federici et al., 2011; Chapter 3). The second pillar highlights the fact that any assessment process has to help designers to include the users' perspective in their mental model. Therefore, the evaluator should act as a mediator between designer and user by analyzing the dialogue between user and technology through a set of integrated evaluation methods. The aim of these integrated evaluation methods is to analyze all the possible variables that could affect the users' experience of the interaction and to report to and discuss with designers how to transform a technology into a psychotechnology (Chapters 4 and 5). The last pillar of our work is based on the fact that any evaluation cannot be considered as a complete process without the involvement of users with disabilities in the assessment cohort. In fact, the analysis of the intrasystemic dialogue carried out by involving users with a disability is a necessary condition for measuring the interaction between people and technologies in all its objective and subjective aspects by representing the whole possible variety of the human functioning (Chapter 6).

This book consists of eight chapters that aim to drive professionals in usability and user experience (UX) analysis to rethink and reorganize their perspective about the assessment of interaction. Moreover, it aims to help designers, manufacturers of technological products, as well as laypeople to understand what an evaluation is, the complexity of an evaluation, and the importance of assessment for the success of a product. In tune with this attempt to drive the reader through complex topics such as the interaction assessment, we focus, in collaboration with other experts, on specific sections (boxes) in which some of the topics presented in this book are discussed in depth and examples are given.

The eight chapters are organized in ascending order from the theoretic to the pragmatic issues of an HCI assessment by moving from the historical and theoretical background to the management of the assessment data and the application of evaluation techniques, as follows:

- *Chapter 1: Brief History of Human–Computer Interaction.* This chapter discusses the historical evolution of HCI and the most important models of interaction evaluation. Starting from an overview of how hardware and software have changed over time, from the 1960s onward, we conclude by discussing some of the latest ideas about the interaction between user and technology—ideas that have brought a significant increase in the development of specific evaluation techniques based on innovative aims and theoretical models. So far, practitioners have not provided the basis for defining a uniform interaction evaluation methodology nor have researchers agreed on standard tools for evaluating and comparing usability evaluation methods. In light of our historical analysis, we first point out how single evaluation techniques lack the possibility of catching the multidimensional aspects of usability, and second, as a consequence, we show the need for an integrated and comparable methodology in order to include the evaluation possibilities of all the different interaction evaluation methods.
- *Chapter 2: Defining Usability, Accessibility, and User Experience.* This chapter aims to present the definitions of accessibility, usability, and UX provided throughout the evolution in the field of HCI. We discuss the international rules of interaction, starting from a historical overview of the different definitions of accessibility and usability. On the basis of these international standards, the usability concept emerges as strongly linked to the accessibility one; first, because, from the evaluation point of view, it is often difficult to distinguish among interaction problems due to usability or accessibility issues and, second, because access and use are hierarchically related. Finally, we discuss UX as a new and evolving concept of HCI. As ISO 9241-210 (2010) suggests, UX is strongly linked to usability and represents the subjective perspective of the interaction system. In fact, as our analysis shows, the current international debate is moving toward a unified standard in which accessibility, usability, and UX concepts will be clearly redefined to highlight their relationships and measurements. Moreover, we propose that users' perception of their interaction with a product (UX) is a dependent variable, based on the access to the interface

(accessibility) and on the use and the navigation of the technology and its contents (usability). Therefore, accessibility, usability, and UX should be considered as three different perspectives of the interaction, and any evaluator should assess these aspects in a hierarchical sequence in order to evaluate interaction completely.

- *Chapter 3: Why We Should Be Talking about Psychotechnologies for Socialization, Not Just Websites.* This chapter discusses the evolution of media and communication technologies in terms of the extension of human psychological abilities and participation opportunities. The discussion underlines how new developments and the success of communication technologies meet psychosocial users' needs (e.g., belongingness, esteem, and self-actualization), fostering direct user participation in the communication process and extending the network of socialization and participation opportunities. We propose the use of the term "psychotechnology for socialization," which replaces the classic "media and communication technology," and we also propose a new classification in which psychotechnologies are not only new kinds of technologies but are also a new user-driven adaptation, integration, and use of common technologies. A psychotechnology is presented as any technological product developed and assessed as an intrasystemic solution that can both facilitate and drive the dialogue between user and device in a specific context of use.
- *Chapter 4: Equalizing the Relationship between Design and Evaluation.* This chapter analyzes the relationship between the design and evaluation processes during the development of a product. We use the psychotechnological construct for showing how important it is to equalize, and concurrently discriminate between, the role of the designers and the role of the evaluators in the product life cycle. We suggest that designers and evaluators, from their individual observation poles of interaction, should share a holistic common perspective in which the components of the interaction, as entities in an intrasystemic dialogue (technology and user), have a concurrent role in defining the interaction experience. We describe psychotechnology as the outcome of the dynamic and reciprocal causation among the components of the interaction system—the technological object and its functioning, the user and his or her subjective experience of the interaction, the environment of use, and the role of this context in the dynamics of the interaction—that cannot be reduced to the device and its interface functioning per se. Finally, we describe the evaluators' role in the product life cycle by harmonizing it with and equalizing it to the role of the designers.
- *Chapter 5: Why We Need an Integrated Model of Interaction Evaluation.* This chapter presents and discusses the IMIE. We define an interaction problem as an interruption in the communication flow between the user and one or more elements of the interface. This gap concerns either the execution of the user action or the feedback of the product, and it can be due to an objective error (machine error) or a subjective error (a difficulty of the user in executing his or her action in the interface or in correctly understanding the feedback provided by the system). In light of this, we describe the

interaction evaluation as the measure of the distance between the developer's and the user's mental models. This distance can be measured only by introducing another external mental model—that of the evaluator. After defining this mental model, we propose that a product be evaluated from two perspectives: (i) objectively, that is, from the perspective of measuring the accessibility, usability, and satisfaction generated by the developer's mental model; and (ii) subjectively, that is, from the perspective of measuring the accessibility and usability of, and satisfaction with, the product in the context of use. Finally, we present an IMIE together with the variables that an evaluator has to take into account in the assessment decision process.

- *Chapter 6: Why Understanding Disabled Users' Experience Matters.* By following the psychotechnology construct and the IMIE, this chapter proposes a wide accessibility approach in which accessibility is considered not as a special need that has to be measured by particular users, but as one of the main variables that an evaluator has to consider for an overall testing of the interaction. Moreover, we propose that the involvement of users with disabilities in the design and assessment of an interaction is a necessary condition. Since disability has to be considered as one way of functioning among the infinite possibilities of human functioning, an evaluator should include people with different abilities when selecting a sample of users. If the aim of evaluators is to support designers in transforming a technology into a psychotechnology, concurrently promoting the goal of the "user interface for all," then evaluators have to gather reliable and generalizable evaluation data. An evaluator can achieve this goal only by testing a large spectrum of human functioning and by including in the sample a wide range of user behavior. In light of this, we discuss the concept of representativeness of the overall population and how the evaluator may invest his or her budget and select a sample of users in the most productive manner. Finally, in order to support an evaluator's selection of interaction test participants, we present a user testing decision flow mechanism, and, on the basis of this, we suggest how practitioners may select people with and without disability for the assessment and monitoring of the sample representativeness of the overall population.
- *Chapter 7: How You Can Set Up and Perform an Interaction Evaluation: Rules and Methods.* This chapter aims to present the way in which an evaluator can set up and manage an IMIE to assess usability and the UX. By moving from the commonsense perspective, this chapter discusses what an evaluation is, in terms of measurements and criteria, in line with international standards. First, we distinguish between interaction assessments on the basis of whether the product has long- or short-term use, and then we define and discuss the main aspects that an evaluator has to take into account when analyzing the UX: the *Kansei* (emotional or affective aspects in Japanese), the quality traits, and the meaningfulness of the product. In line with this analysis, we present an innovative synoptic table that represents and organizes the most common evaluation techniques and measures of the UX and usability. Moreover, we discuss how the evaluator can

organize and use the data obtained using the different techniques by using different approaches to evaluation data management. In particular, we explain how to manage the user testing data and how to determine the number of problems discovered by a sample of users by means of the "grounded procedure" (Borsci et al., 2013), a specific process created for extending the five-user assumption.

- *Chapter 8: Evaluation Techniques, Applications, and Tools.* This chapter aims to present a set of the most common evaluation techniques and their use in the framework of the IMIE. We start by discussing the inspection and simulation methods of the expected interaction (heuristics analysis, cognitive walkthrough, etc.), which allow a practitioner to inspect the product, without the involvement of users, by defining the gaps in the system and the errors in the product functioning. Furthermore, we present qualitative methods and subjective measurements of the interaction (questionnaire and psychometric tools, interview, eye-tracker and biofeedback analysis, etc.), which allow evaluators to observe users' reactions to the problems that they experienced while interacting with a technology. Finally, we discuss the usability testing methods and the analysis of real interaction (thinking aloud, remote testing, etc.), which are an essential step in any evaluation to assess how the functioning of the product is perceived by the user. For all the techniques discussed in this chapter, we show how it is possible to involve users with disabilities in the assessment by specific adapted tools and methods, such as partial concurrent thinking aloud (Federici et al., 2010a,b).

REFERENCES

Borsci, S., Macredie, R. D., Barnett, J., Martin, J., Kuljis, J., and Young, T. (Accepted on July 22, 2013). *Reviewing and Extending the Five–User Assumption: A Grounded Procedure for Interaction Evaluation. ACM Transactions on Computer-Human Interaction (TOCHI).*

Federici, S., Borsci, S., and Mele, M. L. (2010a). Usability evaluation with screen reader users: A video presentation of the PCTA's experimental setting and rules. *Cognitive Processing, 11*(3), 285-288. doi:10.1007/s10339-010-0365-9.

Federici, S., Borsci, S., and Stamerra, G. (2010b). Web usability evaluation with screen reader users: Implementation of the partial concurrent thinking aloud technique. *Cognitive Processing, 11*(3), 263-272. doi:10.1007/s10339-009-0347-y.

Federici, S., Corradi, F., Mele, M. L., and Miesenberger, K. (2011). From cognitive ergonomist to psychotechnologist: A new professional profile in a multidisciplinary team in a centre for technical aids. In G. J. Gelderblom, M. Soede, L. Adriaens, and K. Miesenberger (Eds.), *Everyday Technology for Independence and Care: AAATE 2011* (Vol. 29, pp. 1178–1184). Amsterdam, the Netherlands: IOS Press. doi:10.3233/978-1-60750-814-4-1178.

ISO 9241-210:2010. Ergonomics of human–system interaction—Part 210: Human-centred design for interactive systems. International Organization for Standardization (ISO), Geneva, Switzerland.

Krug, S. (2000). *Don't Make Me Think! A Common Sense Approach to Web Usability.* Indianapolis, IN: New Riders.

Norman, D. A. (1983). Some observations on mental models. In D. Gentner and A. L. Steven (Eds.), *Mental Models* (pp. 7–14). Hillsdale, NJ: Lawrence Erlbaum Associates.

Norman, D. A. (1988). *The Psychology of Everyday Things.* New York: Basic Books.

Stephanidis, C. (1995). Towards user interfaces for all: Some critical issues. In K. O. Yuichiro Anzai and M. Hirohiko (Eds.), *Advances in Human Factors/Ergonomics* (Vol. 20, pp. 137–142). Amsterdam, the Netherlands: Elsevier. doi:10.1016/s0921-2647(06)80024-9.

Stephanidis, C. (2001). User interfaces for all: New perspectives into human–computer interaction. In C. Stephanidis (Ed.), *User Interfaces for All: Concepts, Methods, and Tools* (pp. 3–17). Mahwah, NJ: Lawrence Erlbaum Associates.

Acknowledgments

Sincere thanks go to the authors of the focus sections (boxes)—Massimo Capponi, Maria Laura De Filippis, Giuseppe Liotta, Yousri Marzouki, Fabio Meloni, and Giuseppe Riva—whose contributions have enriched several of the topics discussed in the book. Special thanks go to the publisher, Taylor & Francis Group, for handling this project competently and for supporting the long process of drafting and revising the work. Special thanks also go to the many peer reviewers of the book, who have played a valuable role by guaranteeing the scientific nature and validity of the book.

Authors

Simone Borsci, PhD, is a user experience researcher and analyst with more than ten years of experience in human computer/artifact interaction assessment. He holds a PhD in cognitive psychology from the Sapienza University of Rome and currently works as a researcher at Brunel University of London in the MATCH and MATCH+ projects. His research is focused on different aspects of interaction: the user experience evaluation of interfaces and artifacts, the user preference analysis before and after use, the application of estimation models for determining an optimized sample size for an evaluation test, and the matching between assistive technologies/medical devices and users' needs. He is a member of the CognitiveLab research team at the University of Perugia, Italy. He is also an author or a contributor of more than 30 publications on human–computer interaction (HCI) and user experience (UX) assessment.

Masaaki Kurosu, MA, is a professor at the Open University of Japan. He is also the president of Human-Centered Design Network in Japan. Based on his experience as a usability professional in industry and academia, he proposed the concept of user engineering and the idea of artifact development analysis as well as the new concept of experience engineering. Before joining the National Institute of Multimedia Education that was consolidated to the Open University of Japan in 2009, he was a professor at the Faculty of Informatics of Shizuoka University. Prior to this, he was working at the design center of Hitachi Ltd. and at the Central Research Institute. Professor Masaaki received his MA in psychology from Waseda University. He served as a conference chair in many international conferences and is an author or a contributor of more than 40 books.

Stefano Federici, PhD, is a psychologist. He currently serves as a professor of general psychology and the psychology of disability at the University of Perugia, Italy. He is a member of the editorial board of *Disability and Rehabilitation: Assistive Technology* and *Cognitive Processing* as well as of the Scientific Committee of the International Conference on Space Cognition. He has authored more than 150 international and national publications on cognitive psychology, psychotechnology, disability, sexuality and disability, and usability. He has recently edited with Marcia J. Scherer, a leader in the field of assistive technology assessment, *The Assistive Technology Assessment Handbook*, a cross-cultural handbook that includes contributions from leading experts across five continents. He currently leads the CognitiveLab research team at the University of Perugia.

Maria Laura Mele, PhD, is a psychologist who earned her PhD in cognitive, physiological, and personality psychology from the Interuniversity Center for Research on Cognitive Processing in Natural and Artificial Systems (ECoNA) of the Sapienza University of Rome. Her main research topics are focused on usability and user experience of visual and sonified human–computer interfaces, with a focus on both implicit and explicit cognitive components involved in human interaction processes. She is currently a member of the CognitiveLab research team at the University of Perugia.

Contributors

Massimo Capponi
Department of Human Science and
  Education
University of Perugia
Perugia, Italy

Maria Laura De Filippis
Institute for Bioengineering
Brunel University
Middlesex, United Kingdom

Giuseppe Liotta
Department of Computer Engineering
University of Perugia
Perugia, Italy

Yousri Marzouki
Cognitive Psychology Laboratory
Aix-Marseille University
and
National Center for Scientific Research
Marseille, France

Fabio Meloni
Department of Human Science and
  Education
University of Perugia
Perugia Italy

Giuseppe Riva
ICE-NET Lab
Università Cattolica
and
ATN-P Lab
Istituto Auxologico
Milan, Italy

1 Brief History of Human–Computer Interaction

1.1 HISTORICAL PROGRESS OF EVALUATION MODELS IN HUMAN–COMPUTER INTERACTION SCIENCE

The main idea of this historical review about human–computer interaction (HCI) models is that technology (considered as *téchnê*) has to be understood as an extension of human abilities. Derrick De Kerckhove, director of the Marshal McLuhan Programme in Culture and Technologies, claims that technologies are a "second skin" (1995) able to modify the human mind and extend the senses. In order to understand this concept, we first need to consider that in today's society interactions between humans and systems have become daily actions. In this kind of society, defined as "e-societies," or "information and knowledge society" (Bindé, 2005), people consider access to and use of information as important goods. Second, we must also consider that each dialogue between users and computers is mediated by an interface that uses graphic elements, affordances (Gibson, 1979), and relations between elements. These interfaces indicate to users the actions they should perform in order to achieve a goal. In this sense, the technological product (i.e., the interface) is not only a "means" for communication, but, to a certain extent, also becomes an interlocutor for the user. In order to achieve their goals, users are forced to adapt their skills to the technologies they are dealing with and therefore are also forced to extend and partially change their abilities, transforming the technologies into a "second skin." Without any intent of reductionism, we may consider De Kerckhove's idea of technology as a second skin to be an extreme extension of the distributed cognition concept (Hutchins, 1980, 1995), an extension that is well justified by the extreme relation between human and technology in today's societies. Edwin Hutchins (2001), professor of cognitive science at the University of California, describes the concept of distributed cognition as

> a framework for thinking about cognition which seeks to understand how the cognitive properties of aggregates emerge from the interactions of component parts. It can be applied to cognitive systems at many levels of complexity, from areas of an individual brain to communities of interacting persons. Distributed cognition is sometimes construed as a special kind of cognition that occurs when people are in interaction with one another or with material artifacts. This is only partly correct. Rather than being a kind of cognition, distributed cognition is a manner of thinking about cognition that permits one to examine the relationships between what is in the mind and the world the mind is in. When applied to groups of persons, distributed cognition provides a language for cognitive processes that are distributed across the members of a social group, between people and their material environments, and through time. It attempts

to use an understanding of the social, cultural, and material context of cognitive practices to constrain models of cognitive processes within and among individual minds. (Hutchins, 2001, pp. 2068–2072)

In an information society, the relationship between human and material artifacts (which, in our case, are information and communication technologies [ICTs]) is a wide and pervasive process that changes the way information is accessed and used; indeed, these external relations become internal and symbolic, thus changing users' cognitive processes. As Hutchins (2001) states:

> The notion that cognitive artifacts amplify the cognition of the artifact user is fairly commonplace. If one focuses on the products of cognitive activity, cognitive artifacts do seem to amplify human abilities. A calculator seems to amplify one's ability to do arithmetic, writing down something one wants to remember seems to amplify one's memory. [...] When I remember something by writing it down and reading it later, my memory has not been amplified. Rather, I am using a different set of functional skills to do the memory task. Cognitive artifacts are involved in a process of organizing functional skills into cognitive functional systems. (Hutchins, 2001, pp. 2068–2072)

Hutchins, together with his colleagues at the University of California, James Hollan and David Krish (2000), claims that distributed cognition has a deep impact on HCI:

> Whereas traditional views look for cognitive events in the manipulation of symbols inside individual actors, distributed cognition looks for a broader class of cognitive events and does not expect all such events to be encompassed by the skin or skull of an individual [...] The field of human-computer interaction could certainly benefit from an integrated research framework [...] Taking a distributed cognition perspective radically alters the way we look at human-computer interaction. Traditional information processing psychology posits a gulf between inside and outside and then "bridges" this gulf with transduction processes that convert external events into internal symbolic representations [...] Distributed cognition does not posit a gulf between "cognitive" processes and an "external" world, so it does not attempt to show how such a gulf could be bridged. (Hollan et al., 2000, pp. 175–193)

We will use the idea of technology as a second skin as a conceptual background for our analysis, by endorsing a perspective in which the interaction is a pervasive process of distributed cognition. The second-skin metaphor suggests that any user interacting with any technology is forced into some kind of adaptation that results into a modification of the same user's cognitive processes. However, each different user adapts to the technology in a different way, which reflects in different abilities of learning the system, quality and time of performances, number of problems, and solutions found during the interaction. The users' adaptation is the core cognitive process of the relation between human and technology because it is necessary to grant a satisfactory dialogue, together with two technological conditions: first, the access to the system (accessibility) and second, the opportunity to learn and use the system in a effective way (usability).

The relation between the users' adaptation process and the technological conditions (i.e., access and use) has changed due to the evolution of the hardware and software technology.

By following these evolutionary changeovers, we divide the historical evolution of HCI into four periods, considered as the process in which the conditions for the dialogue between humans and computers have grown up:

- The first period (1950–1963), where the end user of software does not yet exist, because the programmer who creates the interface is, at the same time, the user of the software. In this period, the use of systems is only allowed to an elite (e.g., programmers, specialized, and operators) and the interaction is not through a visual interface, but directly with the functioning of the program through a set of textual commands.
- The second period (1963–1984), in which there is still no distinction between users and programmers, is characterized by an evolution of systems and models of interaction.
- The third period (1984–1998), in which the diffusion of personal computers and the Internet, with the consequent distinction between users and programmers, opens accessibility and usability issues due to increasing demand by nonexpert users to access and use the information on the World Wide Web and to manipulate interfaces.
- The fourth period (since 1998), in which the Web Accessibility Initiative (WAI) of the World Wide Web Consortium (W3C) has released the Web Content Accessibility Guidelines (WCAG), opening up the possibility for designers to share a common framework for developing an accessible user interface. At the same time, in this period, the improvement of technology and the diffusion of computers and mobile devices have extended the roles of the subjects in interaction: the passive customer has become a proactive user. The end users are no longer passive observers of the information on the web, from the side; they can decide to become designers themselves (at least to some extent), as happened with web 2.0 and 3.0 (see for a review, Lassila and Hendler, 2007; O'Reilly, 2007). They can decide to be even more visible and reachable in the virtual and the real world, as has happened through the diffusion of social networks and the use of mobile technologies. This everyday perfusion of hi-tech has led to an extension of De Kerckhove's idea of technology as a second skin, resulting in a world in which the adaptation of people to devices and interfaces has become one of the most important socialization processes in human life.

1.1.1 First Period, from 1950 to 1963: The Programmer Is the User

Since the end of the 1950s, technological and computer tools have been created with specific functions determined by different ideal interaction models elaborated by programmers. The fundamental goal was to get either better calculation performances or better machine functions, with a greater setup for the management and control of technology: the operator/user had to adapt to the formal rules of the system introduced by the designers into the technology, whether the system was a computing device, or an appliance, or industrial machinery.

The operator/user could control the technology with a panel meant to be used only for two operations: the correction of the machinery's functions (i.e., program debugging) and the input of command lines into the system. The interaction was built up following the ideas of the command line interface (CLI). The operator/user was forced to learn the commands and to input them via the keyboard. The interface was substantially textual, and, usually, the interaction was limited to inserting data into the system.

In the early 1960s, the need of a new interaction model started to grow stronger among researchers. This new need was the consequence of the introduction of new hardware elements (Dix et al., 2004) and a redefinition of the industrial operators. Indeed, in this period, the operators of industrial technological products were no longer considered as mere objects embedded in the assembly process but started to be considered as consumers of the production process. This historical step marked the passage from operators to users.

These new perspectives developed the need to improve the conditions of interactive exchange. People were progressively overloaded by physical work. The users interacted with machinery that asked for instructions and transmitted information to the development process. The ergonomic attention moved from a muscular to a perceptive load.

Users sitting in front of radar screens, dashboards, or command panels were involved in new interactions with technology, and, as a consequence, their cognitive workloads were much heavier: attention decreased, while detection time of the signal and answer time increased. In this new scenario, reduction of the number of errors during interaction with the system (especially in a work environment) became a major issue for HCI researchers and practitioners. With the progressive automation of the work process, an ever larger proportion of information, procedures, strategies, and solutions started to be elaborated through machines. In this way, operators were released from a large part of their workload (which was undertaken by the machine) and could better focus on complex cognitive tasks. As a consequence, in the 1960s, ergonomic studies switched their attention from the physical workload and work environment to its psychological and cognitive aspects.

In summary, in this period, the main problem of the relation between users and technology was that only a restricted number of users could access and use the technology. In fact, the interaction was the exclusive right of those elite (i.e., operators) who had been trained and were skilled in nonnatural languages (i.e., programming languages) for interacting with systems in a satisfactory and productive way. In this sense, the accessibility and usability were external conditions of the systems, because all the systems were accessible and usable only to those users that had learned the command lines by adapting to the programming languages; the more a user was skilled in the use of CLI, the more she or he could access and use the system.

1.1.2 Second Period, from 1963 to 1984: Evolution of Human–Computer Interaction Models

In 1963, at the Massachusetts Institute of Technology, Ivan Edward Sutherland developed the first interactive graphical user interface (GUI), Sketchpad. This system consisted of the direct manipulation of graphic objects through an optic pen with which the user could create and move graphic elements, receive graphic feedback, and modify the interface setup (Sutherland, 1964). The idea of direct manipulation contributed to overtaking the CLI and opening new scenarios for HCI, as Sutherland explains: "The Sketchpad system, by eliminating typed statements (except for legends) in favor of line drawings, opens up a new area of man-machine communication" (2003, p. 507).

Graphic interface development changed the relation between users and technology. In fact, the operators manipulating the graphic elements could interact with a system by knowing only the program command lines they needed. In light of this, the concept of manipulation, by reducing the specialized knowledge needed for the interaction, creates a distinction between the programmer (i.e., who creates or manipulates the programming language) and the user (i.e., who interacts only by manipulating the elements of the interface). In 1983, Ben Shneiderman, professor of computer science at the Human–Computer Interaction Laboratory at the University of Maryland, defined the main features of direct interface manipulation in graphic interface:

- "Continuous representation of the object of interest.
- Physical actions (movement and selection by mouse, joystick, touch screen, etc.) or labeled button presses instead of complex syntax.
- Rapid, incremental, reversible operations whose impact on the object of interest is immediately visible.
- Layered or spiral approach to learning that permits usage with minimal knowledge. Novices can learn a modest and useful set of commands, which they can exercise till they become an "expert" at level 1 of the system. After obtaining reinforcing feedback from successful operation, users can gracefully expand their knowledge of features and gain fluency" (Shneiderman, 1983, p. 64; see also Box 1.1).

These principles were further developed by Hutchins et al. (1985). They started from the idea that the interaction quality must be linked to the affordance concept (Gibson, 1979). Affordances are to be understood as all the latent "action possibilities" in the environment that are objectively measurable and independent from the subject's ability to recognize them. Even though affordances are not dependent on the subject's recognition, they are still always related to the actors and their skills. James Gibson's affordance concept was developed to explain subjects' interactions in physical environments, while Hutchins, Hollan, and Norman extended its range to virtual environments, also taking into consideration, along with physical capabilities, other aspects related to HCI such as actors' goals, plans, values, beliefs, and past experiences.

An interface, as a place of functions and variables, is designed for operating on a system, starting from the user inputs (click/query). In a simple virtual environment, users should be able to immediately elaborate messages or recall useful knowledge from their memory.

BOX 1.1   A BRIEF INTRODUCTION TO THE VISUALIZATION OF NETWORKED DATA SETS

GIUSEPPE LIOTTA

INTRODUCTION

Information visualization is a discipline of computer science and engineering whose goal is to design and develop systems and methods to discover, analyze, query, and communicate data by means of diagrams and layouts of various types. In this note, we briefly highlight some of the characteristics of the particularly vibrant area of information visualization with particular attention to network visualization, which is widely used to mine information in large data sets.

One of the main characteristics of the large amount of data coming from today's life and applications is in fact their strong relational nature. Data are conveniently modeled as networks (also called graphs), consisting of entities and their connections (i.e., relationships between pairs of entities). Examples include social networks, computer networks, biological networks, and financial activity networks. These networks are typically (1) extremely large and complex, (2) heterogeneous both in their semantic and in their topological properties, and (3) uncertain and dynamic. Analyzing them with the purpose of rapidly gaining knowledge is therefore a hard task that typically requires intensive HCIs. In this scenario, there is broad consensus that algorithms and software systems for the visual analysis of networks are crucial to support humans in better understanding large data sets, arising from complex phenomena and, in timely, extracting information and taking decisions that may have relevant impacts in a variety of application areas. This has motivated an enormous amount of scientific research in the field of network visualization and network visual analysis, also called graph drawing.

CONCEPTUAL DESIGN OF A VISUALIZATION SYSTEM FOR NETWORKED DATA: THE FUNCTIONAL LAYER AND THE OPTIMIZATION LAYER

At a conceptual level, the design process of an information visualization system for networked data sets has two main ingredients: the functional design and the identification of the readability criteria. The functional design is concerned with the definition of the system architecture, the definition of the software interfaces that manipulate the data, the algorithms that support the analysis, and the efficient use of the data structures. The readability criteria are the rules that a visualization must satisfy in order to easily convey the intrinsic structural properties of the data set, so as to make it easy for the end user to mine the data and hence discover useful information.

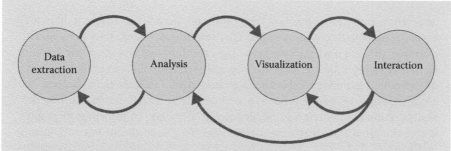

FIGURE 1.1 **(See color insert.)** Conceptual design tasks for the functional layer.

Several different approaches have been used at the functional level design, namely, the functional layer design combines aspects of software engineering, data management, and algorithms engineering. For each such aspect, there is a vast literature and well-established theories and practices in the field of computer engineering and computer science. The interested reader may, for example, refer to Jünger and Mutzel (2004) for a book about software systems devoted to network visualization. Figure 1.1 summarizes the steps that must be undertaken when designing the functional layer. It also shows the interplay between the different tasks.

Concerning the optimization layer, we can distinguish between a classical approach, called researcher-centered approach, and an emerging approach, called user-centered approach. In the researcher-centered approach, the definitions of what are the criteria that the visualization should satisfy in order to guarantee good readability are defined based on the intuition of the researcher who designs the visual interaction between the end user and the data. These criteria are called aesthetics in the literature. Aesthetics translate into a set of geometric constraints that the algorithms computing the visualizations of the data aim at optimizing. In the case of networked data sets, e.g., researchers conjectured in the early 1980s that too many crossings between the edges of the network were a major obstacle for the visual exploration of the data. As a consequence, a rich literature of algorithmic results and combinatorial studies have focused on crossing minimization in graphs (e.g., see Di Battista et al., 1999; Nishizeki and Rahman, 2004). The first cognitive studies confirming that, in fact, crossings are bad for the visual analysis of networks were published more than 10 years later (e.g., see Purchase, 2000; Purchase et al., 2002; Ware et al., 2002).

The user-centered model for the optimization layer was not long ago proposed by Eades, Huang, and Hong in the context of network visualizations (Huang, 2007; Huang et al., 2008). The approach consists of first understanding how end users (and not researchers) would like to read networks in a specific application context and then of designing algorithms that compute visualizations that comply these needs. In their seminal papers, Eades et al. (2008) performed a series of eye-tracking experiments to suggest and refine theories about how the end user perceived different network visualizations with crossing edges. By these observations, they derived, for example, that not only the number of the crossings but also the angle formed by the crossing edges affects the readability. They then executed a series of controlled laboratory experiments to statistically validate their theories. As a consequence of this approach, a new fertile research are in information visualization is rapidly evolving, devoted to the study of drawings of graphs where the crossing edges form large angles (e.g., see the survey in Didimo and Liotta, 2012).

SOME RESOURCES ON THE WEB

We conclude this short note with some pointers to network visualization resources that can be found online:

- The graph drawing e-print archive at the University of Koeln (http://gdea.informatik.uni-koeln.de/).
- The web page maintained by Tamassia (http://www.cs.brown.edu/people/rt/gd.html).
- The web page maintained by Brandes (http://graphdrawing.org/).
- The Wiki for Open Problems page maintained by Marcus Raitne (http://problems.graphdrawing.org/index.php/).
- The section of the "Geometry in Action" pages devoted to Graph Drawing and maintained by David Eppstein (http://www.ics.uci.edu/eppstein/gina/gdraw.html).
- The information visualization material in the web pages of Hanrahan (http://www-graphics.stanford.edu/courses/cs448b-04-winter/).
- The information visualization material in the web pages of Munzner (http://www.cs.ubc.ca/tmm/courses/infovis/).
- The data mining and visualization page of Batagelj (http://vlado.fmf.uni-lj.si/vlado/vladodam.htm).
- The Atlas of Cyberspace at http://www.cybergeography.org/atlas/atlas.html
- The graph drawing page maintained by Stephen Koubourov (http://www.cs.arizona.edu/people/kobourov/gdiv.html).
- The social networks and visualization page maintained by Jonathon N. Cummings (http://www.netvis.org/resources.php).

This memory recall can be divided into two categories stored in long-term memory:

1. *Syntactic knowledge*: This is volatile, easily forgotten unless frequently used, and therefore acquired by rote memorization. This knowledge is system dependent with some possible overlap among systems; for example, "In a text editor, syntactic knowledge—the details of command syntax—include

permissible item delimiters (space, comma, slash or colon), insertion of a new line after the third line (13, 1 3 or 31), or the key stroke necessary for erasing a character (delete key, CONTROL-H or ESCAPE)" (Shneiderman, 1987, p. 65).

2. *Semantic knowledge*: This is largely system independent and acquired through general explanation and example. It is easily anchored to familiar concepts and is therefore stable in the memory. Semantic knowledge represents the functionality (or the concept of the functions) that is hierarchically structured from low-level functions to higher-level concepts. For example,

> in text editors, lower-level functions might be cursor movement, insertion, deletion, changes, text copying, centering, and indentation. These lower-level concepts are close to the syntax of the command language. A middle-level semantic concept for text editing might be the process for correcting a misspelling: produce a display of the misspelled word, move the cursor to the appropriate spot, and issue the change command or key in the correct characters. A higher-level concept might be the process for moving a sentence from one paragraph to another: move the cursor to the beginning of the sentence, mark this position, move the cursor to the end of the sentence, mark this second position, copy the sentence to a buffer area, clean up the source paragraph, move the cursor to the target location, copy from the buffer, check that the target paragraph is satisfactory, and clear the buffer area. The higher-level concepts in the problem domain (moving a sentence) are decomposed by the expert user, top-down into multiple, lower-level concepts (move cursor, copy from buffer, etc.) closer to the program or syntax domain (Shneiderman, 1983, p. 63).

This theoretical model of graphical interaction, in which the specialized knowledge of the programming languages required by users is strongly reduced, gave rise to a new relation between users and technology: Users work with a system through multiple aspects of knowledge as action, objects, and manifold levels of syntactic and semantic knowledge. In this kind of relation, the access to and use of the technology are both conditions linked to the design of the system functioning and to the ability of the users to manipulate the graphical elements. The better a system is designed, the less the knowledge that users have to acquire in order to manipulate/interact with it (i.e., high level of accessibility), and the fewer the problems experienced by users in manipulating system elements (i.e., high level of usability).

Thanks to Shneiderman's work at the Palo Alto Research Center and the subsequent formalization of the GUI, the first window systems were developed in the second half of the 1980s (Smalltalk and InterLisp).

1.1.3 THIRD PERIOD, FROM 1984 TO 1998: PERSONAL COMPUTER AND THE INTERNET ERA

In 1984, at the Massachusetts Institute of Technology, a client/server architecture was produced in order to work with large flexibility on an interactive windows information system. It was named "X Window System." In 1985, the GUI system became available to the general public when the first version of MS-Windows 1.0 was released. Finally, during the 1990s, the WIMP (Windows, Icons, Menus, and Pointer) type of interface became the most used operative system until today.

The transformations in hardware and software over the last 30 years have promoted the development of graphic elements and have imposed the use of an interaction code based on symbolic and spatial elements and not only on a linear language. In fact, in the WIMP interface, the information is spread both by the succession and by the order of content (i.e., the drop-down menus, the toolbars, and the textual guides). At the same time, the information follows the rules of temporality, irreversibility, horizontality, uniformity, causality, and fragmentation of the written language (De Kerckhove, 1995). Users interact with information both through graphic contents and through organization of space and forms (e.g., the aspect of a desktop, the icons, the radial menus, and the interaction through the mouse). Therefore, users must extend their cognitive faculties from logical–analytical, linear, and sequential abilities to figurative, spatial, gestaltic, and circular ones (De Kerckhove, 1995).

Indeed, while in the CLI both the designer and the user were bound by the same communication code, which was logical and analytical (i.e., typed text), in the WIMP the information is also communicated through graphic-spatial codes. The WIMP code does not coincide any more with the system code. The information relevance of an icon, for example, is linked not only to its content and functions but also to its position on the screen or in the environment of the interface. The information content of the CLI was entirely lacking in graphic context, and the facilitations for users' interactions could be reduced to a few ergonomic rules (e.g., size of the screen, size and shape of the fonts, and brightness). On the other hand, in the WIMP model, the content is linked to the graphic-spatial context, thereby introducing greater possibilities for the interpretation of content and environment (position, clarity of symbol, graphic effects, etc.). With WIMP interfaces, the developers' function, in order to guarantee the functionality of the environment, is no longer limited to the verification of the syntactic correctness of the code. In this way, users' interpretative analysis of the code becomes part of the design process itself. The WIMP interaction model reached a twofold goal: It enlarged the concept of computing consumers by making it easy for nonspecialized users to interact with the technology, and it enlarged the computer market by overcoming new business opportunities for the software companies.

This interaction model explicitly proposed that any user, without any specialized knowledge, may access and manage elements of the system by only learning a physical process (point, click, etc.). With respect to the CLI model, users make fewer mistakes and are unburdened of load of any complex cognitive process. By following this approach in the HCI field, the idea was spread that the interaction difficulties experienced by users only depended on system design errors. For more than 20 years, this idea has strongly influenced HCI researchers, who have mostly focused their studies on improving the model of design in order to simplify interaction, underestimating the role of users' needs, expectations, behaviors, and cognitive processes in relation to a system.

This shared idea in the HCI field was formalized, as in the designer's perspective, by Stephen Krug (2000) when, in the first years of the twenty-first century, he clearly stated that the main aim of a good design process was to create an interface that could be experienced by users without thinking about actions.

As we will discuss in Chapter 4, we can claim that both the WIMP model and the designer's perspective were reductive for two main different reasons:

- The WIMP interaction model is more accessible and usable than the CLI model, but it does not ensure accessibility and usability for all users. By overtaking the model of interaction centered on the code, the WIMP interface has increased the number of potential final users of the interactive systems, but it has not ensured that all users have had the same opportunity to access and use the system. Indeed, a large proportion of disabled users has been excluded for a long time from gaining access to computer interaction.
- *The quality of interaction is not only linked to the quality of system design.* The WIMP model aims to reduce the knowledge required by users to interact with a system to a set of physical processes and assumes that a user in interaction is implicitly passive in acting with the system. By following this perspective, a user has only to follow the rules and the relations among the interactive components of the system, so the better the object is designed, the better is the interaction. Today, this passive user perspective has been overtaken, because the evolution of interaction studies, along with the diffusion of technology in everyday life, has shown how users' perspective is important in evaluating and determining the success and spread of technologies and innovation.

Today, ICTs play an essential role in supporting daily life in the digital society. Technologies are used at work, in day-to-day relationships, in dealing with public services, in culture, entertainment, leisure, and when participating in community and political dialogues.

The historical changeover, from the first WIMP computers to the current interfaces accessed by a multiple set of mobile devices, is driven by a complex transformation process of the political, technical, and theoretical perspectives for achieving the aim of social inclusion, formalized only in the first years of twenty-first century with the terms "digital inclusion" or "e-inclusion" (European Commission, 2003; Warschauer, 2003). Digital inclusion was the strategic process for contrasting the digital divide intended as the "gap between those who do and do not have access to computers and the Internet" (National Telecommunication and Information Administration [NTIA], 1999; Warschauer, 2003).

We can define e-inclusion as the process of promoting the ICT used for overcoming social exclusion and for improving economic performance, employment opportunities, quality of life, social participation, and cohesion. The e-inclusion process, as we are going to discuss in the following sections, has led technology to assume an increasing role in everyday life and relations through the evolution of three pillars of HCI:

- The formalization of accessibility standards
- The evolution of usability evaluation methods
- The formalization of the relation between the design process and evaluation process

1.1.4   FOURTH PERIOD, FROM 1998 UNTIL NOW: FROM INTERACTION STANDARDS TO USER INTERFACE FOR ALL

The historical transition from the CLI to the GUI and the diffusion of personal computers open up usability and accessibility problems (Federici and Borsci, 2010). In fact, until 1998, the Internet was considered as a "universal medium" without taking into account neither the individual differences of users, much less the interaction barriers that prevent people with disabilities to access the interfaces, nor the digital divide (NTIA, 1999).

However, the expansion of technology in everyday life opened up at least two problems: The first was how to share and promote standards in order to guarantee equal access and use of technology and information for all users; and, consequently, the second problem was how to involve all kinds of users in this process of technology diffusion, avoiding interaction barriers.

In order to understand how these two main problems were addressed, we have to look at, on the one hand, the political decisions and policies promoted in the world by different national and international organizations and, on the other hand, the diffusion and the agreement of the researchers and practitioners on usability evaluation methods and design philosophy.

1.2   POLITICAL MOVEMENT AND THE STANDARDS: ACCESSIBILITY AS THE FIRST PILLAR

The promotion of the accessibility standards is strictly related to both the diffusion of policies on human rights and disabled users' access and participation in societies.

The United Nations (UN), as well as other international organizations, has been promoting human rights recognition for people with disabilities for a long time. In 1975, the "Declaration on the Rights of Disabled Persons" was promulgated, proclaiming equal civil and political rights for people with disabilities (UN, 1975). The first coherent strategy was developed, in 1981, during the International Year of Disabled Persons, resulting in the adoption of the World Programme of Action for people with disabilities (1983–1992). This program recognized that

> there is a great variation from some countries with a high educational level for disabled persons to countries where such facilities are limited or non-existent. There is a lack in existing knowledge of the potential of disabled persons. Furthermore, there is often no legislation which deals with their needs and a shortage of teaching staff and facilities. Disabled persons have in most countries so far not benefited from a lifelong education. (UN, 1982)

With the finalization of the World Programme of Action, it was at once evident that no international legal instrument for the safeguarding of the rights of "handicapped" persons existed, apart from those relative to discrimination for reasons of gender and race. Therefore, following the recommendations of the World Programme of Action relative to "handicapped" persons, the UN General Assembly adopted, in 1993, the Standard Rules on the Equalization of Opportunities for Persons with Disabilities (Lemay, 1994).

In the same year, the Vienna Declaration on Human Rights reaffirmed that "all human rights and fundamental freedoms are universal, and therefore must absolutely include persons with disabilities" and "put the active participation of persons with disabilities in all the aspects of civil society explicitly in a context of human rights" (UN, 1993).

The Standard Rules present the directives of social change that should allow all citizens, without exception, to take part in an equal manner in society life.

Progressively, the Standard Rules became the international instrument and the control mechanism for guaranteeing the respect of human and civil rights through their application and their effectiveness. They introduced a fundamental principle, applicable to any process for receiving equal treatment: equal opportunities. From the beginning, the policy debate about the knowledge society was connected to social progress and it mostly focused on potential benefits and risks that could affect vulnerable groups of people, including the disabled.

Only in the last years of the 1990s, when the Internet became a shared technology in information societies, the problem of disabled people's access to information was taken into consideration by institutions. The legislative movement for the promotion of accessibility began in the US Congress by voting Section 508 in 1998, which amends the *Rehabilitation Act* (U.S. Congress, 1973) requiring that all public websites (federal agencies and institutions) must be accessible according to criteria defined in the act. In this period, the WAI, a department of the W3C, developed accessibility guidelines for the web. The first version of these rules was published in 1999 (see for a complete review Brewer, 2004), and they relate to WCAG, web browsers (UAAG), and Web Authoring Tool Accessibility Guidelines (ATAG).

The European Commission only joined the legislative movement in 2001, recognizing the accessibility guidelines of the W3C-WAI as the *de facto* standards in its resolution of 13 July on e-learning (European Union, 2001). The European Commission endorsed the importance of ICT for education and training. Additionally, an e-learning action plan was developed to coordinate European activities concerning the use of ICT in education. The commission stated that e-learning would shortly become mainstream in education and training systems (European Union, 2001).

In 2003, following a resolution of the European Parliament (European Commission, 2012b), all European websites had to meet at least Level 2 of the WCAG rules. Many European countries, after the 2003 promulgated laws requiring the electronic services of their public sector to be accessible to persons with disabilities, introduced the accessibility concept in national legislations.

In this sense, not only accessibility but also "e-accessibility," considered as "improving access of people with disabilities to the knowledge-based society" (European Union, 2003a), became central in order to grant "equal opportunities for pupils and students with disabilities in education and training" (European Union, 2003b). Thus, e-inclusion refers to the need to make sure that everyone in society can benefit from the opportunities offered by new ICT. E-inclusion is about closing the gap between those who can access ICT and those who cannot.

In 2005, the European Commission launched a new policy framework, embracing all aspects of the information, communication, and audiovisual sector. The idea was to seamlessly join individual policy initiatives into a coherent strategy. This framework is called "i2010—A European Information Society for growth and employment." It provides the broad policy guidelines for what we call the emerging "information society" in the years up to 2010 (European Commission, 2003). i2010, following the idea that access and use of ICT is a growing need in the information society, endorses a philosophy of accessibility and usability for all.

This philosophy is centered on the political diffusion of all the standards able to grant the diffusion of Internet use (e.g., W3C guidelines and design principles). In this way, i2010 aims to

1. Establish a single European information space—i.e., a truly single market for the digital economy so as to fully exploit the economies of scale offered by Europe's 500 million-strong consumer market
2. Reinforce innovation and investment in ICT research, given that ICT is a major driver of the economy
3. Promote inclusion, public services, and quality of life—in other words, extend the European values of inclusion and quality of life to the information society

Inclusion and accessibility are the pillars of the i2010 initiative on the information society and are closely related to other European policies, namely, social inclusion, education and culture, and regional development (European Commission, 2008).

At the same time, in 2006, the Convention on the Rights of Persons with Disabilities was released by the UN, where it is declared that "States shall take appropriate measures to ensure [...] access to information and communication including systems and information technology and communication" (UN, 2006). This Convention on the Rights of Persons with Disabilities, along with the document entitled "Some facts about persons with disabilities" (UN Enable, 2006), reported the following

- Around 10% of the world's population, or 650 million people, live with a disability.
- Eighty percent of persons with disabilities live in developing countries.
- The World Bank estimates that 20% of the world's poorest people are disabled and tend to be regarded in their own communities as the most disadvantaged.
- Ninety percent of children with disabilities in developing countries do not attend school.
- An estimated 386 million of the world's working-age people are disabled. Unemployment among the disabled is as high as 80% in some countries. Often employers assume that people with disabilities are unable to work.

The policies against the e-exclusion in information societies are a main topic in order to have an "accessibility for all" that means creating access to the web, to education, and to job possibilities for people with or without disabilities (UN Enable, 2006), so reducing the digital divide.

The United States had an important role in the diffusion of the accessibility idea. According to Section 508, approved in 1998, all electronic and information technologies of federal agencies must be accessible to people with disabilities. This law sets the standards for American web and software accessibility and has its roots in the Workforce Rehabilitation Act approved in 1973 in order to overcome the barriers for disabled people. In June 2006, a draft recommendation was made to the Information Organization, Usability, Currency, and Accessibility Working Group (IOUCA). The Department of Rehabilitation recommended that states' websites should meet both web accessibility standards.

Today, as the World Health Organization (WHO and World Bank, 2011) recently reported, the diffusion of guidelines and regulation standards, considered as a level of quality accepted as the norm, is the most important action against e-exclusion in order to create an enabling environment. The possibility of a ubiquitous access to the web by mobile phone and other portable technologies has changed the concept of the digital divide that now refers "not only to physical access to computers, connectivity, and infrastructure but also to the geographical, economic, cultural and social factors – such as illiteracy – that create barriers to social inclusion" (WHO and World Bank, 2011, p. 172).

Accessibility is a current central issue not only for public institutions but also for private companies that have to enlarge their e-business by reaching all kinds of consumers. In this sense, improvement of the accessibility standards is a priority for knowledge societies. In order to answer this priority, in 2008, W3C-WAI published a draft of the second version of the accessibility guidelines (see Box 1.2).

1.3   USABILITY AND DESIGN PHILOSOPHY: THE SECOND AND THE THIRD PILLARS

It is a worth remarking that ICTs, in a wide sense, are today a human second skin that allow a ubiquitous access to information. The users of this second skin are every day becoming more selective consumers and, at the same time, more predisposed to the use of different technologies, with a growing set of expectations about, and need to be satisfied by, their use of these technologies. In e-societies, the evaluation of these products, and in particular the evaluation of users' interaction with the systems, has become the main way to diffuse the ICT.

In this sense, not only the accessibility but also the usability and the relation between the design and the process of the evaluation are pillars of the e-inclusion. We define an interaction evaluation as the assessment process able to guarantee access and use of technology in a satisfactory way, comprising (1) the evaluation of the accessibility and conformance to the standards and (2) the evaluation of the usability experienced by the users. Today, this process is even more centered on users' perspective and, as we are going to discuss in Chapter 5, the involvement of disabled people in creating standards, developing systems, and evaluating the interaction is a necessary condition for achieving the aim of the e-inclusion.

BOX 1.2   FROM WCAG 1.0 TO WCAG 2.0

MASSIMO CAPPONI

The World Wide Web is an essential component of the Information Society. Tim Berners-Lee, the inventor of the World Wide Web, once said that "the power of the web is in its universality" and that "access by everyone regardless of disability is an essential aspect" (W3C-WAI, 2012).

First, "accessible" means "reachable" (Diodati, 2007) (and not reachable with a hitch, like a snow-covered mountain top, but easily reachable without too much effort, like an entry-phone set at the correct height). Moreover, "accessible" means reachable physically, by our body, as well as mentally, by our mind, or comprehensible. In this sense, "accessible" means something that can be easily reached by our body as well as something that can be easily understood.

A second way to think of accessibility, often called "e-accessibility," is to think about the use of ICTs—in other words, not only about web technologies but also about standard office applications, information retrieval, user interface, educational software, and so on. As a matter of fact, the European Commission promotes e-accessibility in order to ensure

> people with disabilities and elderly people access ICTs on an equal basis with others [...] this includes removing the barriers encountered when trying to access and use ICT products, services and applications" (European Commission, 2012a).

Accessibility is about World Wide Web access, as well as about websites that can be designed to be more accessible by conforming to certain design principles established by the international community.

Since the World Wide Web was first activated, web accessibility has always been very important. A common definition regards how a website can be accessed by different users in different contexts. The European Commission's website claims that "Web accessibility means that everyone including people with disabilities can perceive, understand, navigate, and interact with the Internet, and they are offered the possibility to contribute to the society." Moreover, "Web accessibility is both a question of technical standards and how you build your web site, but it is also a question of political goals and securing equal rights for everyone" (European Commission, 2012b).

The "Rehabilitation Act of 1973," a U.S. federal law concerning the human rights of people with disabilities, is the first public document to have addressed the topic of disabilities from a computer applications point of view. Section 508 in particular, added in 1986 and amended in 1998, affirms certain principles meant to eliminate barriers in information technology and to make electronic and information technology applications accessible to people with disabilities, especially with regard to web applications.

Section 508 of the Rehabilitation Act of 1973:

a. A text equivalent for every non-text element shall be provided (e.g., via "alt," "longdesc," or in element content).
b. Equivalent alternatives for any multimedia presentation shall be synchronized with the presentation.
c. Web pages shall be designed so that all information conveyed with color is also available without color, for example from context or markup.
d. Documents shall be organized so they are readable without requiring an associated style sheet.
e. Redundant text links shall be provided for each active region of a server-side image map.
f. Client-side image maps shall be provided instead of server-side image maps except where the regions cannot be defined with an available geometric shape.
g. Row and column headers shall be identified for data tables.
h. Markup shall be used to associate data cells and header cells for data tables that have two or more logical levels of row or column headers.
i. Frames shall be titled with text that facilitates frame identification and navigation.
j. Pages shall be designed to avoid causing the screen to flicker with a frequency greater than 2 Hz and lower than 55 Hz.
k. A text-only page, with equivalent information or functionality, shall be provided to make a web site comply with the provisions of this part, when compliance cannot be accomplished in any other way. The content of the text-only page shall be updated whenever the primary page changes.
l. When pages utilize scripting languages to display content, or to create interface elements, the information provided by the script shall be identified with functional text that can be read by assistive technology.
m. When a web page requires that an applet, plug-in or other application be present on the client system to interpret page content, the page must provide a link to a plug-in or applet that complies with § 1194.21(a) through (l).
n. When electronic forms are designed to be completed on-line, the form shall allow people using assistive technology to access the

information, field elements, and functionality required for completion and submission of the form, including all directions and cues.
o. A method shall be provided that permits users to skip repetitive
navigation links.
p. When a timed response is required, the user shall be alerted and
given sufficient time to indicate more time is required.

Source: United States Congress, Section 508 of The
Rehabilitation Act, Public Law 29 U.S.C. 794d, 1998, http://www.
section508.gov (retrieved September 15, 2013).

Of course, as the Internet has grown, its structure and the way we interface
with the World Wide Web has been modified; since the Internet has become an
essential tool, the W3C—a not-for-profit international community created in
1994 whose main aim is to standardize web technologies and languages—has
dealt with the issue of web accessibility in an effort to ensure access to websites
in a manner that is easier than before. They have also sought to establish technical standards regarding markup languages and communications protocols.

Those who can be helped by the application of accessibility principles are,
according to W3C, individuals with vision problems, hearing problems, and
cognitive disabilities. On the other hand, the people being addressed by these
accessibility rules are, for the most part, web developers.

Making a website accessible allows it to more readily satisfy other categories, as well, some of which go beyond those listed earlier; as a matter of fact,
many users may be able to access and operate the Internet in conditions and
contexts that are very different, reducing the number of ways to enjoy web
contents. In such a case, an accessible website would be understood as allowing many classes of users to browse web content, including

- People with physical and/or cognitive disabilities
- People who encounter difficulties similar to those encountered by peo-
ple with physical and/or cognitive disabilities (i.e., those who work in a
noisy environment or who do not know how to speak a foreign language)
- People using obsolete hardware and/or software, and very slow
Internet connections

The WAI, a section of the W3C, has put forth guidelines to help web developers
in constructing accessible websites, resulting in three standards: one for authoring
tools, one for user agents (browsers and assistive technologies), and one for content:

- ATAG are a set of guidelines for the developers of web content–
authoring tools such as simple HTML editors, tools that export content to be used on the web (e.g., Word Editor in order to export data
in HTML), tools that have multimedia files as an output, web content
management systems, etc.

- User Agent Accessibility Guidelines (UAAG) are a set of guidelines geared toward user agent developers (as well as the developers of web browsers and multimedia players) that aim to make user agents accessible to users with disabilities.
- WCAG 1.0 (Chisholm et al., 1999) and WCAG 2.0 (Caldwell et al., 2008) are a set of guidelines meant to ensure web content is accessible to people with disabilities. They are useful in making web content more accessible on other devices as well, including smartphones and other mobile devices. WCAG have been recognized as an international standard, and they form the foundations of related laws in many countries.

As stated earlier, WCAG documents explain how to make web content more accessible to people with disabilities, whereas web "content" generally refers to the information on a web page or a web application.

WCAG 1.0

Version 1.0 of the WCAG was published and became a W3C recommendation on May 5, 1999. While Section 508 is law, compliance with the WCAG more broadly is completely voluntary, although many national laws in a number of countries refer to WCAG. They have long been seen as a landmark for web developers involved in easing access to websites.

WCAG 1.0 Guidelines:

Guideline 1. Provide equivalent alternatives to auditory and visual content.

Guideline 2. Don't rely on color alone.

Guideline 3. Use markup and style sheets and do so properly.

Guideline 4. Clarify natural language usage.

Guideline 5. Create tables that transform gracefully.

Guideline 6. Ensure that pages featuring new technologies transform gracefully.

Guideline 7. Ensure user control of time-sensitive content changes.

Guideline 8. Ensure direct accessibility of embedded user interfaces.

Guideline 9. Design for device-independence.

Guideline 10. Use interim solutions.

Guideline 11. Use W3C technologies and guidelines.

Guideline 12. Provide context and orientation information.

Guideline 13. Provide clear navigation mechanisms.

Guideline 14. Ensure that documents are clear and simple.

Each guideline includes, among other things, a list of checkpoint definitions.

Each checkpoint has a priority level assigned by the Working Group based on the checkpoint's impact on accessibility

[Priority 1]
A web content developer *must* satisfy this checkpoint. Otherwise, one or more groups will find it impossible to access information in the document. Satisfying this checkpoint is a basic requirement for some groups to be able to use web documents.

[Priority 2]
A web content developer *should* satisfy this checkpoint. Otherwise, one or more groups will find it difficult to access information in the document. Satisfying this checkpoint will remove significant barriers to accessing web documents.

[Priority 3]
A web content developer *may* address this checkpoint. Otherwise, one or more groups will find it somewhat difficult to access information in the document. Satisfying this checkpoint will improve access to web documents.

There are three levels of conformance to WCAG 1.0 (Chisholm et al., 1999): ·

> Conformance Level "A": all Priority 1 checkpoints are satisfied;
> Conformance Level "Double-A": all Priority 1 and 2 checkpoints
>   are satisfied;
> Conformance Level "Triple-A": all Priority 1, 2, and 3 checkpoints
>   are satisfied.

WCAG 2.0

The web has recently changed in a very substantial way, with new ways of interaction and new communication technologies. This has made it essential to establish a new set of rules and best practices to move the international and online communities toward a new understanding of web accessibility:

> It's no longer an HTML-only world. It has evolved into an exciting, compelling medium for providing innovative services. One of the major goals of WCAG 2.0 was to describe the requirements for web content accessibility in technology neutral language so that it could be applicable to any W3C or non-W3C technology, such as CSS, SMIL, SVG, XML, PDF, or Flash in addition to HTML and XHTML. A second major goal of WCAG 2.0 was to ensure that the requirements are all objectively testable so that policy makers can adopt them unchanged. (Reid and Snow-Weaver, 2008, p. 109)

WCAG 1.0 had been drawn up when web pages were designed mainly through the use of HTML, and every aspect of the interface was edited through cascading style sheets (CSS). What the W3C Working Group was looking for was a universal formula, one able to satisfy the needs of users with disabilities in a general and multipurpose way.

It took a long time to write these new guidelines, as the web is continuously growing in a "dramatic" and difficult-to-conceive of manner. After a long period of debate among experts in the field of website development, WCAG 2.0 guidelines were published as a W3C Recommendation on December 11, 2008. The following box is a list of principles and guidelines:

WCAG 2.0

Principle 1: *Perceivable*—Information and user interface components must be presentable to users in ways they can perceive.

1.1 Provide text alternatives for any non-text content so that it can be changed into other forms people need, such as large print, braille, speech, symbols or simpler language.

1.2 Provide alternatives for time-based media.

1.3 Create content that can be presented in different ways (for example simpler layout) without losing information or structure.

1.4 Make it easier for users to see and hear content including separating foreground from background.

Principle 2: *Operable*—User interface components and navigation must be operable.

2.1 Make all functionality available from a keyboard.

2.2 Provide users enough time to read and use content.

2.3 Do not design content in a way that is known to cause seizures.

2.4 Provide ways to help users navigate, find content, and determine where they are.

Principle 3: *Understandable*—Information and the operation of user interface must be understandable.

3.1 Make text content readable and understandable.

3.2 Make web pages appear and operate in predictable ways.

3.3 Help users avoid and correct mistakes.

Principle 4: *Robust*—Content must be robust enough that it can be interpreted reliably by a wide variety of user agents, including assistive technologies.

4.1 Maximize compatibility with current and future user agents, including assistive technologies.

The 12 guidelines provide the basic goals that authors should work toward in order to make content more accessible to users with different disabilities.

The guidelines are not testable, but provide the framework and overall objectives to help authors understand the success criteria and better implement the techniques.

Success Criteria—For each guideline, testable success criteria are provided to allow WCAG 2.0 (Caldwell et al., 2008) to be used where requirements and conformance testing are necessary such as in design specification, purchasing, regulation, and contractual agreements. In order to meet the needs of different groups and different situations, three levels of conformance are defined: A (lowest), AA, and AAA (highest).

Many criticisms have been directed toward WCAG. Given the hundreds of pages of associated technical documentation, Clark commented that the WCAG 2.0 were "overlong," unreadable, and impossible to understand, and he claimed that, "the fundamentals of WCAG 2 are nearly impossible for a working standards-compliant developer to understand" (Clark, 2006). Moreover, WCAG have often been criticized by experts in the fields of usability and HCI (Godwin-Jones, 2001; Kelly et al., 2007; Ribera et al., 2009), and by associations of persons with disabilities. Four main criticisms have been put forth:

- "They are not based on a statistically validated research of users.
- They do not deal with the needs of persons with cognitive disabilities and the elderly.
- They are not comprehensible for a typical webmaster.
- They encourage webmasters to seek easy compliance rather than real accessibility" (Termens et al., 2009, p. 1172).

The path blazed by WCAG 2.0 goes in search of an accessibility that is compatible with every web interface—not only with contemporary technology but also with the future ones regardless of the techniques and languages involved. This is why the most important difference between WCAG 1.0 and WCAG 2.0 is the latter's focus on technology independence. In this way, WCAG 2.0's criteria for success in effect correspond to WCAG 1.0 checkpoints, with one very important difference (Diodati, 2007): while WCAG 1.0 checkpoints were somewhat ambiguously defined and not universal, making it impossible to define specific criteria by which to verify their implementation, success criteria have been designed to be testable. They are "Yes/No" statements; the levels of WCAG 2.0 are analogous to the WCAG 1.0 notion of priorities, but more precise.

Furthermore, certain techniques have been joined to success criteria, allowing them to verify whether or not a website could be made accessible according to the WCAG 2.0 success criteria.

Finally, we can say that the WCAG are an important step toward the improved accessibility of the World Wide Web, but accessibility must be considered alongside usability. Kelly, for example, has said that

> the WAI's definition of accessibility makes it much closer to usability: content is accessible when it may be *used* by someone with a disability [...] therefore the appropriate test for where a Web site is accessible is whether disabled people can use it, not whether it conforms to WCAG or other guidelines. (Kelly et al., 2005, p. 49 [italic in original])

Though WCAG 2.0 are a useful tool for governments and institutions, they are only a first step toward true accessibility, which can only be achieved through user-centered design (Ribera et al., 2009).

In order to explore the historical evolution of both the usability evaluation and the relation between the design and the evaluation process (i.e., the last two pillars), we will follow two different steps: First, we shall analyze the evolution of the usability studies from the 1980s, following the historical presentation of one of the most referenced historical and comparative analyses provided by Rex Hartson, Terence Andre, and Robert Williges (2003). Second, we shall analyze the evolution of different design approaches from the first conceptualization (e.g., the human factor evaluation) to the most enhanced and widely adopted design philosophies.

1.3.1 FROM A FRAGMENTED SET OF USABILITY EVALUATION METHODS TO THE NEED FOR A UNIFIED EVALUATION APPROACH

The historical evolution of the methods for assessing usability was driven by two parallel goals. On the one hand, researchers and practitioners worked to increase the reliability and the validity of the evaluation data in order to optimize HCI. On the other hand, in order to accomplish the designers' needs, they had to look for methods capable of decreasing the time and costs of the evaluation process. In the period between 1980 and today, we can identify at least three main different evaluation approaches: subjective evaluation (i.e., user based), the evaluation of experts through the standards (i.e., expert based), and predictive evaluation by a model of user behavior (i.e., model based). We shall closely analyze the different kinds of evaluation methods in Chapter 8, while in this section we provide an analysis of the historical needs that have driven their development.

In the 1980s, laboratory usability testing quickly became the primary usability environmental setting for examining a new or modified interface. These evaluations were focused on measure, in a controlled environment: the speed, accuracy, and errors of users' performances by different user-based evaluation methods. Developers considered laboratory testing as a way to minimize costs of service calls and increase sales through the design of a more competitive product, by minimizing risk and creating a historical record of usability benchmarks for future releases (Rubin and Chisnell, 2008). The user-based evaluation methods, such as verbal protocols (Ericsson and Simon, 1984, 1987), critical incident reporting (del Galdo et al., 1986), and user satisfaction ratings (Chin et al., 1988), are mainly focused on identifying the problems experienced by a sample of users during an interaction for improving the system. Although these kinds of methods obtained significant successes by providing reliable data for the optimization of software interfaces, the developers still considered the costs of evaluation testing too expensive, compared with the benefit provided by reducing the problems in the system.

In the 1990s, in order to decrease the costs and time required for traditional usability testing with user-based methods, practitioners explored two different kinds of methodology that could be used by developers with the prototypes in an early design process (Bradford, 1994; Marchetti, 1994): the expert-based and the model-based evaluation methods.

- The expert-based evaluation that involved interaction experts (e.g., practitioners and design experts) in an evaluation by a system analysis through a set of questions based on design principles. Some of the most popular expert-based methods include guidelines for the evaluators based on the rules of the interaction design (Smith and Mosier, 1986), heuristic evaluation (Nielsen and Molich, 1990), cognitive walkthroughs (Lewis et al., 1990; Wharton et al., 1992), usability walkthroughs (Bias, 1991), formal usability inspections (Kahn and Prail, 1994), and heuristic walkthroughs (Sears, 1997).
- The model-based methods introduced an ideal model of the human process of information elaboration capable of representing human perception and elaboration of external stimuli and of predicting human performance during interaction with the technology (John and Kieras, 1996b). Model-based methods were used as a predictive measure of users' interaction in order to optimize the system. Among the model-based evaluation techniques, GOMS (goals, operators, methods, and selection rules) is one of the most popular. GOMS was developed in 1983 by three pioneers of HCI: Stuart Card, a senior research fellow at Xerox PARC; Thomas Moran, a distinguished engineer at the IBM Almaden Research Center; and Allen Newell, a researcher in computer science and cognitive psychology at the RAND Corporation (see Card et al., 1983). It consists of the measure of the difference between the time of the actions estimated by the model and real users' actions during interaction with a system. Another model, closely related to GOMS (see Box 1.3), is the cognitive complexity theory (CCT) (Bovair et al., 1990), which predicts performances and learning times of users during an interaction with a certain technology. At the same time, it may be necessary to underline the important role played by the application in the HCI field of the mathematical law developed by Paul Fitts (1954). This law is a model of human movement that predicts the time required for a subject to rapidly move to a target area, expressed as a logarithmic function of the distance to the target area and its size. Fitts' law was applied in different studies of HCI and, in particular, for computing the index of performance in the interaction movements when manipulating the interfaces with different kinds of mouse units and of pointers (MacKenzie, 1992).

BOX 1.3 GOMS EVALUATION TECHNIQUE

SIMONE BORSCI AND MARIA LAURA DE FILIPPIS

In 1983, Card et al. (1983) defined a general model of human interaction with a system, called the model human processor (MHP). In the MHP, the user is considered as an elaborator of information that can be measured by analyzing the time of his or her performance in accomplishing a specific task via an interface. The most well-known application of MHP in an interface effectiveness assessment is called the CMN–GOMS model (John and Kieras, 1996a), which stands for Card, Moran, and Newell–goals, operators, methods, and selection rules. This model, which represents the original conceptualization of a family of predictive techniques, is known as the GOMS model (John, 1990; John and Kieras, 1996a,b; Kieras, 1988). A GOMS model assumes that during an interaction (1) a user has to reach a specific goal (goals); (2) this goal can be reached by performing a set of actions in a certain amount of time (operators); (3) the user, in achieving the goal, must perform the actions in a sequence (methods); and (4) if in the interface a user can reach a goal by performing more than one possible sequence of actions (i.e., more than one method), the user must select one sequence of actions over the others (selection rules).

Bonnie E. John, assistant professor of computer science at the Carnegie Mellon University, and David Kieras, professor in electrical engineering and computer science at the University of Michigan (1996a), suggested that a GOMS model results in an engineering model of human performance that produces a priori quantitative predictions of performance, in terms of execution time, learning time, and errors, which can be used by designers for improving the effectiveness of the interface. In particular, the original conceptualization of the GOMS model (i.e., CMN–GOMS) assumes that the user's actions during an interaction can be categorized into three main kinds of elementary operators: (1) motor actions, such as put the hand on the mouse; (2) perceptual actions, such as visually searching for the icon that has to be clicked; and (3) cognitive actions, such as think/decide if moving the pointer over the icon (Card et al., 1983; John and Kieras, 1996a).

This distinction between motor, perceptual, and cognitive operators is a common base of all the variants of the original CNM–GOMS that have been developed during the evolution of the HCI field. Following the proposals of John and Kieras (1996a) from their analysis of the GOMS model family, we can identify three main variations of the CNM–GOMS model:

- The first variation is the keystroke-level model (KLM) proposed by Card, Moran, and Newell (1980). The KLM is a simplified version of the CMN–GOMS model that can be used by evaluators for analyzing solely those actions that a user must perform for achieving a goal (i.e., operators), without consideration of the user's goals, methods, and selection rules.

- The second variation is the natural GOMS language (NGOMSL), proposed by Kieras (1988). The NGOMSL incorporates a more rigorous procedure than the other variations. In fact, according to this kind of GOMS, the evaluator must express in a formal and logical syntax all the components of the user interaction (i.e., GOMS), in order to assess not only the user's performances but also the time taken by the user in learning the correct procedure and reaching the goal.
- The last variation is the cognitive perceptual motor–GOMS (CPM–GOMS) proposed by John (1990). The CPM–GOMS extends the premise of the classic GOMS model; assuming that during the interaction, a user can perform actions (motor, cognitive, and perceptual) not only sequentially, as proposed by the CMN–GOMS, but also in parallel. In light of this, the CPM–GOMS allows an evaluator to make quantitative predictions of a user's interaction in performing in a parallel way the actions required in order to achieve the goal.

Each variation of the CMN-GOMS has a specific set of advantages and limits. For instance, an evaluator is forced to use NGOMSL in order to test the time spent by a user in learning the correct procedure of interaction. Although it is more costly than other variations in terms of the time spent by an evaluator for the analysis, it is the only model that can be used for predicting and analyzing the user's learning time (for a complete review on the GOMS family advantages and disadvantages, see John and Kieras, 1996b).

In order to assess the interface's effectiveness, independently of the selected variation of the GOMS model, the evaluator must assign an expected time to each action that a user must perform in order to achieve the task (John and Kieras, 1996a). Usually, the expected time is defined by the evaluator on the basis of previous research. For instance, in order to assign a time for the motor operator "put hand on the mouse" in a drag and drop task, an evaluator can fix the expected time as 320 ms with a range of 214–400 ms, by following the indications from experimental studies on similar tasks (see Baber, 2004). By using these empirical standards of time (for a global review on empirical standards, see John, 1990), an evaluator can define an expected time for a user's performance in terms of operators for doing an action. In light of this, an evaluator has a benchmark (for a global review on GOMS procedure for evaluation, see John and Kieras, 1996a) by which to analyze the difference between the observed time spent by a cohort of users in achieving a goal in a system and the time of user's performance modeled by the evaluator through a GOMS technique. For example, analyzing the effectiveness experienced by the users against an expected model, or for comparing the user's performance in interaction with two different models of the same technology. For instance, the evaluator may use the GOMS for analyzing the differences in the interaction performance of a sample of users between an old and a new version of a mobile phone, by using the expected time of task performance as a parameter for establishing which model (old or new) best allows the users effective interaction.

In Table 1.1, we propose an example of a CNM–GOMS application, created by using the data of John and Kieras (1996a), in which the user's task is to highlight and clear an arbitrary word in a text by using the mouse functions of a word processor.

In light of our discussion, we can consider a GOMS model as a powerful evaluation technique for improving the effectiveness of interaction on the basis

---

TABLE 1.1

Example of a CMN–GOMS Analysis of the Following Task: "Highlight and Clear a Word in Text"

Goal: Cut-Arbitrary-Text

	Expected time (seconds)
• Goal: Highlight-Word	
Method:	
Move-cursor-to-word	
Double-click-mouse-button	
Verify-highlight	
Selection rule: highlight-text	
• Goal: highlight-arbitrary-text	
Actions/operators:	1.10
Move-cursor-to-beginning	0.20
Click-mouse-button	1.10
Move-cursor-to-end	0.48
Shift-click-mouse-button	1.35
Verify-highlight	
• Goal: Issue-cut-command	
Actions/operators:	1.10
Move-cursor-to-edit-menu	0.10
Press-mouse-button	1.10
Move-cursor-to-cut-item	1.35
Verify-highlight	0.10
Release-mouse-button	
Total time predicted	6.98

Note: The overall predicted time for the task is 6.98 s, following the standard time of operators identified by John and Kieras (1996a).

of simulation of a user's behavior. Nevertheless, as Yvonne Rogers et al. (2011) claim, GOMS is not a conclusive and realistic assessment but it is only a useful tool for measuring the effectiveness of the interface. In fact, first, GOMS does not consider the efficiency and satisfaction of the interaction, and second, as a human model, GOMS considers all the users as elaborators of information, discarding the individual differences and the variables that could affect the interaction, such as the users' cognitive workload, attitudes, expectations, and functioning (Rogers et al., 2011; Tonn-Eichstädt, 2006).

Both the expert- and the model-based evaluation, from the evaluators' point of view, have decreased the costs of usability assessment and have also provided a more objective evaluation than the user-based assessment. However, these methods totally exclude the real user from the evaluation that significantly affects the reliability of the evaluation data for the developers.

By considering the different methodologies developed since the 1980s, we can state that evaluation was a very diversified and fragmented field in which practitioners were far from settled in a uniform process, and nowhere near agreeing on a standard for evaluating the systems. In 1998, in order to overcome the problem of a fragmented evaluation approach, Wayne Gray and Marilyn Salzman (1998) strongly supported the introduction of comparative studies in the usability evaluation field. They proposed that only the application of a comparative evaluation and of a rigorous experimental methodology could lead to a future formalization of several standard rules for a usability evaluation capable of unifying the different evaluation approaches. A subsequent international debate of researchers and practitioners approved this idea (see Olson and Moran, 1998).

The need for a unified approach of the different evaluation methods driven by a rigorous experimental methodology was well summarized in 2001 by Andrew Dillon, dean of the School of Information and professor of psychology at the University of Texas:

> Finally, there are good reasons for thinking that the best approach to evaluating usability is to combine methods—e.g., using the expert-based approach to identify problems and inform the design of a user-based test scenario, since the overlap between the outputs of these methods is only partial, and a user-based test normally cannot cover as much of the interface as an expert-based method (2001, p. 1111).
>
> According to the latest studies in the scientific literature, the integration of evaluation models emerges as the only possible solution in order to take into account, in the evaluation process, the totality of aspects involved in the interaction.

Today, the debate on usability measurements is centered on the possibility of evaluation method integration and the role played by subjectivity in the assessment of HCI.

1.3.2   DESIGN PHILOSOPHY

When we talk about design philosophy, we mean a framework created for helping and guiding designers to take into account all factors (i.e., accessibility and usability) and all actors involved during an interaction. In this sense, a design framework defines the success of a technology. In fact, even if the success of a technology could depend on many factors (functions, aesthetic, etc.), the most important one, as Jakob Nielsen (1993), user advocate and principal of the Nielsen Norman Group, suggests, is the user interface, which could be considered the more important part of technology. The user interface decides the success of the product because it allows users to experience the technology in a good or in a bad way. Bearing that in mind, we could underline that not only a good design process but also a proper evaluation strategy is part of a complete technological design philosophy. In fact, both the development process and the evaluation techniques have to work together in order to drive the developers' team to design a technology that is experienced by all users in a satisfactory way, which is the ideal goal of design. In order to achieve this ideal goal, it is necessary for a product to satisfy two ideal conditions:

1. The technology has to be accessible to everybody in order to fulfill the universal access condition. The term "universal access" is usually linked to the U.S. Communications Act of 1934 on the access of telecommunication technologies such as telephone, telegraph, and radio services. It tried to ensure adequate facilities at reasonable charges, especially in rural areas, and prevent discrimination on the basis of race, color, religion, national origin, or sex. As Shneiderman claims (2000), when the term "universal access" has been applied to computing services, the greater complexity of interaction immediately makes it clear that providing access for all is not sufficient without ensuring successful usage.
2. The technology has to be usable to everybody in order to fulfill the universal usability condition. The term "universal usability" was defined by Shneiderman (2003) as an approach to design that is focused on enabling all citizens to succeed using communication and information technology in their tasks.

By using the more extensive conceptualization of Nigel Bevan (2001), we could refer to these two ideal conditions as "quality in use for all."

The design process of interaction has been approached in different ways during the evolution of the HCI field, from the engineering and aesthetical approach to the application of the cognitive science paradigm (see Stephanidis, 2001). However, all such approaches cannot be considered as a design philosophy because they do not aim to drive the designers to achieve the quality in use for all, but are only focused on designing a system that operates without shortcomings (i.e., without interactive problems).

Considering a design philosophy as a framework for achieving the quality in use for all (i.e., the ideal goal of interaction design), we could identify at least three main design philosophies that have been developed in the history of HCI:

1. *The user-centered design (UCD)*: The UCD is the first pioneering design philosophy that tried to drive the designer to fulfill the two ideal conditions.
2. *The universal design (UD)*: The UD includes the UCD but can be considered as a more formalized philosophy than the UCD. The UD was

introduced in the HCI field in the middle of the 1990s, when there was a growing need for policies and guidelines capable of granting universal access.

3. *The user interface for all (UIA)*: The UIA was developed in order to solve the problems and overcome the criticism and the shortcomings of the UD. It includes the design philosophy mentioned earlier.

The term UCD was first originated in Donald Norman's research laboratory at the University of California in the 1980s (Norman and Draper, 1986). The UCD is a design process characterized by a cycle of tests and retests of the technology. In the first series of tests, run in order to optimize the interface, experts analyze how users are likely to use the prototype of the interface. In this first step, experts try to simulate the behavior of a common user following the guidelines of a users' model. Then, in the second series of tests, users are involved in a prototype analysis in order to further identify interface problems and to allow a redesign of the information architecture. Following the result of these two different cycles of tests (one carried out by experts and one by users), the UCD model is able to take into account the needs and the abilities of the users in order to optimize the interface, rather than forcing users to adapt themselves to an interface strictly dependent on the developers' model.

The UCD today is one of the most frequently used design processes, but when Norman proposed it in 1986, this perspective was considered to be only a theoretical aim rather than a real process, mostly because the process of test and retest proposed in the UCD was considered expensive if compared with the more linear processes of product design, test, and release. Only in the 1990s, when the diffusion of accessibility and usability was universally recognized as a right to be respected, we can identify the first guidelines proposed by several institutions and disciplines in order to solve the interaction problem. As M. Mirza et al. (2012) underline:

In the United States the first structured guidelines codifying accessibility of the built environment, known by the acronym ADAAG (Americans with Disabilities Act Accessibility Guidelines), were created in 1990 (U.S. Access Board, 2004). Likewise, other countries around the globe have developed accessibility standards, some of which are informed by legislation (Dion et al., 2006). In Europe, through the work of the European Institute for Design and Disability (EIDD Design for All Europe, 2004) network, the *Build for All reference manual* was created in 2006 in order to organize and promote accessibility within the built environment (Build for All project, 2006). Build for All aims to "enable all people to have equal opportunities to participate in every aspect of society. To achieve this, the built environment, everyday objects, services, culture and information – in short, everything that is designed and made by people to be used by people – must be accessible, convenient for everyone in society to use and responsive to evolving human diversity" (Build for All project, 2006; EIDD Design for All Europe, 2004). Although these standards and policies were primarily geared toward promoting accessibility for people with

disabilities, the current international trend has progressed toward a broader definition of the population that could benefit from "accessible" environments. This broad-
ening definition of the user population is expressed in the philosophy of UD. (Mirza
et al., 2012, pp. 68–69)

In this sense, the philosophy of UD is the result of different theoretical perspectives
embodied in the work of different institutions that have tried, by different multidisciplinary approaches, to answer the same needs of access and use for all.

UD, known also as Design for All or inclusive design in the HCI field, implicitly
includes the UCD philosophy. The term UD was first used in the United States by
Mace, who defines it as follows: "Universal design is an approach to design that
incorporates products as well as building features which, to the greatest extent possible, can be used by everyone" (1985). This term identifies a framework for developing solutions to meet the needs of all end users (Knecht, 2004).

As Constantine Stephanidis (2001) claims, UD is often criticized for two main
reasons. On the one hand, because the idea of a Design for All is just an ideal condition that cannot be truly realized but only used as an ideal goal for a user-centered
approach in order to provide products that can address the possible range of human
abilities, skills, requirements, and preferences. This argumentation is well summarized by the motto "many ideas that are supposed to be good for everybody aren't
good for anybody" (Lewis and Rieman, 1993, pp. 12–13). On the other hand, UD is
considered too costly for the benefits it offers (Stephanidis, 2001).

For these reasons, Stephanidis (1995) developed the concept of UIA following the
results of several research initiatives in international projects such as ACCESS and
AVANTI (see Box 1.4).

As Stephanidis underlines (2001), the UIA framework pursues a threefold aim:

1. *Help the designers to improve a UCD*: The UIA framework is focused on
   users' evaluation, by assuming that a UCD provides a new insight into how
   interactive systems can be developed. Such insight aims to replace the tech-
   nocentric practices of the current paradigm with a human focus, which will
   help and guide designers to achieve access and use for all, as the two ideal
   conditions of the *quality in use for all* (Bevan, 2001).
2. *Drive designers in user interface development*: The UIA framework
   describes the useful architectural model and the development tools and
   techniques for the designers.
3. *Define the evaluation cycle*: The UIA framework proposes a formative and
   summative evaluation in an iterative development cycle in which the main
   role in the evaluation is played by the users' evaluation in the specific context of use assessed through different UEMs.

Nowadays, the UAI design philosophy, as we will discuss in Chapter 4, is the only
framework able to include the UD and UCD perspective by taking into account the
context-oriented design, the different user requirements, and the adaptable and adaptive interactive behaviors.

BOX 1.4   ACCESS AND AVANTI PROJECT: INTERNATIONAL INITIATIVES TOWARD USER INTERFACE FOR ALL

MARIA LAURA DE FILIPPIS AND SIMONE BORSCI

The user interface for all (UIA) is an overall and ideal goal of the interactive systems process of development, and it involves issues pertaining to context-oriented design and diverse user requirements as well as adaptable and adaptive interactive behaviors (Stephanidis, 1995, 2001). The UIA's aim can be achieved by designers and evaluators only by a specific and pragmatic methodology for the development and assessment of a user- and use-adapted interaction. This methodology, called unified user interface development, was defined in the 1990s on the basis of the results of two international projects: the TIDE ACCESS and the AVANTI project.

The TIDE ACCESS project, funded by the European Commission from 1994 to 1996, aimed to provide "new technological solutions for developing user interfaces, facilitating unified access to computer-based applications by users with different characteristics, abilities and preferences" (CORDIS, 1994). The overall achievement of the ACCESS project has been the development of specific applications for users with speech-motor, language-cognitive impaired, and visual impairment by a unified user interface development methodology. This methodology was embedded in a platform of toolkits that drove the designers in developing interfaces adapted to the individual user's characteristics and needs. As Stephanidis and Emiliani (1998) have suggested, the ACCESS project defined the concept of UIA as an applicative aim, in tune with the idea of Design for All, that can drive developers in focusing their attention during the design of the interface on the accessibility and quality of the interaction and on the individual abilities, skills, requirements, and preferences of the user population. In particular, the ACCESS project proposed the first application of a unified development methodology for designing a product as a vehicle to efficiently and effectively serve the goal of UIA. This methodology was created for unifying several aspects of user interface design in a set of tools that a designer can use for developing an interface that will not require a redesign or a customization (Stephanidis, 1997) by creating an interface that is able to adapt itself to all the possible users' needs anytime and anywhere (Figure 1.2).

As Stephanidis has underlined (2001), the ACCESS project represented the first international effort toward the UIA, and many accessibility initiatives, industrial companies, and nonmarket institutions have endorsed its outcomes, such as "development of nonvisual interaction metaphors, encapsulation of alternative dialogue patterns, platform abstraction, and generation of user interface implementation through executable specifications rather than programming" (Stephanidis, 2001, p. 9). Whereas the ACCESS project was only focused on the user's access to the information, only in the AdaptiVe

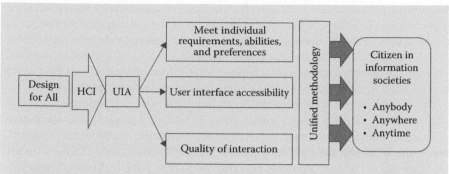

FIGURE 1.2   (See color insert.) Conceptual application of the UIA aim in the design process. The designer can reach the goal of design for all by pursuing the UIA aim. By means of the unified methodology and taking into account the simulated accessibility, the quality of interaction, and the user's needs, abilities, and preferences, the designer can define an interface for any kind of user of information societies that can be used anywhere and anytime. (Adapted from Stephanidis, C. and Emiliani, P.L., Design for All in the TIDE ACCESS Project. Paper presented at the *TIDE '98*, Helsinki, Finland, 1998, http://www.dinf.ne.jp/doc/english/Us_Eu/conf/tide98/164/stephanidis_emiliani.html)

and Adaptable iNteractions for multimedia Telecommunication applIcations project (AVANTI)—funded by the European Commission within the ACTS program from 1995 to 1998 (CORDIS, 1995)—was the unified user interface development methodology applied for designing an interface in a context of UCD by iterative phases of evaluation and redesign. The main aim of the AVANTI project was to develop and evaluate a distributed and adaptable information system that provides hypermedia information about a metropolitan area for different kinds of users (Fink et al., 1996). The AVANTI project outcome consisted in an adaptable system in which the user interface

> dynamically tailor[s] itself to the abilities, skills, requirements and preferences of the users, to the different contexts of use, as well as to the changing characteristics of users, as they interact with the system. The AVANTI UI also features integrated support for various "special" input and output devices, along with a number of appropriate interaction techniques that facilitate the interaction of disabled end-users with the system. (Stephanidis et al., 1998, p. 156)

Finally, the model of information architecture proposed by the AVANTI project represents the first concrete example of UIA.

1.4   MERGING DESIGN AND EVALUATION OF INTERACTION: AN INTEGRATED MODEL OF INTERACTION EVALUATION

The relatively brief evolution of the interaction studies is closely related with the evolution of the technology. As we have seen, each technology evolution has resulted in an enrichment of the interaction functions, and, at the same time, it increased the complexity of use for the users. Our historical analysis has allowed us to understand how this growing complexity of the relation between user and technology was approached by practitioners in order to reduce the distance between the end users and the designers. All the accessibility and usability standards (i.e., the standard rules and the UEMs), together with the design philosophies, have found their main goal in reaching the ideal conditions of universal access and usability. Nevertheless, all these efforts have never accomplished a real integration of the design and the evaluation perspective.

The design and the evaluation processes are, still now, two separate steps that could work together in a design project cycle. In fact, in a project cycle, the design approach tends to fill all the steps by reducing the assessment to a secondary moment, even if the UCD and the most recent UIA philosophy have clearly focused on the shortcomings of the design process in taking into account the real users. These philosophies remark the users' need for adaptable interfaces, the importance of the context of use, and of the necessity of creating samples composed of different kinds of users in user experience (UX) tests.

We should regard the design and the evaluation perspective as two opposite points of view pursuing the same aim: the success of the technology. While the designers try to develop a tool by thinking to a user model, the evaluators try to rethink the object from the point of view of the users:

1. *The designers' perspective*: This perspective can be well summarized by a motto: the better the system works, the better the interaction will be. As Steve Krug (2000) claims in his famous work, *Don't Make Me Think: A Common Sense Approach to Web Usability*, a user has a good interaction experience only when the interface is "self-evident" (Krug, 2000), i.e., when the user cannot "perceive" the interface. The implementation of a "self-evident" interface should be considered as one of the most important issues to be solved when it comes to creating a good system (i.e., a good architecture of information). Krug's assumption relates closely to the designer perspective. However, even though a well-designed interface can only be achieved by considering the properties of the object, the evaluation process also needs to take into account other dimensions of the interaction. In particular, since the goal of the evaluation process is to measure the HCI, the user's point of view somehow needs to be integrated into the evaluation methodologies. Krug's work intends to provide developers with the methods for creating "successful" systems; the author expresses the "success" of a system by using the metaphor of "good navigation" or of "navigation without barriers." This navigation corresponds to his motto "don't make me think."

2. *The evaluators' perspective*: This perspective is focused on "what the user thinks" (or thought) about the system. Following Krug's perspective, the user "should not think" because the developer should have already thought about the possible barriers that could occur during the interaction; from the evaluators' perspective, the sole simulation carried out by the developers during the design process cannot be enough to create a fully accessible and usable system. In this sense, since users must judge the system they are interacting with, for an evaluator the user has to be considered as a "thinker" of the system.

When considering these two opposite viewpoints, a project cycle in which the design and evaluation perspectives are not equalized cannot provide a successful technology. In order to equalize the role of the design and of the evaluation in a project cycle, we think that it is not sufficient to propose a new design perspective able to include the evaluation, as the UCD and the UIA do. Trying to equalize the role of both design and evaluation phases by a design perspective, indeed, implicitly means that the design philosophy should include the evaluation (i.e., the design has priority over the evaluation). By avoiding this false counterbalance, we propose an adaptable model of evaluation capable of integrating the designers' and the evaluators' perspectives, defining and separating their roles independently from the project cycle and from the design perspective endorsed by the developers.

Our work is not focused on the developers' view, but it takes into account all the actors involved in the evaluation process:

- Expert evaluators who are supposed to detect those barriers that "usually" prevent the interaction
- Users who evaluate to what extent a detected barrier is preventing their navigation
- The coordinator of the evaluation (meta-evaluator) who integrates results coming from the expert-based tests with those coming from the user-based tests by performing an evaluation of the evaluation (meta-evaluation), for example, indicating which problems detected by the expert evaluators are real ones, i.e., those problems that were also detected during the user-based tests

In order to equalize the role of the design and the evaluation perspectives, we shall propose a "user-driven" process capable of observing the user's behavior during the actual interaction with the system; in this sense, our perspective on the evaluation of HCI readapts Krug's concept of a "self-evident" interface and focuses on "when the user thinks" rather than "when he or she does not think."

Our user-driven model is called the integrated model of interaction evaluation (IMIE). This model is an adaptable evaluation perspective that can be integrated into any kind of project cycle and can work with any kind of design perspective (see Chapters 4 and 5).

In the IMIE, the goal of the evaluation process is to assess the overall interaction, considering both the subjective and the objective dimensions engaged in the intrasystemic dialogue between the user and the technology. The perspectives and the models we are going to propose should be considered as a new methodological synthesis of the interaction assessment in the HCI field.

2 Defining Usability, Accessibility, and User Experience

2.1 INTRODUCTION: ACCESSIBILITY, USABILITY, AND USER EXPERIENCE IN HUMAN–COMPUTER INTERACTION

The definitions of accessibility, usability, and user experience (UX) are the most important issues of every discussion centered on human–system interaction. These three conceptual dimensions of the interaction define the qualitative and quantitative aspects that guide the design, judgment, assessment, measurement, and implementation of the system–user interaction.

The concept of accessibility refers to how a technological product can be used by people regardless of their disability, abilities, attitudes, and skills for accessing and reaching information and their goals (Roulstone, 2010; W3C-WAI, 2006). If we consider the concept of accessibility in relation to that of usability, however, the two can be regarded as aligning in a temporal order—i.e., people first access the artifact and then they use it. In other words, the accessibility is just the possibility and the ease of accessing the artifacts. On the other hand, usability describes how the use of a system is perceived by the user. As Federici and Borsci (2010) have claimed, the usability evaluation is the process for assessing the

> quality of communication (interaction) between a technological product (system) and a user (the one who uses that technological product). The unit of measurement is the user's behaviour (satisfaction, comfort, time spent in performing an action, etc.) in a specific context of use (natural and virtual environment as well as the physical environment where communication between user and technological product takes place). (Federici and Borsci, 2010, p. 1)

In this sense

> the usability concept and its measurement are strictly connected to that of accessibility [...] and the space of the problem, shared by the users, in which the interaction takes place (user–technology interaction). (Federici and Borsci, 2010, p. 1)

In addition to the aforementioned statement of meanings, alternative definitions are also provided by the International Standard Organization (ISO). For example, in ISO 9241-210, which updates ISO 13407 (ISO, 1999), accessibility is defined as the "usability of a product, service, environment or facility by people with the widest range of capabilities" (ISO, 2010, p. 1). This definition, which is in turn based on ISO 9241-171 (ISO, 2008), highlights the fact that accessibility as a construct can be considered a part of usability and that, at the same time, it has to be considered as different from usability in its wider scope—i.e., in terms of diversity among people. On the other hand, the concept of usability has formerly been defined by the well-known and widely applied ISO 9241-11 as: "the extent to which a product can be used by specified users to achieve specified goals with effectiveness, efficiency, and satisfaction in a specified context of use" (ISO, 1998, p. 2). This definition describes the different dimensions of usability by defining: (1) effectiveness as "the accuracy and completeness with which users achieve specified goals," (2) efficiency as "the resources expended in relation to the accuracy and completeness with which users achieve goals," and (3) satisfaction as "the freedom from discomfort, and positive attitudes towards the use of the product"; in addition, the context of use is described as "users, tasks, equipment (hardware, software and materials), and the physical and social environments in which a product is used" (ISO, 1998, p. 2). The ISO 9241-11's usability definition was also quoted in the ISO 13407 (ISO, 1999), and subsequently amended by the ISO 9241-210 (which revised the ISO 13407) to, "the extent to which a system, product or service can be used by specified users to achieve specified goals with effectiveness, efficiency, and satisfaction in a specified context of use" (ISO, 2010, pp. 1–2). The difference is in the target having been widened to include the system and the service as well as the product. A more recent concept shared in the HCI field is that of UX. It is considered to be a holistic perspective on how a user feels about using a system. We can consider the UX as a meta-analysis of the user interaction with the system focused on the user's perceptions of and about the accessibility and usability he or she has experienced in accessing, using, and manipulating a system. UX results in a sort of extreme subjective perspective that does not consider the real technological functioning of the system but rather the subjective perception, the memorization and the categorization of the interactive elements, and the reaction of the user to a certain technology. In this sense, the UX is more focused on as a marketing measure of the system's success in a certain population of users when they use the technology in real-world settings.

We propose a perspective in which the three conceptual dimensions of accessibility, usability, and UX point out (1) a hierarchical relationship between the concepts (accessibility, usability, and UX) and (2) a model evaluation process.

1. Accessibility, usability, and UX are necessary requirements of the interaction in the same hierarchical and sequential order (from accessibility through usability to arrive at the UX), without which the intrasystemic relationship between user and technology is hampered. From the side of the interaction, without an acceptable level of accessibility, a system cannot be considered truly usable, because some people with specific needs

are excluded by the interaction. At the same time, without a good level of both accessibility and usability, users cannot have a great UX in interacting with a system. In this sense, the interaction dimensions are in a hierarchical order.

2. The hierarchical and sequential relationship among accessibility, usability, and UX suggests a three-step evaluation process: (1) It starts from an objective perspective on the object of the intrasystemic relationship (technology) that turns into an evaluation of features of the technological functioning (accessibility); (2) It goes through a subjective perspective on the interaction and on the use of the technological elements through the assessment of the usability of multidimensional aspects (effectiveness, efficiency, and satisfaction); and, (3) It ends with an overall assessment of the object and interaction from a user perspective (UX). From our point of view, accessibility, usability, and UX are three different perspectives that an evaluator adopts in sequence while assessing the intrasystemic relationship between user and system.

Upholding this perspective, we shall define accessibility, usability, and UX as features of interaction that have to be designed to pursue an interface for all and accomplish universal design aims, and as phases that compose the evaluation process of the interaction as well.

In the following sections, we explore the most widely known definitions of accessibility, usability, and UX and their hierarchical relationship in order to enrich the evaluator's point of view on what should be evaluated for across each of these three dimensions. The multistep evaluation model that results from the hierarchical relationship of accessibility, usability, and UX is presented in Chapter 4.

2.2 CONCEPT OF ACCESSIBILITY

As was discussed in Chapter 1, the concept of accessibility evolved with the growth of the Internet. Throughout the Internet's history, different definitions of accessibility have been proposed, which have sought to spread the idea of access as a right. These definitions, however, never identified the dimensions under which accessibility was being assessed. We can say that today, although the concept of accessibility is largely defined, there is still no shared and unique definition of accessibility, but only a set of definitions which coexist. We can identify three main definitions of accessibility, representing different perspectives on accessibility along the evolution of the Internet:

- The first definition of accessibility was proposed in the 1990s by Berners-Lee, developers of the Internet protocols of communication and director of the W3C, in his autobiography written together with the senior editor at Scientific American, Mark Fischetti, as follows: "The art of ensuring that, to as large an extent as possible, facilities are available to people whether or not they have impairments of one sort or another" (Berners-Lee and Fischetti, 1999, p. 231). According to this definition, accessibility has to be considered a dimension of the websites' interfaces for guaranteeing and extending the possibilities that disabled people may access.

- The second definition of accessibility was provided by the WAI group of the W3C, and extended the Berners-Lee definition. According to the WAI definition, accessibility has to be considered the possibility for people with disabilities to "perceive, understand, navigate and interact with the web" (W3C-WAI, 2006).
- The third definition of accessibility was provided by the ISO 9241-171, which defines accessibility as the "usability of a product, service, environment, or facility by people with the widest range of capabilities" (ISO, 2008, p. 2).

Web accessibility means the possibility for people with disabilities to access wanted information. Since the definition of accessibility provided by the ISO has shown a link between this construct and that of usability, in HCI studies disabled users' needs and abilities in the interaction process have become a central issue that must be addressed in order to respect the idea of a universal design granting accessibility and usability for all.

As discussed in Chapter 1, we can divide the evolution of the concept of accessibility into three periods that broadly follow the evolution of the web:

1990–1999: In this period, the Internet is considered a "universal medium" without taking into account the interaction of peoples with disabilities. Only in the last years of 1990s, when the Internet became a shared technology in information societies, were the needs of disabled people taken into consideration by institutions. The legislative movement began in the United States with a measure voted on in 1998, Section 508, which required all public websites (i.e., those for federal agencies and institutions) to be accessible according to the criteria defined in the Act. In this period, the W3C-WAI, as discussed in Chapter 1, developed the accessibility guidelines for web. The first version of these rules, relating to the Web Content Accessibility, was published in 1999.

1999–2008: The European Commission joined the legislative movement only in 2001, recognizing the accessibility guidelines of the W3C-WAI as the de facto standards. In 2003, following a resolution passed by the European Parliament (European Commission, 2012b), all European websites were required to meet at least Level 2 of W3C-WAI's rules. Since 2003, many European countries have passed additional legislation that requires that the electronic services of their respective public sectors be accessible to persons with disabilities, introducing the accessibility concept in national legislation.

2008–present: Since 2006, the *Convention on the Rights of Persons with Disabilities*, published by the UN, has stated that, "States Parties shall take appropriate measures to ensure to persons with disabilities access to information and communication including systems and information technology and communication" (UN, 2006, art. 9). A draft of the second version of the accessibility guidelines of the W3C-WAI was published in late 2008. The diffusion of web technology on mobile phones and other portable technologies has made accessibility a central business issue for private companies, and not only for public institutions. As discussed earlier, researchers' efforts to define and spread the concept of accessibility during the evolution of the web technologies have produced a set of definitions without a unified understanding of "accessibility" and in need of clarification as to how it has been assessed. We can state that, although the rules pertaining to accessibility such as the WCAG 2.0 clearly indicate what an expert is expected to check for in measuring accessibility and describe how to assess the features of a product, they do not provide a clear, unified definition of accessibility. In sum, from an evaluative point of view, a high level of accessibility to technology is just the first step in creating a positive interactive environment between users and system. Developers can be confident that the system will be somehow accessible by adhering to the established guidelines in designing the system; in order to identify both level of accessibility and any usability problems experienced by users, however, an evaluation process is also required. In order to evaluate the achievement of or adherence to the standard rules, experts should carry out an assessment of interactions with the system, with the participation of a mixed panel of users with different kind of disabilities and with different sets of assistive technologies. This kind of evaluation process is necessary to provide designers with data about the accessibility problems needing to be solved in order to ensure adherence to the guidelines and that they have met different users' needs.

2.3 USABILITY: FROM THE SMALL TO THE BIG PERSPECTIVE

Over the last 30 years, many different definitions of usability have been proposed to keep up with transformations to technology and the subsequent changes to the user–technology interaction design process. As Chou and Hsiao, both of Taiwan University (2007), have stated:

> "Usability" is a well-known and well-defined concept in human-computer interaction research, referring to the extent to which the user and the system can "communicate" clearly and without misunderstanding through the interface. (2007, p. 2041)

We cannot totally endorse the idea of Chou and Hsiao, however, that usability is a well-defined concept; in fact, in the historical evolution of the HCI field, there has been more than one useful definition that researchers and practitioners have claimed as the definition of usability.

Following the analysis of the evolution of usability definitions provided by Kurosu (2007) and based on the discussion of the ISO working group, we shall divide the usability definitions into two main approaches: small usability and big usability.

Small usability: This approach, common in the HCI field, defines usability as a multidimensional concept encompassed by the following dimensions: effectiveness, efficiency, learnability, flexibility, memorability, errors, and satisfaction (Hix and Hartson, 1993; Jordan, 1994; Nielsen, 1993). This is a functional approach that defines the dimensions of usability in order to set standards for identifying problems with and in the to-be-evaluated systems. If usability is defined as a multidimensional measure able to evaluate only the "lacks" of the system, then the evaluation goals concern only the possibility of improving the negative aspects of the interface. In this case, Kurosu speaks about the "small" or "non-negative concept of usability" (2007, p. 580).

The small usability approach is well represented by the ISO/International Electrotechnical Commission (IEC) 9126, first proposed in 1991 and revised by a four-part distinction in 2001 (ISO/IEC 9126-1, 9126-2, 9126-3, 9126-4). ISO/IEC 9126-1 defines usability as the "understandability, learnability, operability and attractiveness" (2001, p. 9) of the system, considering it to be focused on the quality of the technology instead of on the quality of the interaction. This definition highlights the fact that small usability concerns any kind of approach in which assessing usability means ameliorating the features of the system.

Big usability: The small usability approach was overcome in 1998, when usability was redefined by ISO 9241-11 in a manner that shifted the focus of usability from the features of the technology to the quality of the interaction between the user and the technology, as follows: "the extent to which a product can be used by specified users to achieve specified goals with effectiveness, efficiency, and satisfaction in a specified context of use" (1998, p. 2). Today, the ISO 9241-11 is accepted as the main reference for the definition of usability and, since it refers to this construct as the relationship between effectiveness, efficiency, and satisfaction in a context of use, it clearly explicates the link between usability and user's ability to achieve goals. In particular, the definition provided in ISO 9241-11 assumes that usability is measured by the quality of the user's interaction, instead of by the quality of the technology features (as would be the case in small usability).

Kurosu (2007) rewords ISO 9241-11's usability definition as a "big usability" concept centered on user's goal achievement instead of on the identification of the "non-negative" aspects of the interface.

> It is important that the effectiveness and the efficiency are not only related to the "non-negative" aspects but also the positive aspects of artefacts. Regarding the effectiveness, the artefact can become usable by minimizing the difficulty of use. But at the same time, the artefact can become usable providing the function that will solve the user's problem and make it easier to achieve the goal. Regarding the efficiency, the usability will be improved by changing the interaction procedure in order to shorten time of operation. But it could be improved by the faster CPU. (Kurosu, 2007, p. 582)

Kurosu and Hashizume (2012) have recently connected the big usability approach to the UX construct, proposing that satisfaction is included not only in usability but also as an important variable of the UX concept. The authors state that the relationship between usability and the UX is similar to variables in a function where the quality traits of the interaction—including usability—correspond to independent variables, and variables such as satisfaction act as dependent variables (Kurosu and Hashizume, 2012). In a causal relationship such as this, the quality traits of the interaction (of a good level of usability and a positive UX) affect user satisfaction. Moreover, in Kurosu and Hashizume's (2012) study of three different types of interaction behavior—goal-oriented behavior, process-oriented behavior, and state-oriented behavior—they have shown that satisfaction is not the unique dependent variable or the unique result of the quality traits of the interaction:

> Because the usability is closely related to the goal achieving behavior, it is accept-able that ISO 9241-11 included satisfaction in its definition of usability. But because the satisfaction is also influenced by other traits such as reliability, safety, aesthetic aspects, etc., the concept of satisfaction should be considered as a top-most evaluation concept in terms of the goal achieving behavior including the pragmatic aspects and the hedonic aspects. (Kurosu and Hashizume, 2012)

We should clarify that the big usability approach proposed by Kurosu, and later extended by Kurosu and Hashizume (2012), plays an important role in clarifying the relationship among the different dimensions of usability defined in the ISO 9241-11 (i.e., effectiveness, efficiency, and satisfaction). For Kurosu and Hashizume (2012), the user's satisfaction is a dependent variable of efficiency and effectiveness, and, at the same time, the efficiency of the interaction is hierarchically dependent on the effectiveness dimension. In fact, the measuring of efficiency presupposes that users achieve the goal with a certain degree of effectiveness.

2.3.1 USABILITY: TOWARD A UNIFIED STANDARD

By following the ISO modifications over time, we have defined the small and big usability approaches, the shared definition of usability, and its assessment dimensions (i.e., effectiveness, efficiency, and satisfaction) by analyzing the differences between these concepts. Nevertheless, defining usability is not sufficient to explain the relationship between accessibility, usability, and UX as hierarchical. In fact, it is necessary to define not only what usability is and how to assess it, but also what is the relationship between accessibility and UX. In order to better understand this point, we have to consider two recent standards: the ISO 9241-210 (2010) and the ISO/IEC 25010 (2011).

The ISO 9241-210 (2010) is an evolution of the ISO 13407 (1999), and it defines the human-centered design for interactive systems, concurrently formalizing the UX concept. This ISO clearly underlines the fact that the usability of the system is a necessary condition for the UX. We shall discuss this relationship between usability and UX in Section 2.5.

The ISO/IEC 25010 (2011), which revises the ISO 9126-1 (2001), analyzes the concept of quality in use by presenting usability as a dimension that affects the quality of the interaction (Figure 2.1). This ISO proposes a specific model of product quality, linking usability and accessibility (Figure 2.2). In fact, accessibility is considered one of the main characteristics of a product for guaranteeing usability. In light of this, we can say that the hierarchical relationship between accessibility and both usability (ISO 25010) and UX (ISO 9241-210) is clearly specified by the standards, albeit not explicitly formalized.

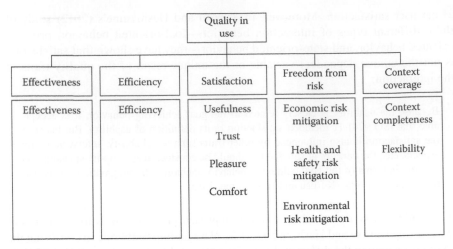

FIGURE 2.1 Quality in use model which shows the five main variables of quality in use: effectiveness, efficiency, satisfaction, freedom from risk, and the context coverage. (From ISO/IEC 25010, Systems and software engineering—Systems and software quality requirements and evaluation (SQuaRE)—System and software quality models, 2011.)

Even though we cannot attempt to forecast the actions of international experts, we can hypothesize that the formalization of the relationship between accessibility, usability, and UX in a new ISO—one able to harmonize ISO 9241-11, ISO 9241-201, and ISO 25010—could be one of the most probable future scenarios of the HCI discussion. We synthesize our hypothesis in Figure 2.3 by proposing a graphic representation of the connections shared by the first standards from the 1990s through to those in effect today, which suggests that the next step taken by the international community could be to propose a unified standard through a revision of ISO 9241-11.

What we aim to underline is that one piece of evidence emerges when we consider usability as a measure of the interaction while taking into account the complexity of its historical evolution: usability cannot be achieved without an accessible system. Indeed, while from the technical point of view we could design a usable interface that is not accessible at all (e.g., a flash website that is not optimized following the accessibility guidelines), from the interaction point of view, the usability of a system cannot be observed without some degree of accessibility. For instance, if a blind user were hampered in accessing web page contents by the fact that these are fully conveyed through visual media, an evaluator would not observe any positive level of usability of the system.

In light of this, whereas "accessibility refers to the environmental characteristics of entrance/exit movements" (Federici et al., 2005, p. 781)—i.e., no entrance to system, no level of usability of system—usability refers to the use and interaction of the system in which the user is entered. In this sense, the evaluator can assess the usability only after the accessibility problems of the interface have been solved and the system is considered to be accessible.

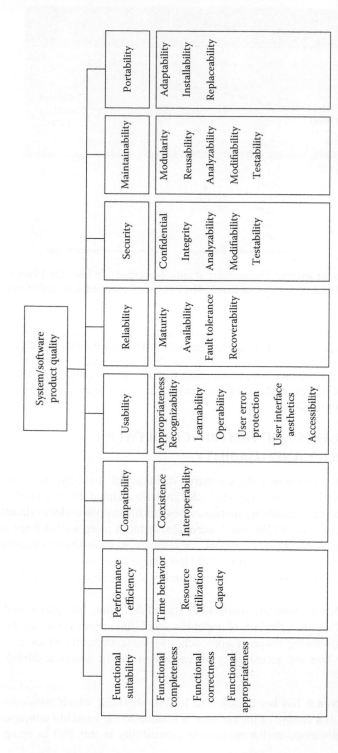

FIGURE 2.2 Product quality model which shows the eight important quality features of a product: functional sustainability, performance efficiency, compatibility, usability, reliability, security, maintainability, and probability. In this model, accessibility is considered one of the main user needs that must characterize the product when measuring usability. (From ISO/IEC 25010, Systems and software engineering—Systems and software quality requirements and evaluation (SQuaRE)—System and software quality models, 2011)

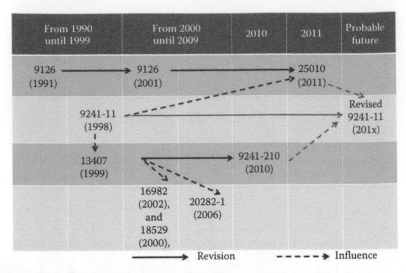

From 1990 until 1999	From 2000 until 2009	2010	2011	Probable future

——————→ Revision   - - - - -→ Influence

FIGURE 2.3   (See color insert.) The usability standards relationship from the 1990s until today, and the possible future revision of ISO 9241-11 to create a unified standard of usability. The solid arrows indicate the recent standards that have replaced the old ones, while the dashed arrows show the influence of the old standards on the most recent ones. The figure, by moving from the concept of quality in ISO 9126-1 (2001), shows the concurrent evolution of the usability concept in the relationship between ISO 9241-11 (1998), ISO 13407 (1999), and ISO 25010 (2011). At the same time, ISO 13407, by defining the human-centered design process, has strongly affected ISO 16982 (2002), 18529 (2000), 20282-1 (2006), and 9241-210 (2010). All of these standards should be summarized in the coming years into a single ISO, most likely the revision of 9241-11.

2.4   RELATIONSHIPS AND DIFFERENCES BETWEEN ACCESSIBILITY AND USABILITY

As discussed earlier, there is nowadays a shared definition of usability, provided by ISO 9241-11 (1998), whereas as Borsci et al. (2012b) have claimed, there is no shared and unique definition of accessibility that describes the dimensions under evaluation. Moreover, as Borsci et al. (2012b) noted, accessibility has a more well-defined and shared method of assessment—as is evident, for instance, in accessibility guidelines (e.g., the WCAG 2.0)—while the usability field has a large set of assessment methods with different outcomes, costs, and levels of reliability (e.g., heuristic and the GOMS analysis).

While the usability assessment, thanks to its shared definition, has increased during the evolution of the HCI, the lack of a specific set of dimensions for accessibility has produced the following range of approaches in the community of evaluators looking to identify how the accessibility of interaction can be assessed during an evaluation process:

1. The first approach has been suggested by ISO 9241-20, which considers accessibility as a feature of the product in relation to the usability concept, whereas we discussed earlier mentioned accessibility in this ISO as being

defined as, "the usability of a product, service, environment or facility by people with the widest range of capabilities" (ISO, 2009, p. 2). According to this perspective, accessibility is considered to be a dimension in an inclusive dependence with the usability one.

2. Another common approach in HCI is to define accessibility as a right of people to have access to information. Accessibility is linked to the rights of "access" to a wide "range of services, information, cultural exchanges, identity reaffirmations and social transactions [...] seen as a basic right of citizens in many advanced society contexts" (Roulstone, 2010, p. 9). In particular, ensuring web accessibility means that "people with disabilities can use the web. [...] More specifically [they] can perceive, understand, navigate, and interact with the web" (W3C-WAI, 2006). According to this approach, accessibility is an independent dimension of the interaction.

It is important to underline that the two approaches previously illustrated are the results of the historical evolution of the accessibility concept, and that accessibility is an issue that is growing along with Internet technology and the need to include disabled users in the resultant information societies. It is therefore quite comprehensible that accessibility is considered to be a right and that, at the same time, the achieving of accessibility guidelines is considered an important part of accessibility analysis, as well. Nevertheless, as Nicoletta Di Blas, Paolo Paolini, and Marco Speroni state:

> W3C guidelines only guarantee "technical readability," i.e. the very fact that screen readers can work; they do not ensure at all the fact that the Website is "accessible" by blind users, in the sense that blind users can effectively access it. (2004, p. 1)

In light of this, the guidelines' achievement of guaranteeing the right of access is only the first step of accessibility analysis. The second one, as Di Blas et al. (2004) have suggested, consists of assessing the "usable accessibility" experienced by the user.

As Federici and Borsci have claimed, the relationship between accessibility and usability in the assessment cannot be superficially reduced to an objective–subjective distinction.

> [A]ccessibility and usability are not understood as characteristics of two separate interacting entities but rather as one intrasystemic relation, where both object and subject are just moments in a multiphase process of empirical observation. This prevents the existence of user-less technological products thereby guaranteeing that the accessibility of a machine refers only to the possible entrance and exit of a signal needed to fulfil the task for which it was designed, and that it is in constant relation either to its designer or to its user. In this sense, a machine cannot be accessible and yet unusable at the same time. (Federici and Borsci, 2010, p. 2)

As already pointed out, accessibility and usability have to be considered as two interrelated means, in a hierarchical relationship, of detecting interaction problems from different evaluative perspectives.

During an evaluation of the interaction, it is difficult to distinguish between accessibility and usability issues. As we illustrate in Figure 2.4, during the assessment, the accessibility and usability problems can be seen as two overlapping sets, which would include three categories, as follows:

- "Problems that only affect disabled people, which can be termed "pure accessibility" problems;
- Problems that only affect non-disabled people, which can be termed "pure usability" problems;

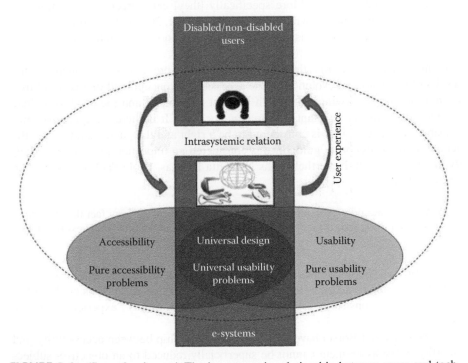

FIGURE 2.4   (See color insert.) The intrasystemic relationship between users and technology. UX is represented as the user perspective in the intrasystemic relation of action and feedback with the system. The universal design properties that comprise the system are obtained by the intersection of the accessibility and usability of the system. According to Petrie and Kheir (2007), the universal usability problems represent interaction problems of usability and accessibility that are encountered by all kinds of users in a bad intrasystemic relation, due to a bad universal design. When the problems affect mostly disabled people's interaction, we may use the term "pure accessibility problems"; when the problems do not pertain to disabled users' interaction, we may use the term "pure usability problems." Between these two extremes, however, there are many different degrees of interaction problems that affect the UX of disabled and nondisabled users. (From Federici, S. and Borsci, S., Usability evaluation: Models, methods, and applications, in Stone, J and Blouin, M (Eds.), *International Encyclopedia of Rehabilitation*, Center for International Rehabilitation Research Information and Exchange (CIRRIE), Buffalo, NY, pp. 1–17, 2010, retrieved from http://cirrie.buffalo.edu/encyclopedia/article.php?id = 277&language = en)

- Problems that affect both disabled and non-disabled people, which can be termed "universal usability" problems (Horton, 2005; Lazar, 2007; Shneiderman, 2003). Accessibility problems were not a complete sub-set of usability problems" (Petrie and Kheir, 2007, p. 398).

In summary, we can say that accessibility problems are not a subset of usability problems, nor are usability problems a subset of accessibility problems. In fact, during the assessment of the interaction, accessibility and usability are used as two interrelated means of detecting interaction problems from different angles, and, therefore, they have to be considered to be in a hierarchical relationship.

As we discussed in Section 2.3.1, both the level of accessibility and usability define the UX with the system. In fact, from an interaction point of view, the only way to grant the success of the technology, and therefore a highly positive UX, is to control at least the "accessibility" and "usability" variables. In light of this, as we shall discuss in the following section, the evaluation of UX has to be considered to be a holistic process, one that allows practitioners to assess how users rate and interact with the system by taking into account their feelings and judgments, thus providing an indirect and subjective measure of the accessibility and the usability of the system.

2.5 USER EXPERIENCE

In the 1990s, Donald A. Norman et al. (1995), researchers at the Apple Computer Inc., defined the UX concept as a user perspective on pleasure, value, and performance during an interaction with a system. Only 3 years later, Norman provided a complete explanation of this concept by defining UX as

> all aspects of the user's interactions with the product: how it is perceived, learned and used. It includes ease of use and, most important of all, the needs that the product fulfills. (Norman, 1998, p. 47)

Although Norman's definition remains one of the most referenced, there are currently at least 27 definitions of UX, which have been provided in the last 15 years by different authors, companies, and associations and as reported on Allaboutux. org's (http://www.allaboutux.org/ux-definitions) list of UX definitions, created by a team of experts lead by Virpi Hannele Roto, principal scientist on UX at the Nokia Research Center of Helsinki. This number of proposed definitions suggests that, on the one hand, there is growing interest in the UX concept by the companies and the HCI community, whereas, on the other hand, it underlines that there is still no unified and shared definition of the concept that satisfactorily identifies all of the assessment dimensions of the UX.

Only recently, in 2010, did international experts try to summarize all of the existing definitions into one single standard, in ISO 9241-210 (2010), by indicating the main dimensions that have to be considered for assessing the UX. This ISO defined the UX as a

> person's perceptions and responses resulting from the use and/or anticipated use of a product, system or service

NOTE 1 User experience includes all the users' emotions, beliefs, preferences, perceptions, physical and psychological responses, behaviours and accomplishments that occur before, during and after use.

NOTE 2 User experience is a consequence of brand image, presentation, functionality, system performance, interactive behaviour and assistive capabilities of the interactive system, the user's internal and physical state resulting from prior experiences, attitudes, skills and personality, and the context of use.

NOTE 3 Usability, when interpreted from the perspective of the users' personal goals, can include the kind of perceptual and emotional aspects typically associated with user experience. Usability criteria can be used to assess aspects of user experience. (ISO, 2010, p. 3)

The definition provided in ISO 9241-210 highlights the fact that UX is a subjective dimension of the interaction that can be measured through both a short-term assessment measuring specific aspects such as comfort and pleasure in use and a long-term follow-up analysis—i.e., 6–12 months after product installation—measuring aspects such as well-being and satisfaction of use that emerge once the user has acquired a specific competence of use. Moreover, the definition underlined a strong link between UX and usability, thereby supporting our notion of a hierarchical relationship existing among accessibility (i.e., access to the system), usability (use/navigate/explore the system when it is accessible), and UX (experience the system when it can be accessed and used).

In the international debate, many authors (Hassenzahl and Tractinsky, 2006; Law et al., 2007) have underlined the fact that it is difficult to discern what pertains to usability measures and what pertains to UX measures. As Hellen Petrie, professor of Human–Computer Interaction at the University of York, and Nigel Bevan, research manager at Serco Usability Services and National Physical Laboratory, has summarized, there are some areas in which UX goes beyond usability, illustrated as follows:

- "*Holistic*: As previously discussed, usability focuses on performance of and satisfaction with users' tasks and their achievement in defined contexts of use; UX takes a more holistic view, aiming for a balance between task-oriented aspects and other non-task-oriented aspects (often called *hedonic* aspects) of e-system use and possession, such as beauty, challenge, stimulation, and self-expression.
- *Subjective*: Usability has emphasized objective measures of its components, such as percentage of tasks achieved for effectiveness and task completion times and error rates for efficiency; UX is more concerned with users' subjective reactions to e-systems, their perceptions of the e-systems themselves and their interaction with them.
- *Positive*: Usability has often focused on the removal of barriers or problems in e-systems as the methodology for improving them; UX is more concerned with the positive aspects of e-system use, and how to maximize them, whether those positive aspects be joy, happiness, or engagement" (Petrie and Bevan, 2009, p. 300).

Nowadays, the international debate over the definition of UX is still ongoing, and it is even more focused on defining those measures of the UX that distinguish it from measures of usability. In 2010, in order to unify the concept and measures of UX, a total of 30 usability professionals and experts joined together in a workshop held in Dagstuhl, Germany, which has been summarized by Virpi Roto and colleagues in a White Paper (Roto et al., 2011). This White Paper (Roto et al., 2011) underlines the fact that three factors may influence the level of UX: the context around the user and system, the user's state, and the system properties:

1. *The context around the user and the system*—In the UX domain, the level of UX is dependent upon the context and it may change independently from the system when the context changes. The context is the environment in which users interact with the system, such as the social environment (i.e., interacting alone or with other people), the physical environment of use, the task context (i.e., the level of attention and cognitive workload required to achieve the task), and the technical and information context.
2. *The user's state*—The subject of the interaction is a cognitive system in relation to a designed system. In this sense, the UX represents the subjects' point of view of the intrasystemic relation between them and the system. The quality of the UX is dependent upon the persons' motivation to use the product, their mood, the current mental and physical resources available, and the users' expectations.
3. *The system properties*—Viewed from a UX perspective, the image of the system as it is perceived by users is a highly influential variable. Different factors influence how users experience the properties of the system: the designed properties of the technological functioning (i.e., accessibility, the usability perceived by users), its aesthetics, its ability to allow and maintain personalization (i.e., the properties that the user adds or changes in the system or that are consequence of its use), and how users perceive the brand or manufacturer image.

In summary, we can say that although ISO 9241-210 does define UX, there is still little agreement of the variables that affect the UX and its measurements. At the same time, it is clear that UX is not an independent feature of the interaction but, as we have proposed, has a hierarchical relationship to both accessibility and usability. In fact, as Borsci et al. (2012b) have stated:

> Although the accessibility and the usability refer to the quality of the device and system in access and in use that can be described objectively, the concept of UX relates to such subjective aspects as an expected experience, and perception and memory on the part of the user. In other words, quality traits such as usability and reliability can be regarded as independent variables whereas the UX is a dependent variable that will be influenced by the quality traits of devices and systems to be used. This means that consideration of the quality traits alone will not necessarily lead to a good UX. We should consider something more to achieve a better UX. This stance of putting an emphasis on the resulting UX is better than just focusing on the quality traits (Borsci et al., 2012b, p. 338).

In conclusion, we can say that ISO 9241-210 strongly emphasizes the fact that it is not possible to obtain a reliable UX evaluation by analyzing only the functionality of the system or by testing the interaction only in an experimental setting since UX is an interaction dimension that can be measured only in real contexts of use by users with a long-term experience of interaction.

2.5.1 STEPS OF UX: FROM THE EXPECTATIONS OF THE USERS BEFORE PRODUCT PURCHASE TO THE FINAL IMPRESSION OF THE PRODUCT

As we underlined in the previous section, the UX is nowadays an evolving concept, as the variables that affect its evaluation still must be clearly defined. As Kurosu and Ando (2008; see also Kurosu, 2010) have suggested, although the theoretical framework regarding UX is not yet complete, according to ISO 9241-210 (2010), it is possible to identify at least four main phases of UX, from the acquisition of a product through to the follow-up. This four-phase model is based on the idea that people may change their stance in moving from consumer to user, before and after the purchase of a technology (Kurosu and Ando, 2008; see also Kurosu, 2010), as is illustrated in Figure 2.5. In the four-phase model, UX is thus observed from the user's point of view, since it represents the progression of people interested in purchasing a product (consumers) to users that have acquired a certain degree of experience in use (informed users):

- *Phase 1: Subject as a consumer.* In the first phase, people shape their expectations of devices and systems in both subjective ways (e.g., simple desire) and objective ways (e.g., foreseeable usage). Such expectancies may be based on various pieces of information obtained through such ephemera as advertisements and TV commercials, as well as websites, journal articles, and information from friends. Thereafter, people obtain an impression of a

Expectancy (subjective and objective) based on various information sources	Impression based on the trial use	Evaluation based on accumulated interactions in the real context	Impression based on the memory trace after the waste
(Consumer)	(Purchaser)	(User)	(Post-user)

Time ⟶

FIGURE 2.5 The four-phase model of UX forms the user's perspective. In phase 1, the person is interested in purchasing a product (consumer) and recruits specific information about the technology on the basis of his/her level of motivation, experience in use, and expectation. Then, in phase 2, the purchaser starts to interact with the new product, becoming a user. After a period of use, in phase 3, the user acquires a certain degree of experience, becoming an informed user. Finally, in phase 4, the informed user can look for a new product that can satisfy his or her increased motivation, experience in use, and expectation of interaction. (From Kurosu, M. and Ando, M., The psychology of non-selection and waste: A tentative approach for constructing the user behavior theory based on the Artifact Development Analysis, Paper presented at the *74th Annual Convention of Japanese Psychological Association*, Osaka University, Osaka, Japan, 2008, http://www.wdc-jp.biz/jpa/conf2010/)

device and a system that may be based on a trial use of the product (if they can test it), or on the base of the information and experience they have with a similar product (if they cannot test it). If the consumer is both interested in and motivated toward purchasing the product, they may become a purchaser (see Figure 2.5).

- *Phase 2: Subject as a purchaser.* After the purchase, people become users and start interacting with the system in a real context. Usability testing, as a summative evaluation, measures what corresponds to this second phase.
- *Phase 3: Subject as a user with experience.* The repetitive interactions in a real environment will be stored in the user's memory, thus forming an evaluation of the system. In this phase, during which the user has a certain degree of experience gained over a period of time, usually 6–12 months, it is possible to measure the UX by a short-term or a long-term evaluation (ISO 9241-210, 2010).
- *Phase 4: Subject returns to a consumer role with an increase of his or hers' competence as a user.* After having used the device and the system, there still remains a trace in the user's memory about that type of technology. This information will serve as a basis for searching out a new device or system as a consumer in the next cyclical stage.

These four phases will form a spiral structure, from consumer to informed consumer (see Figure 2.5).

Kurosu and Hashizume (2012) have recently transformed the four-phase model into a UX model able to guide evaluators during UX assessment (see Figure 2.6). In their model, Kurosu and Hashizume explore each phase in which people become

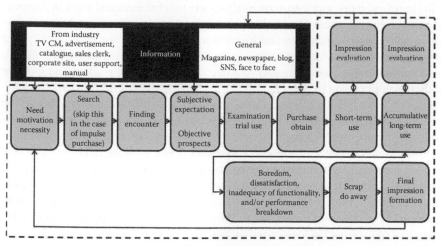

User experience

FIGURE 2.6 (See color insert.) Overall stages of the UX. In line with the four-phase model of UX (Figure 2.5), the model proposes the overall stages over time that can affect the UX assessment. (From Kurosu, M. and Hashizume, A., *Describing Experiences in Different Mode of Behavior—GOB, POB and SOB*, Paper presented at the *Kansei Engineering and Emotion Research: KEER '12*, Penghu, Taiwan, China, May 22–25, 2012.)

purchaser, user, and informed user (see Figure 2.6) by analyzing it from the evaluators' point of view, in order to describe all the variables that can affect UX, from the motivation to purchase to the final impression on the product.

The model proposed by Kurosu and Hashizume (2012) is currently the first comprehensive representation of all the variables that, in line with ISO 9241-210, an evaluator must consider in assessing the UX. The UX model proposes 10 variables that an evaluator has to consider when assessing UX (see Figure 2.6). The first three variables of the UX model concern the motivation for searching out and purchasing the product: (1) the user needs, inducted or reinforced by the information that the users know or have received through media; (2) the user motivation created by his or her experience; and (3) the reason for acquiring the product (necessity). These variables determine the kind of product that people are looking for (search and find or encounter). The final purchase is determined by the distance between (4) the subjective expectations and (5) the objects' features as perceived by users (if such is possible, for instance through a trial use period). As in phase 1 of the four-phase model, by following these steps people become purchasers.

Once the product has been obtained, the purchaser starts the interaction and, as in phase 2 of the four-phase model, it is possible to evaluate the short-term use by considering (6) the effectiveness, (7) the efficiency, (8) the satisfaction (i.e., usability), and (9) the overall impression of the user about the interaction with the product on the bases of his or hers' expectations as created through the collecting of information regarding the product.

As previously discussed when describing phase 3 of the four-phase model, since users require long-term use of a product to accumulate a certain degree of experience in its use, only then is it possible to (10) assess their impression about the interaction with the product.

In summary, short- and long-term analyses are two fundamental steps in composing a final UX assessment (the final impression), which provides to evaluators information on the user satisfaction and his or her opinion about the functionality and performance of the product. Of course, in line with phase 4 of the four-phase model, this final impression guides the user to a decision: discard the product and look for another one or proceed in using it.

The UX model of Kurosu and Hashizume (2012) describes the variables of the assessment that, in the relevant literature, are considered to be valid by the international experts; the methods as to how to perform the assessment, however, are not discussed in this model. Currently, UX assessment is a growing field in which new methods for assessing the interaction (such as the eye-tracking methodology) and usability methods and techniques (such as the thinking aloud technique) are used to obtain an overall analysis of an interaction system by comparing the evaluation as performed by its users with a low degree of experience with the product (short-term use) to that of users with a long experience of use (long-term use).

2.6　CONCLUSION

In this chapter, in line with the international debate of HCI experts and following the evolution of standards, we have described and analyzed different definitions of accessibility, usability, and UX, suggesting that in order to fully investigate all aspects of the intrasystemic dialogue between user and technology, an evaluation process has to consider the three dimensions of accessibility, usability, and UX in a hierarchical and sequential order.

By discussing the international literature, we proposed that evaluators have to take into account accessibility as the first dimension to be analyzed, because it pertains to the possibility for users to access the virtual space and materially achieve and manipulate the information. We discussed the fact that, although accessibility is a right from an ethical and political point of view, most evaluators actually consider accessibility as nothing more than a necessary condition for the interaction.

Moreover, our analysis has shown that the accessibility concept is strongly linked to the usability one—first, because, from the evaluation point of view, it is often difficult to distinguish between interaction problems (due to usability or accessibility issues) and, second, because access and use are logically linked together by international standards (i.e., ISO 9241-20, 2009). We proposed that the current international debate is moving toward a unified standard (see Figure 2.3) in which the accessibility, usability, and UX concepts will be clearly redefined to highlight their relationships and measurements.

Finally, we discussed UX as a new and evolving concept of the HCI. As ISO 9241-210 (2010) suggests, the UX is strongly linked to usability and it represents the subjective perspective of the interaction system. As we have proposed, the users' perceptions of their interactions with a product (UX) is a dependent variable of the possibility to access the interface (accessibility) and use and navigate the technology and its contents (usability).

Therefore, accessibility, usability, and UX have to be considered as three different perspectives of the interaction, and any evaluator should assess these aspects in sequence in order to produce a complete interaction evaluation.

We shall discuss an integrating evaluation model for assessing the interaction in Chapters 4 and 5, while in the next chapter, we shall discuss the object of the interaction (the system) by introducing the new concept of "psychotechnology," in order to clarify the relation between users and technology in an intrasystemic perspective.

3 Why We Should Be Talking about Psychotechnologies for Socialization, Not Just Websites

3.1 INTRODUCTION: THE PSYCHOTECHNOLOGICAL EVOLUTION

Since its first release, the World Wide Web (W3) has had a complex and rapidly changing evolution involving the development of the different functions developed over the last 20 years. Web data pass through a structure, which is organized into networks distributed over different physical allocation nodes; this structure is characterized by a high plasticity, which facilitates data processing and provides users with sets of "unified" information, thanks to the hypertext transfer protocol (HTTP) network protocol.

The so-called "web era" began in the early 1990s and started from an idea Tim Berners-Lee had, which was in response to the need for a platform-independent system to share scientific documentation in electronic format. Therefore, the first version of the web was not intended to be for everyone, but it was developed for the transmission of information and for communication between a few researchers at the European Organization for Nuclear Research (CERN) (Gillies and Cailliau, 2000). Since 1993, thanks to the liberalization of the Berners-Lee's project for the public, Internet traffic has doubled, on average, every year (Coffman and Odlyzko, 2002; Odlyzko, 2003), and the web has thus become the main channel for sending and receiving information. The way to transmit information has evolved gradually from a static mode to a dynamic one, toward what is now defined as the Semantic Web (Wikipedia contributors, 2012f), which is a digital environment in which the contents are associated with metadata allowing the automatic management of interconnected semantic information (Wikipedia contributors, 2012c). The last 20 years have seen a significant increase in the opportunity to access the web. In 2011, about one-third of the world's population had regular access to the Internet

(International Telecommunication Union, 2011), and their great confidence in Information and Communication Technology (ICT) has led to the need for a more personalized—and not just individualized—management of it. With the growth of a "knowledge society," the need for a more interactive web has increased together with the necessity of active participation and easy management of its contents; this is the case for the so-called "Web 2.0," a platform, which allows the network capabilities to be matched to the user's needs. Different from its first version, Web 2.0 is not a technological invention, but instead it is a "symptom" of a cultural revolution or, in other words, the outcome of a social insight corresponding to a reconfiguration of the web's original functions of use. As stated during a brainstorming session at a conference at O'Reilly Media, the "Web 2.0 is an attitude not a technology" (Davis, 2012; O'Reilly, 2007); it is an attitude acquired as a result of users' adaptation to and learning about the functioning of Web 1.0. Therefore, the growing expertise of web users led to the necessity of a platform interconnecting the several functions of the Web 1.0, in order to meet individuals' need for an active participation in content creation and sharing. The Web 2.0 phenomenon can be understood as the result of a technological evolution that does not disregard the users' experience of the Internet. We call this cultural process a psychotechnological evolution, with psychotechnology meaning any "technology that emulates, extends, amplifies and *modifies* sensory-motor, psychological or cognitive functions of the mind" (Federici et al., 2011, p. 1179; Federici and Scherer, 2012a; Miesenberger et al., 2012, p. 180).

Starting from the definition of the concept of psychotechnology and what differentiates it from artifacts, Chapter 3 describes the evolution of ICT in terms of psychotechnologies for socialization, highlighting their role in the extension of human psychological abilities, and in terms of socialization and participation opportunities.

3.2   WHAT IS PSYCHOTECHNOLOGY?

The word "psychotechnology" is not a neologism. Since 1991, it has been used in the study of media theory to explain the dynamics of the interaction between people and technology, according to which technology is an object that is able to extend the cognitive functions by acting as an electronic sensory extension of the user's central nervous system, thus amplifying and extending the human mind (De Kerckhove, 1991, p. 132). Derrick De Kerckhove (1995) proposed the first definition of psychotechnology in *The Skin of Culture*:

> I have coined the term "psychotechnology," patterned on the model of biotechnology to define any technology that emulates, extends or amplifies the powers of our minds. [...] Telephone, radio, television, computers and other media combine to create environments that, together, establish intermediate realms of information processing. These are the realms of psychotechnologies. (1995, p. 5)

According to De Kerckhove, it is especially with interactive and adaptable media* such as the Internet that the realms of psychotechnologies become places in which a collective memory becomes constitutive of an "augmented mind," that is, a mind that is "externalized, shared, multiplied, accelerated, random accessed and generally processed connectively outside our heads" (De Kerckhove, 2010, p. 9).

Since 1991, the new communication technologies have evolved and specialized with a rate of increase that is much faster than for the previous two decades (Wikipedia contributors, 2012a). Compared to other ICTs, the web has had a preferential evolution, so that other technologies and services that, until then, were characterized as being for different aims and functions have been redesigned by following a web-based approach (Jenkins, 2006); these include voice and telephony technologies (e.g., VoIP, or voice over Internet protocol) or educational services (e.g., Wikis for online collaboration or sharing content). During the years in which the dream of bringing a computer into every home (Microsoft Corporation, 2012) was becoming a reality, when Berners-Lee's goal of "making the web accessible to everyone" (W3C–World Wide Web Consortium, 2012) started to be recognized as a political necessity, the concept of psychotechnology was revised under a new systemic perspective in line with the cultural revolution that was taking place in the domain of the human functioning—that is, the biopsychosocial model emerged (Federici and Scherer, 2012a; Federici et al., 2012b) (see Box 3.1).

Starting from an intrasystemic approach, a new definition of psychotechnology has been set out by Stefano Federici who reread the interaction process between person and technology by considering that the outcome of this relation is more than

---

* Actually, any technology can be considered as a psychotechnology insofar as it has influenced and modified human behavior and cognition. Therefore, it would be simplistic to imagine that psychotechnology refers only to those digital products that use the Internet. De Kerckhove himself talks about the invention of the alphabet too as a psychotechnology that was followed, in his historical reconstruction, by the printing machine, the telegraph, the television, and the computer. In an even broader sense, the phylogenetic history of the human being is associated with the invention of psychotechnologies. As Francoise Audouze claims,

> since the beginning of prehistoric archaeology, tools have been associated with prehistoric humans (called *Homo faber* by philosophers). The different stages of *Homo* have been related to their material culture, essentially lithic industries (assemblages of typical stone tools) that were the only artifacts to survive in number (1999, p. 828 [italics in original].).

In 1964, André Leroi-Gourhan constructed a theory that related the evolution of human beings and their culture to the exteriorization of physical and mental functions:

> The whole of our evolution has been oriented toward placing outside ourselves what in the rest of the animal world is achieved inside by species adaptation. The most striking material fact is certainly the "freeing" of tools, but the fundamental fact is really the freeing of the word and our unique ability to transfer our memory to a social organism outside ourselves (1993, p. 235)

More recently, Bernard Stiegler (1992) called "epiphylogenesis" the phenomenon of a new relation between the human organism and its environment mediated by the use of technology (see Box 3.1). Finally, as Jared Diamond—professor of geography and physiology at the University of California, who won the Pulitzer Prize in 1998 with the book *Guns, Germs and Steel*—convincingly demonstrated, the possession of new and advanced technologies, rather than racial differences, within human societies, rooted in environmental differences, can explain much of the course of human history.

BOX 3.1   THE BIOPSYCHOSOCIAL MODEL AND RECIPROCAL TRIADIC CAUSATION

STEFANO FEDERICI AND FABIO MELONI

The biopsychosocial model of health and individual functioning, promoted by the World Health Organization and endorsed by the *International Classification of Functioning, Disability and Health* (ICF; WHO, 2001), considers disability as the complex and multideterminate outcome of three main factors: the individual's health condition, personal factors, and environmental factors. The triadic reciprocal causation of these factors has replaced the etiological perspective of linear development that, from an altered state of health, leads to disability. In the biopsychosocial model, disability, understood as both a limitation of an individual's abilities and a restriction in social participation, is certainly related to a health condition, conventionally regarded as pathological; however, it is not necessarily considered to be caused by the same health status as that in the linear model of the previous classification of disability published in 1980, the *International Classification of Impairments, Disability and Handicaps,* known by the acronym ICIDH (WHO, 1980). Within the ICIDH, disability (and/or handicap) is the direct result of an impairment of the individual *"that limits or prevents the fulfilment of a role that is normal (depending on age, sex, and social and cultural factors) for that individual"* (WHO, 1980, p. 29 [italics in the original].), according to a model based on linear causality and relations between an independent variable and a dependent one (Federici et al., 2012b) as shown in this sequence taken from the *Introduction* of the ICIDH (WHO, 1980, p. 11):

$$Disease \rightarrow impairment \rightarrow disability \rightarrow handicap$$

According to this model, more commonly called the medical/individual model, disability, and within ICIDH, handicap too—a term that during the revision process from ICIDH to ICF was abandoned, in response to the requests from the English-speaking countries that considered the term handicap to be both stigmatizing and discriminatory (Federici and Meloni, 2010a)—is described as a manifest consequence of a pathological health condition. As a consequence, the ICIDH's categories describe different structural and functional impairments, and different disabilities and handicaps resulting from impairment. In contrast, the ICF does not classify disability as a direct consequence of a disease, but as an individual's specific, temporary or permanent, way of "functioning" in a given context. Therefore, it can be argued that "ICF does not classify people, but describes the situation of each person within an array of health or health-related domains" (WHO, 2001, p. 10).

The origins of the biopsychosocial model date back to the proposal put forward by psychiatrist George Engel in 1977 for integrating the dominant social and psychological variables within the medical model:

> The dominant model of disease today is biomedical, and it leaves no room within its framework for the social, psychological, and behavioural dimensions of illness. A biopsychosocial model is proposed that provides a blueprint for research, a framework for teaching, and a design for action in the real world of health care. (Engel, 1977, p. 130)

Engel made the leading theoretical contribution to building the biopsychosocial model, identified in von Bertalanffy's General Systems Theory (von Bertalanffy, 1950). According to this approach, the unifying principles in the scientific context are not understood by a reduction to smaller units; instead, it is the nature of its organization that explains a scientific phenomenon. It is not sufficient to divide a scientific phenomenon into a simpler unit of analysis and study such units one by one; instead, it is necessary to study the interrelations among these units.

> As a result, human beings are also seen as systems ecologically plunged into multiple systems (Gray et al., 1969). In the biopsychosocial model, the definition of the state of health or illness is therefore the outcome of the interaction of processes that operate at the macro level (e.g., the existence of social support for depression) and the processes that operate at the micro level (e.g., biological or biochemical derangements). (Federici et al., 2012b, p. 12)

According to the biopsychosocial model, the factors that affect an individual's functioning are interconnected elements of a system (Figure 3.1), which have properties that are not readily apparent from the properties of the individual elements (Rydin et al., 2012).

> Thus, it is impossible from this perspective to isolate disability from the functioning of an individual and vice versa, or rather hypothesize one without the other, not only at the level of social organization but also at the level of a single individual. Disability implies functioning and vice versa. When I. K. Zola in "Toward the Necessary Universalizing of a Disability Policy" (1989) expresses hope for the demystification of the "specialness" of disability and the admission that "people with a disability have long been treated as an oppressed minority" (p. 19), he assumes a conception of disability that is fluid and contextual: "Disability is not a human attribute that demarks one portion of humanity from another (as gender does, and race sometimes does); it is an infinitely various but universal feature of the human condition" (Bickenbach et al., 1999, p. 1182). The issue of disability for individuals "is not whether but when, not so much which one, but how many and in what combination" (Zola, 1993, p. 18). (Federici et al., 2012b, p. 12)

Triadic reciprocal causation (Figure 3.1) is a term introduced by Albert Bandura (1986) to refer to the mutual influence between three sets of factors.

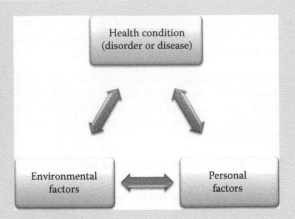

FIGURE 3.1 Reciprocal triadic causation between the components of ICF according to the biopsychosocial model: "There is a dynamic interaction among these entities: interventions in one entity have the potential to modify one or more of the other entities." (From World Health Organization (WHO), *International Classification of Impairments, Disabilities, and Handicaps. A Manual of Classification Relating to the Consequences of Disease*, WHO, Geneva, Switzerland, p. 26.)

Applying Bandura's theory to the biopsychosocial model, the fact that the three entities (health condition, environmental factors, and personal factors) affect each other does not mean that they have the same weight (Bandura, 1997). Not only, then, is the model of a linear causality within the ICIDH superseded by a transactional model in which the elements are in a reciprocal causation (the term causation is used herein with the meaning of functional dependence between events; Bandura, 1997), but the weight that the health conditions (disorders or diseases) can exert on disability may, under certain conditions, be minimal compared with, for example, the effect of environmental factors:

> A problem with performance can result directly from the social environment, even when the individual has no impairment. For example, an individual who is HIV-positive without any symptoms or disease, or someone with a genetic predisposition to a certain disease, may exhibit no impairments or may have sufficient capacity to work, yet may not do *so* because of the denial of access to services, discrimination or stigma. (WHO, 2001, p. 21)

According to the ICF, technologies, when viewed as a systematic process, method, or an artifact designed to solve problems posed by the environment, are set within the context of the individual operating components (health condition, environmental factors, personal factors) as facilitators for improving individual functioning. To the extent, then, that a technology is produced with the specific goal of assisting a person with disability, it can be defined as an assistive product or technology (WHO, 2001, p. 164). In this sense, the definition of technology can be traced back to what the philosopher of science

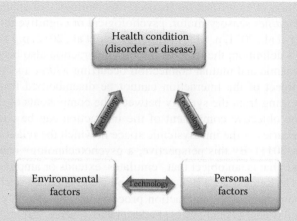

FIGURE 3.2　Reciprocal triadic causation between the components of ICF according to the biopsychosocial model and the role of the technology.

Bernard Stiegler proposed could be seen in the relation between the human being and its technology, namely, a phenomenon of epiphylogenesis, a new relation between the human organism and its environment: lithic technology and tools are preserved beyond the life of the individual who produced them and determine the relation of the human being with the environment, thus conditioning a part of the selection pressure (Stiegler, 1992).

As shown in Figure 3.2, then, the technology itself arises as product that modifies human behavior, in that it determines the relationship with the environment (e.g., by placing itself as a facilitator that reduces barriers); it assigns meaning to the environment (e.g., because it makes the environment accessible to the human experience and, therefore, usable: a particular stone may begin a wheel); it expresses meanings about individuals (the introduction of writing, by changing the way of human communication, gives new meanings to individuals who mediate their communication by writing, for example, separating them into the illiterate and the literate); it is a method of an organism–environment interaction (a square as a real meeting place and a square as virtual reality, such as a social network, are two ways of interaction determined by the introduction of two different human technologies); and, finally, it is a behavior (the use of specific technology requires the acquisition of new skills that produce culturally determined human behavioral skills: hunting and fishing, agriculture, urbanization, etc.).

In these circumstances, it is easy to see how the biopsychosocial model of human functioning and the transactional theory of reciprocal triadic causation provide a theoretical framework within which we may include and develop the definition of psychotechnologies. In fact, technology, by its nature, originated from the human psyche, but it also determines the relation of the human being with its environment, and affects part of the selection pressure by modifying its creator.

the simple addition of an artifact for its user: "technology that emulates, extends, amplifies and *modifies* sensory-motor, psychological or cognitive functions of the mind" (Federici et al., 2011, p. 1179; Miesenberger et al., 2012, p. 180). According to the Federici's definition, the user–technology interaction also becomes characterized by a dynamic and mutual connection occurring *within* a subjective space, in which the object of the interaction cannot be disembodied from the human experience emerging from the synergy between the components of the system. In other words, the objective component of the interaction can be considered only within the boundaries of the intrasystemic space in which the relationship evolves (Federici et al., 2011). By this perspective, a psychotechnology is not an icon of the human mind, that is, an object that "emulates, extends or amplifies the powers of our mind" (De Kerckhove, 1995, p. 5) keeping its functions unchanged, but it is an *active* component of the interaction process that can also modify the functions of the mind (Federici et al., 2011; Federici and Scherer, 2012a; Miesenberger et al., 2012).

Since the theoretical approach underlying the concept of psychotechnology supports the idea of active externalism concerning "the active role of the environment in driving cognitive processes" (Clark and Chalmers, 1998, p. 27), it is related to the extended mind theory according to which "mental states, including states of believing, could be grounded in physical traces that remained firmly outside the head" (Clark, 2010, p. 43). According to Richard Menary, "it is not simply that the external features, to which the organism is interactively linked, have a causal influence on the cognitive processing of the organism; rather, the interactive link *is* the cognitive processing" (Menary, 2010, p. 2). The user–technology interaction is here considered more than a relationship based on emerging affordances (Gibson, 1979), since it is also a dynamic process that is mainly characterized by a mutual relationship in which psychotechnology shares and modifies the features and the functions of the mind. Kyle Jasmin and Daniel Casasanto (2012) found that the meanings of words in English, Dutch, and Spanish are related to the way people type them on the QWERTY keyboard. Words with more right-side letters were rated as more positive in valence, on average, than words with more left-side letters. This is what Jasmin and Casasanto call the "QWERTY effect." This effect was observed to be strongest in new words coined after QWERTY was invented, and it was also found in pseudowords.

> Typing is a special kind of motor action. Performing motor actions fluently generally leads to positive feelings and evaluations. (Oppenheimer 2008; Ping et al. 2009). Therefore, if letters on one side of the keyboard can be typed more fluently than letters on the other side, motor fluency could mediate relationships between the locations of letters on the QWERTY keyboard and the valence of the words they compose (i.e., the positivity or negativity of their meanings) (Jasmin and Casasanto, 2012, p. 2).

The QWERTY keyboard technology is an extension of a hand action, and the way people use their hands also influences the way they represent abstract ideas with positive and negative emotional valence (Casasanto, 2011). The universal spread of the QWERTY keyboard has affected not only the action of the manual articulators used for typing words, but the meaning of words. It is a psychotechnology.

The modifying role of psychotechnology is indeed related to its ability to directly take part of the working memory processes, and in doing so, it both enhances and enriches the information flow and, at the same time, modifies the knowledge stored in the long-term memory. According to the cognitive approach to memory, the process of storing information in the mind is a dynamic one, so that any "new incoming information is related to and transformed by preexisting knowledge structures" (Schacter, 1989, p. 689). Moreover, any newly learned information interferes with and impedes the recall of previously learned information, thereby transforming preexisting knowledge structures (Underwood, 1957). The human memory is not like a library where the books are packed closed to one another. Newly learned information in the human memory is like a new book that is placed on the shelf; it is partially rewritten so that it fits with the content of adjacent books, and they are rewritten to fit with its content. Any new book modifies the contents of the library's books and any copy of the same book changes itself to adapt to the material stored in the library (Baddeley et al., 2009). Newly learned information competes with older memorized information, and the more recent association wins out, making it impossible to remember earlier associations (Reitman, 1971). Since the media is the message (McLuhan, 1964), a new technology is not just the skin of a culture, emulating human cognitive systems (De Kerckhove, 1995), but much more, it is a new content, a new association interfering with previous one, and modifying old stored messages (Wohldmann et al., 2008).

> "The medium is the message" because it is the medium that shapes and controls the scale and form of human association and action. The content or uses of such media are as diverse as they are ineffectual in shaping the form of human association. Indeed, it is only too typical that the "content" of any medium blinds us to the character of the medium. (McLuhan, 1964, p. 9)

The human being, indeed, is not someone who ignores how he or she manipulates the world. Neglecting this relationship fails to realize that not just the medium but the human being itself will be transformed (Galimberti, 2002). Any psychotechnology is a medium of systems of symbols, which are organized by rules, restrictions and knowledge possibilities that force users to make cognitive and cultural modifications and adaptations (Miesenberger et al., 2012), and it is a way to guide users to a cognitive and cultural readaptation of the environment system. Federici et al. (2011) claim that, as artifacts, the media play

> a key role in the evolution of the species by allowing human beings to specialize their abilities through the symbols, the restrictions and the knowledge possibilities which any *psycho*technology brings. (Bruner, 1977)

> Psychotechnologies allow us to process the information they provide by reconfiguring and restructuring the relations within the user's experience, thus becoming both a cause of the insight process—which is close to the concept of affordance (Gibson, 1979, p. 1179)—and a "place" for the whole synchronous perception of a meaningful gestalt. (2011, p. 1179)

Since psychotechnologies act as sensory extensions of the user's central nervous system (De Kerckhove, 1995), since they play a constitutive part in the subjective space of the interaction (Federici et al., 2011), and since the dynamic and mutual relationship between users and technologies shares and modifies the functions of the mind (Miesenberger et al., 2012), media and communications technology can be considered as a "mirror" of human mind, which both modifies the constitution and evolution of the personality traits of its users and, at the same time, owes its functional and structural change to the sensory-motor, psychological, or cognitive functions of the mind it reflects.

Given these theoretical considerations, when an expert in human factors aims to analyze and evaluate the interaction between a user and a technology, he or she necessarily has to embrace a methodology that goes beyond the mere summative analysis of subject (i.e., the user) and object (i.e., the technology) by taking into consideration the mutual and dynamic system arising during the interaction. In this sense, simply talking about, for instance, "websites" or "social networks" (or any other technology *per se*) does not clarify the object of study. We need a comprehensive term that acts as a résumé of the complexity of the whole interaction system, and this is the reason why we introduce and recommend adopting the intrasystemic term "psychotechnology" in human–computer interaction.

In the following paragraphs, we shall demonstrate how recent studies are oriented toward a perspective where personality traits are influenced by ICT and vice versa, confirming a psychotechnological view of the mutual influence of the person and technology.

3.3 FROM ARTIFACTS TO PSYCHOTECHNOLOGIES

In the 1970s, on the basis of classical ergonomics, cognitive psychology, and artificial intelligence, a new discipline called cognitive ergonomics emerged with the advent of personal computers. Cognitive ergonomics were born with the aim of developing and/or improving artifacts to provide easy-to-use technologies in the work setting. Therefore, the methods and techniques of cognitive ergonomics aim at evaluating the cognitive process (e.g., perception, attention, memory) that result from the interaction between a person at work and an artifact system, which is a set of objects made by human work or natural elements of the environment, with their interactions occurring in time and space (Karwowski, 2000). Artifacts are objects created by assembling human-made elements or by changing the physical world in some way to both aid and lead to an improvement in the human work performance (Lambie, 2006). The difference between the concept of "object" and "artifact" lies in the function for which the item has been created or modified by means of materials found in nature. In cognitive ergonomics, the concept of artifact is necessarily related to the concept of affordance (Gibson, 1977, 1979) or cultural constraints (Norman, 1988, 1990), which refers to the relationship connecting either the natural or cultural properties of the world and an actor—applied to the working context. As Donald Norman (1991) claims:

> Artifacts pervade our lives, our every activity. The speed, power, and intelligence of human beings are dramatically enhanced by the invention of artificial devices, so much so that tool making and usage constitute one of the defining characteristics of our species. Many artifacts make us stronger or faster, or protect us from the elements or predators, or feed and clothe us. And many artifacts make us smarter, increasing cognitive capabilities and making possible the modern intellectual world. (Norman, 1991, p. 17)

In particular, Norman uses the term "cognitive artifact" to refer to any "artificial device designed to maintain, display, or operate upon information in order to serve a representational function and that affects human cognitive performance" (Norman, 1991, p. 17). The main role of cognitive ergonomics is hence to analyze person–artifact interaction in the working environment, taking into account (1) both the cognitive and behavioral effects arising from the interaction system and (2) the activities and skills needed to improve productivity and effectiveness, while at the same time (3) avoiding any cognitive or physical overload (Federici et al., 2005). In cognitive ergonomics, the interaction system is observed in the light of the Norman's mental/conceptual model theory which claims that three models are involved during an interaction process: the user's mental model, the image of the system, and the conceptual model of the system (Norman, 1983). The mental/conceptual model theory is based on the postulate that the number of interaction problems occurring during a task increases with the distance between the mental and the conceptual models of the system (Norman, 1983). Therefore, in cognitive ergonomics, the dynamics of the interaction are characterized by a dualistic reciprocity between two poles—the user system and the artifact system:

> Every artifact has both a system and a personal view, and they are often very different in appearance. From the system view, the artifact appears to expand some functional capacity of the task performer. From the personal view, the artifact has replaced the original task with a different task, one that may have radically different cognitive requirements and use radically different cognitive capacities than the original task. (Norman, 1991, p. 22)

According to this perspective, the interaction between a user and a cognitive artifact is then composed of two opposite components: a personal/subjective one, namely, the user and an objective one, that is, the artifact. However, this approach does not take into account the role of socioenvironmental components involved in the interaction system. In fact, the methods and techniques used in cognitive ergonomics for the evaluation of a technology such as, for example, an electronic wheelchair, take into account the functions of the artifact with respect to the functional and physical characteristics of end users, but they do not allow practitioners to systematically evaluate the emotional and socioenvironmental impact on the interaction system. Hence, the model underlying the cognitive ergonomics approach does not provide evaluation methods to systematically investigate a fundamental component of the interaction, that is, the role of the milieu and its influence on the user's life.

In the 1980s, together with cognitive ergonomics, researchers started to talk about usability, a new analytical paradigm that was aimed at investigating "the extent to which a product can be used by specified users to achieve specified goals with effectiveness, efficiency and satisfaction in a specified context of use" (ISO, 1998, p. 2) (see Chapter 1). The usability field involved—at least in the early stages (see Section 1.1.3)—the application of methods and techniques borrowed from cognitive ergonomics and applied to different contexts that are not limited only to the work environment.

However, since 1998—during the fourth period of the historical evolution of the human–computer interaction (see Chapter 1)—the usability field has gradually drifted away from the theoretical approach of cognitive ergonomics and has started to increasingly focus both on a third part of the interaction system, the socioenvironmental context, and the complexity of the user system by taking into account also his or her needs and peculiarities. Together with this change of perspective, the experts in human factors introduced a new term, "user experience" (UX), to refer to "a person's perceptions and responses that result from the use or anticipated use of a product, system or service" (ISO, 2010) (see Chapter 2). UX is about how people experience the interaction with a technology:

> The way it feels in their hands, how well they understand how it works, how they feel about it while they are using it, how well it serves their purposes, how well it fits into the context in which they are using it, and how well it contributes to the quality of their lives. (Alben, 1996, p. 13)

According to Marc Hassenzahl and Noam Tractinsky (2006), UX can be described as

> a consequence of a user's internal state (predispositions, expectations, needs, motivation, mood, etc.), the characteristics of the designed system (e.g., complexity, purpose, usability, functionality, etc.) and the context (or the environment) within which the interaction occurs (e.g., organizational/social setting, meaningfulness of the activity, voluntariness of use, etc.). (Hassenzahl and Tractinsky, 2006, p. 95)

As the two previously exposed explanations of UX highlight, the main purpose of UX evaluation and design is both to enhance the relationship between a user and a product/service and to provide as delightful experience as possible to people interacting with an interface.

Taking a different approach from the dualistic view proposed by cognitive ergonomics, the human factors field adopted a new perspective to explain the dynamics of interaction, the intrasystemic one, which identifies a reciprocal triadic causation between the components of the user–technology interaction, that is to say, the user, the technology, and the socioenvironmental system. According to this new perspective, talking about "artifacts" as components of the interaction system no longer fits with the theoretical model underlying usability, since it reflects a dyadic perspective of interaction that considers the interaction system as the result of a simple addition of a subjective component—the user system—and an objective component—the technological system—(Federici and Borsci, 2010; Federici et al., 2005) (see Figures 3.3 and 3.4).

The UX approach investigates three components, namely, the person, the technology, and the environmental dimensions, "as a whole and complex system in which object (system) and subject (user) are a part of a composite and dynamic empirical observation process within a specific environment" (Miesenberger et al., 2012, p. 183). Since "the object cannot be considered *per se* because it always falls out of the human experience" (Miesenberger et al., 2012, p. 180), this book will adopt the term "psychotechnology" instead of "artifact" to refer to any technology that plays an

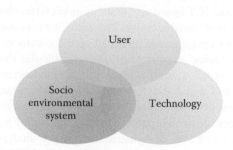

FIGURE 3.3 **(See color insert.)** Reciprocal triadic causation between the components of the user–technology interaction.

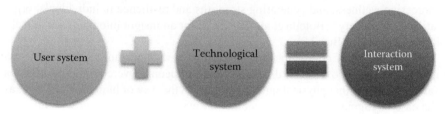

FIGURE 3.4 **(See color insert.)** Dyadic perspective of interaction between a subjective component and an objective one.

active role in the contexts of use by emulating, extending, amplifying, and modifying the cognitive functions involved during the interaction (Federici et al., 2011). In this way, the psychotechnological perspective supplants the cause-and-effect perspective of cognitive ergonomics by embracing an intrasystemic approach to explain the dynamic and mutual interaction emerging within the user–technology system. The outcome of this interaction is considered to be more than the sum of its components; it is a gestaltic phenomenon emerging from the human experience of the technology (Mele and Federici, 2012b). In our evaluation model (see Chapter 4), we propose a perspective that goes beyond the additional or dyadic evaluation of subjects' experience and objects' performance by using integrated methods and techniques, which allow practitioners to analyze the whole system in its dynamic complexity. Hence, we propose the umbrella term "psychotechnologies" to refer to any kind of technology, such as websites or social networking sites, whose interaction components can be fully understood only by following an intrasystemic evaluation approach.

3.4 PSYCHOTECHNOLOGIES FOR SOCIALIZATION

It is widely accepted that, together with personal identity, social identity is a constitutive part of the concept of self and is determined by the social groups that individuals belong to (Abrams and Hogg, 1990; Erikson, 1959; Tajfel, 1978). Social identification is hence related to the perception of belonging to a human aggregate and it is strictly related to "intragroup cohesion, cooperation, and altruism, and positive evaluations of the group" (Ashforth and Mael, 1989, p. 26). In accordance with the social identity theory, since media and communication technologies represent a digital intergroup platform, we can consider ICT-based applications as social environments involved in the development process of social identity. Therefore, we propose the use of the term "psychotechnologies for socialization" instead of the commonly used "media and communication technologies" to refer to all the technologies that have a role in the cognitive and affective processes or that are involved in the development of individuals' attitudes, beliefs, and social activities. Social networks, mashups, blogs, Wikis, file-sharing repositories, discussion boards, instant messaging, and other third-party applications are "places" in which perceived sociostructural beliefs can influence certain intergroup behaviors, as demonstrated in many studies on the impact of ICT on people and society (e.g.: Manago et al., 2008; Sheldon, 2009; Siibak, 2009; Zarghooni, 2007) and on positive technology; or in other words, "the scientific and applied approach for improving the quality of our personal experience with the goal of increasing wellness, and generating strengths and resilience in individuals, organizations, and society" (Botella et al., 2012, p.1; for an insight into the positive technology approach see Box 3.2).

With the spread of communication platforms, new opportunities for social participation have been possible for different groups of people, overcoming the attitudes toward the barriers that physical interaction puts in the way of human interaction, as in the case of stigma; that is, the phenomenon whereby an individual with an attribute is deeply discredited by his or her society and is rejected as a result of the attribute (Goffman, 1963). Sociocultural barriers are considerably reduced, especially those blocking the participation of disabled users in the social media, since in a digital space communication passes primarily through channels that allow users to filter personal information according to their discretion. According to Erving Goffman (1963), "when a stranger comes into our presence [...] first appearances are likely to enable us to anticipate his category and attributes, his social identity" (Goffman, 1963, p. 3). In a way that is different from physical communication—where it is the body and its special features that introduce the person in the interaction space—users in digital communication have the option to choose their own representation through an avatar, or through a certain description of themselves. On the one hand, the individual's freedom to choose not to expose their body through the medium of communication helps to overcome a visible stigma; but on the other hand, this choice is likely to totally conceal the body and then lead to the individual being regarded as a member of a social group other than the real one, "such as a different race, ethnicity, social class, gender, intelligence, age and/or disability status, generally with the purpose of gaining social acceptance" (Renfrow, 2004; Sánchez and Schlossberg, 2001)" (Wikipedia contributors, 2012e). However, it is also true to say that through communication tools such as instant messaging, users whose stigmatizing attributes are immediately evident are more likely to have social and emotional experiences which might otherwise be significantly hampered if the evident impairment were immediately visible face to face (Federici, 2002; see also Box 3.3).

Internet use has been found to affect the well-being by decreasing loneliness and depression significantly and, at the same time, significantly increasing perceived social support and self-esteem (Shaw and Gant, 2002), especially among people with physical disabilities (for a review of the effect of the Internet on well-being among adults with physical disabilities see Cheatham, 2012).

BOX 3.2   POSITIVE TECHNOLOGY

GIUSEPPE RIVA

Positive psychology is a nascent discipline whose broad goals are to understand human strengths and virtues, and to promote these strengths to allow individuals, communities, and societies to flourish (Aspinwall and Staudinger, 2003; Seligman and Csikszentmihalyi, 2000). Here, we suggest that it is possible to combine the objectives of positive psychology with enhancements of Information and Communication Technologies (ICTs) toward a new paradigm: Positive Technology (Botella et al., 2012; Riva et al., 2012; Wiederhold and Riva, 2012). The final aim is to use the technology to manipulate and enhance the features of our personal experience with the goal of increasing wellness, and generating strengths and resilience in individuals, organizations, and society. Positive psychology identifies three characteristics of our personal experience—affective quality, engagement/actualization, and connectedness—that serve to promote personal well-being. In the proposed framework, positive technologies are classified according to their effects on these three features of personal experience (Botella et al., 2012; Riva et al., 2012; Wiederhold and Riva, 2012):

- *Hedonic*: Technologies used to induce positive and pleasant experiences;
- *Eudaimonic*: Technologies used to support individuals in reaching, engaging, and self-actualizing experiences;
- *Social/Interpersonal*: Technologies used to support and improve social integration and/or connectedness between individuals, groups, and organizations.

Hedonic technologies, the first dimension of Positive Technology, include all the technologies used to foster positive emotional states. According to the model of emotions developed by James Russell (2003), it is possible to modify the affective quality of an experience through the manipulation of "core affect," a neurophysiological category corresponding to the combination of valence and arousal levels that endow the subjects with a kind of "core knowledge" about the emotional features of their experience. The "core affect" can be experienced as freefloating (mood) or attributed to some cause (and thereby begins an emotional episode). In this view, an emotional response is the attribution of a change in the core affect given to a specific object (affective quality). Simply put, a positive emotion is achieved by increasing the valence (positive) and arousal (high) of core affect (affect regulation) and by attributing this change to the contents of the proposed experience (object). Key arguments for the usefulness of positive emotions in increasing well-being have been recently provided by Barbara L. Fredrickson (2001, 2004) in what she called the "broaden-and-build model" of positive emotions. According to

Fredrickson, positive emotions provide the organism with nonspecific action tendencies that can lead to adaptive behavior (Fredrickson, 2001).

Eudaimonic technologies, the second dimension of Positive Technology, include all the technologies used to support individuals in reaching, engaging, and self-actualizing experiences. The theory of flow, developed by Positive Psychology pioneer Mihaly Csikszentmihalyi (1990), provides a useful framework for addressing this challenge. Flow, or optimal experience, is a positive and complex state of consciousness that is present when individuals act with total involvement. The basic feature of this experience is the perceived balance between high environmental opportunities for action (challenges) and adequate personal resources in facing them (skills). Some researchers have drawn parallels between the experience of flow in virtual reality and the sense of presence, defined as the subjective perception of "being there" in a virtual environment (Riva, 2009; Riva and Mantovani, 2012; Riva et al., 2011). From the phenomenological viewpoint, both experiences have been described as absorbing states, characterized by a merging of action and awareness, loss of self-consciousness, a feeling of being transported into another reality, and an altered perception of time (Waterworth et al., 2010). Further, both presence and optimal experience are associated with high involvement, focused attention, and high concentration on the ongoing activity (Marsh, 2003).

The final level of Positive Technology, the social and interpersonal one, is concerned with the use of technologies to support and improve the connectedness between individuals, groups, and organizations. However, an open challenge is to understand how to use technology to create a mutual sense of awareness, which is essential to the feeling that other participants are there, and to create a strong sense of community at a distance. John Short, Ederyn Williams, and Bruce Christie (1976) define "social presence" as the "degree of salience of the other person in a mediated communication and the consequent salience of their interpersonal interactions" (p. 65). Conventional computer-mediated communicative tools, such as email or text-based chat, are regarded as having lower social presence and social context cues when compared to face-to-face communication. However, different authors have suggested that it is possible to manipulate the technological experience to enhance social presence and thereby improve different mediated activities such as online learning, e-commerce, and health care. Moreover, in a recent paper, Maurizio Mauri et al. (2011) used different physiological data—skin conductance, blood volume pulse, electroencephalogram, electromyography, respiratory activity, and pupil dilation—to evaluate the affective experience evoked by the use of Facebook. The biological signals revealed that Facebook use can evoke a psychophysiological state characterized by high positive valence and high arousal (core flow state). These findings support the hypothesis that the successful spread of social networks might be associated with a specific positive affective state experienced by users when they use their account.

BOX 3.3   MIND, BODY, AND SEX IN CYBERSPACE*

STEFANO FEDERICI

In the following focus section, we report the interview of an Italian homosexual man, Armando, aged 35, with motor disabilities, who uses an Internet chat client to overcome the emotional distress of his condition of physical disability when meeting new people. For Armando, the chat room begins a cyberspace where the body image of the person is relativized, leaving the body in the background, and favoring that the soul rises up without the evident physical impairment preventing a human relationship.

The unexpected testimony of Armando is surprising in the way in which it brings into question the dominant vision of male homosexuality linked to the fetishized worship of the sculptural shape of an Apollonian body or, to an increasing minority, related to the maniacal deformity of a depraved person. The intelligent use of cyberspace, the healthy recognition of the personal qualities that outweigh the physical deficits, makes of the testimony of Armando a good *vademecum* for those who take refuge in the diversity of their own or others' sexuality as behind a screen of disrespect and lack of acceptance.

As a music critic and musicologist, Armando collaborates with several Italian newspapers and magazines for which he writes specialized and divulging articles about music. He is also a consultant for some record companies and some TV networks.

Armando gives us a serene testimony of his sexual life as a gay person, and he strongly believes in the advantages of this condition. Furthermore, his passion for telematics introduces us to that way of sexual approaching, communication of personality, and sexual interest that allow him to overcome geographical distances and communicate beyond the physical appearance, with the unique power and depth of the written language.

[Interviewer, (I)]: How did you live your sexual identity and drives? *What kind of difficulties did you find? Do you think that the condition of disability has increased your difficulties?*
[Armando, (A)]: Certainly, there were some difficulties related to my illness; it would be foolish to deny it! Despite this, I think, I was pretty lucky because I had already had my first sexual intercourse at 16, even though I was disabled then, although less severely than today.

---

* This box was drawn from the book by Stefano Federici (2002) *Sessualità alterabili. Indagine sulle influenze socioambientali nello sviluppo della sessualità di persone con disabilità in Italia Alter-*able sexuality: Survey of socio-environmental influences in the development of the sexuality of people with disabilities in Italy] pp. 237–248.

[I]: What kind of sexual intercourse *did* you have?

[A]: Homosexual relationships with my peers. Roughly, between 16 and 23 years old, I had sex with three or four guys, with one of which I also had a long-lasting relationship.

[I]: Were all *of them* able-bodied guys?

[A]: Yes, they were all able-bodied!

[I]: Have you ever had sexual experiences with other *people with* disabilities?

[A]: No, I haven't and didn't look for them.

[I]: Neither you weren't sought for, were you?

[A]: No, I wasn't. However, there wasn't the opportunity as I didn't attend many social or care associations for disabled people.

However, I had a relationship with a person who had experienced a serious illness and this suffering certainly brought us closer. He was a person who had suffered a serious form of cancer. At 20 years old, he had been given 3 months to live. Then, after a treatment abroad, he had a relapse and then was miraculously healed—I do not believe in miracles, but in this case the adverb may be used—miraculously healed after a prophylaxis of chemotherapy. We were connected by a strong sense of life, sharing the same way of knowing what is important in life (if there is something important in addition to life!?). And, probably more than me, he looked death in the face. Nevertheless, he was a person living in a positive way, with the ability, that sometimes is also acknowledged to me, to target the point and not be distracted by side things compared to what is the pleasure of living.

[I]: Would you mind telling me which are the core values that you shared? *What did you use to talk about?*

[A]: Well… If I think about the reason that led our relationship to a premature end—actually not so premature, since it lasted 6 months—the reason was that we didn't really share many common interests more than the existential one, namely, the adherence to that kind of life. But sharing the same values wasn't enough to keep up a relationship between two people who didn't attend the same places for many reasons, who didn't have the same interests and who then had some difficulties in living two different parallel lives. The values we shared were values—actually I don't know if they were really values—that we showed each other with gestures of love and tenderness. More than anything, a certain emotional depth tied us. I'm realizing that it is not easy at all to rationalize it, because I don't think that there was anything in particular, anything so defined, even in the field of disease. There was a common sense that certain values, such as certain appearances which are important to other people, were not so important to us.

[I]: For instance?

[A]: The cutest thing that someone told me in my life was that he didn't care at all that I was in a wheelchair. That was definitely a very rewarding thing: he didn't consider it a relevant variable to stay with me or not. Indeed, that wasn't the reason why we broke up.

[...]

[I]: Being forced to move in a wheelchair, how and where do you have contacts with the gay world? And where do your personal meetings occur?

[A]: As I already told you, I had my first gay relationships when I was 16, when I was not yet in a wheelchair. At that time, I had my first encounters in some concert halls. The music world is very popular with gay people... Since I was a teenager, I have had the opportunity to enter in homosexual circles. During these years, I met many homosexual persons regularly, so I became convinced that the musical channel was a good opportunity! Then came the telematic channel, which I would not limit only to the Internet: I would say the telematic knowledge in general. I think certainly that the electronic medium is for reaching specific users interested in certain topics and, of course, in this specific case also to sexuality, including homosexuality.

[I]: "ICT channels" such as Internet chat, for instance?

[A]: Internet chat rooms are spaces where people can talk, meet, or exchange opinions about any kind of things, also aimed, if you wish, at sexual encounter. Meetings via chat were for me a very interesting experience: Internet chat rooms are an extraordinary communication medium! If well used, Internet chat offer the possibility to enter into simultaneous contact with people geographically far away but who have similar interests, as well as with very close people with whom you didn't realize you shared the same interests; it is an opportunity that sounds amazing, especially if you think that I had already started using it 7 years ago. From this point of view, telematics has greatly enriched my life.

[I]: In what way?

[A]: Well, I met many people who became dear friends. After meeting by telematic channel, we met each other; with some of them I had some form of more or less close relationship, while with others I developed friendships that lasted several years and that, I think, I can define as deep. Due to my job, I have to travel to Italy quite often and, every time I go, I meet people with whom the first encounter was telematic, and later I can verify for myself knowledge that at first was just via cable.

[I]: Do you think that the telematic medium *gives people a false reality* compromising *their experience?*

[A]: The telematic medium offers a really deep but sectorial view of other people. Generally, you know something about the person that, at

first glance, you wouldn't tell face to face. But it lacks many other details that are immediately verifiable when you meet each other. So, you cannot know if someone talks looking at the ground or in the eyes, or the way he dresses, before meeting him. What is often missing is the social connotation and, well, the character of the person. We can overcome such limitations with experience: after talking to dozens and dozens of people, you begin to guess at some typical features.

[I]: When you say you "talked" in a telematic way, what does that mean?

[A]: Written: written communication answering to written communication coming up live, in real time.

[I]: This limitation due to written communication does not allow immediate or easy guessing *of some of the individual's main characteristics*, the way he dresses, his...

[A]: ... it erases the differences!

[I]: It erases certain differences.

[A]: And therefore gives many other chances to a disabled person, because it allows the physical appearance to be relativized and, then, you can put into play a series of powers of the individual that would be overshadowed by the first physical impression. This happens also when looking for a sexual relationship. If I want to pick someone and go to a club, I would certainly have a much smaller chance than doing the same thing in a telematic way, because via computer I have the opportunity to highlight a number of my personal features...

[I]: ...that at the disco would be immediately denied by your appearance?!

[A]: Exactly!

[I]: In that case, doesn't the electronic *way* favor too much and in an insane *way* a *fantasmatic* wait for the other, causing it to project expectations onto the other, expectations that cannot be met in reality? Isn't the physical encounter likely to be even more disappointing and more frustrating than the initial difficulty in appearing the way we are, even with a disabled body?

[A]: Well, that can be true. Except that telematics also permit images to be sent, so the impact of our physical appearance is never entirely new. But I recognize that there are some differences between the image that you make out of a person and the person himself once encountered. But the point is that the image of the person itself is to be relativized, that is—even if one doesn't want to make distinctions between soul and body—through telematics it is the soul that passes and, thus, the body stays in the background at the meeting time; however, there are a number of things that the person already knows about you and that are now acquired. All of these can only facilitate mutual understanding.

[I]: Is the number of disabled people who use the online tool to communicate and meet other people high?

[A]: No, it isn't. It is very low, at least in my experience.

[I]: However, *do* you believe that a disabled person chatting would *admit to being* such?

[A]: Maybe yes, and he wouldn't conceal it from me, since I declare it.

[I]: And has that happened?

[A]: Yes, because normally I don't hide being a disabled person, even if it isn't the first thing I say; but it is never the last.

In literature, there are a growing number of studies examining both (1) the personality characteristics associated with social networking sites use and (2) their impact on identity construction. Taken together, the studies, described in the following, show how personality traits can be considered as being influenced by ICT and vice versa.

3.4.1 Studies on Personality Characteristics Associated with Social Networking Sites

The study of the role of psychological factors in influencing people's use of technology platforms is a recent topic. In order to predict attitudes and behaviors, many researchers in the management and psychology fields have adopted the five-factor model of personality, a standard personality trait measure that provides a taxonomy of the personality through five personality factors: extraversion, agreeableness, conscientiousness, emotional stability, and openness to new experiences (Costa and McCrae, 1992; John et al., 2008). In order to understand why some people use Facebook—one of the most widely known social networking sites that currently has more than 500 million registered users (http://www.facebook.com)—more frequently than others, Kelly Moore and James C. McElroy (2012) recently carried out a study involving 219 undergraduate students. The subjects' personality and their reported usage of Facebook were analyzed by means of a survey, and the resulting data were combined with users' Facebook data:

In terms of Facebook usage, less emotionally stable (neurotic) individuals report spending more time on Facebook, while more emotionally stable and more introverted users report more frequently going to Facebook to keep up with friends. All of the personality factors are related to regret, with the exception of openness to new experiences, with more agreeable, more conscientious, more emotionally stable and less extraverted users reporting greater levels of regret for inappropriate content. (Moore and McElroy, 2012, p. 272)

The results produced by Moore and McElroy confirmed and improved the findings of previous studies, which were limited only to surveys of Facebook users without accessing their actual Facebook profiles (Amiel and Sargent, 2004; Correa et al., 2010; Gangadharbatla, 2008; Hamburger and Ben-Artzi, 2000; Ross et al., 2009). For example, a study conducted in 2011 by Tracii Ryan and Sophia Xenos found that "Facebook users tend to be more extraverted and narcissistic, but less conscientious and socially lonely, than nonusers" (2011, p. 1658), and that frequency of use and preferences for specific features seem to be related to neuroticism, loneliness, shyness, and narcissism. The study of Moore and McElroy combines objective data analysis performed on participants' Facebook profiles with subjective data obtained by means of a survey, and the results obtained in this work better explain the relationship between personality factors and Facebook usage than the findings of previously mentioned studies.

Moreover, starting from a systematic review of the existing literature on the psychological factors contributing to Facebook use, Ashwini Nadkarni and Stefan G. Hofmann (2012) recently proposed a model suggesting two primary needs that motivate people to use Facebook: (1) the need to belong and (2) the need for self-presentation. According to the authors, "demographic and cultural factors contribute to the need to belong, whereas neuroticism, narcissism, shyness, self-esteem and self-worth contribute to the need for self-presentation" (Nadkarni and Hofmann, 2012, p. 243). All the previously mentioned studies highlight that the different features provided by Facebook (e.g., Wall, Chat, applications, and games) seem to be able to gratify their users according to their personality traits (Ryan and Xenos, 2011).

3.4.2 STUDIES ON SOCIAL NETWORKING SITES AND IDENTITY CONSTRUCTION

In recent years, different authors have examined the role of media and communication technologies in the socialization processes, with particular attention to the analysis of the presentation of the self on social networks (e.g., Ellison et al., 2007; Manago et al., 2008; Salimkhan et al., 2010; Sheldon, 2009; Siibak, 2009; Zarghooni, 2007). A recent qualitative study shows how the digital language used for self-disclosure and self-representation on social networking might impact upon identity development. The authors found that users construct a shared social space in which images and multimedia become integrated into the sense of self. Through social networks, users create a narrative of social identities connecting past and present social selves (Salimkhan et al., 2010). Starting from the self-discrepancy theory of Tory Higgins (1987, 1991), Andra Siibak (2009) investigated the different self-domains involved in identity management through the virtual space of the Internet. Siibak analyzed the habits of self-presentation of young people in digital online environments and found that the creation of a profile on a social networking site is distinctly socially driven. The expectations of the reference group are an important factor influencing the visual impression management in social networking sites, as the digital profiles are constructed and reconstructed based on the values associated with "the ideal self" or "the ought self" (Siibak, 2009). Computer-mediated communication allows "hyper-personal" relationships to be developed, involving similar feelings of intimacy as those experienced in face-to-face relationships (Walther, 1996). Just as happens in face-to-face relationships, social attraction seems to influence self-disclosure, predictability, and trust between social network users. A study conducted on Facebook revealed that the users who find other users socially attractive are also able to predict their attitudes, values, and beliefs (Sheldon, 2009). In her study, Pavica Sheldon (2009 #4339) extended the uncertainty reduction theory developed by Berger and Calabrese (1975 #4344) to explain the uncertainty reduction in face-to-face relationships to digital communication environments. "As the amount of verbal communication between strangers increases, the level of uncertainty for each interactant in the relationship will decrease. As uncertainty is further reduced, the amount of verbal communication will increase" (Berger and Calabrese, 1975, p. 102). Sheldon found that the same axioms can be applied to profile-to-profile relationships in social networking: "the more Facebook users talk, the less uncertainty they experience and are able to like each other more" (Sheldon, 2009).

All the previous studies have confirmed that the psychotechnologies for communication constitute a virtual and synchronous space through which cognitive and affective functions of mind are emulated, extended, modified, or sometimes amplified, as evidenced in a recent study by Kaveri Subrahmanyam (2007), who compared the new behaviors of adolescents emerging from the use of online forums, chat rooms, and blogs with those described in the physical world. The virtual world seems to be a place in which the same issues emerge as those belonging to the physical world, and the behaviors connected with these issues are sometimes played out with higher intensities than in the physical world (Subrahmanyam, 2007). Moreover, viewing one's own social networking profile is often related to the enhancement of self-esteem, suggesting that "selective self-presentation in digital media, which leads to intensified relationship formation, also influences impressions of the self" (Gonzales and Hancock, 2011, p. 79).

However, some of the studies previously described—which apply personality factors such as the Big Five to clinical categories (for the first test of the Big Five in a largely illiterate indigenous society, refer to Gurven et al., 2012)—beg some questions. Since psychological taxonomies have been classified for application in natural environments, are they valid for analyzing human behaviors in other environments too? In other words, are the traditional classification standards still suitable for the evaluation of human behaviors when the environment of the interaction changes? Is it appropriate to describe behaviors in virtual environments by means of constructs that have been standardized in natural environments, for example, "extroversion"? The psychotechnological approach allows practitioners to study and analyze new kinds of interaction in environments that are different from the traditional ones. In fact, in contrast to the approach of positive technology, the psychotechnological approach does not analyze the effect of a technology on human behavior by considering it as an object *per se*; instead, the psychotechnological perspective considers artifacts as a systemic object. For example, the Social Web, in its functions and purposes, does not exist outside its intrasystemic environment of use, in other words, outside its users and their peculiarities and contexts of interaction. As for a public square, the primary function of social web is as a community place in which people share and build up relationships. In this sense, analyzing this environment without also taking into account the whole interaction system would be like studying the role of a public square in social relationships without considering the people, their needs, and their shared culture. Therefore, just as a public square without people filling it up becomes only an empty place, so the social web (and any other technology) without its users does not phenomenologically exist.

Since the object of observation in psychotechnology is the whole "person–technology" interaction system, it has to be analyzed not as a "simulation" of one unique reality, but as another kind of perceived reality corresponding to another kind of environment. In other words, we consider that technology is "molar" environment and not simply a "molecular" one (Koffka, 1935), and as a new ambient with its own unique proprieties and constitutive components. Psychotechnologies can hence be compared to the behavioral environment concept proposed by Koffka, of a new system resulting from the convergence between the physical environment and the phenomenal one (Koffka, 1935). It is not possible to describe and analyze the object by only taking into account its *objective* reality: the object *per se* is unknown. It is known only as a *percept*, a component of a meaningful *gestalt* emerging from the dynamic relationship between the elements of the system. Therefore, we suppose that if the environment of analysis changes, so do the personality factors involved and how they can be evaluated. In fact, if even one of the elements of a systemic environment changes, the whole system will obtain a new, different equilibrium. Since we cannot anticipate in which way and how much the systemic environment will change, the psychotechnological approach considers the factors related to the interaction system as independent variables of a measure that is not still standardized for that context/environment of interaction.

When we talk about psychotechnologies for socialization we are referring to technologies that are linked to psychosocial users' needs (such as their belongingness, esteem, and self-actualization needs), since they allow users to both directly participate in the communication process and extend their socialization and participation opportunities by influencing "three specific features of our experience—emotions, engagement, and connectedness—that serve to promote adaptive behaviors and positive functioning" (Botella et al., 2012, p. 1). Psychotechnologies such as the web, cell phones, and computer technologies are to be considered as agents of socialization enhancing relationships by means of social media (e.g., Facebook, YouTube, Flickr, Twitter), blogs, feeds, RSS, and tags.* At the same time, user-driven adaptation and integration processes are responsible for the evolution of the

---

* Of course, we do not want to disregard the negative use of technologies that can lead people to conditions of emotional discomfort and to behavior comparable to alcohol abuse, drug abuse, exercise abuse, and gambling. Recently, the concept of Internet addiction has grown in terms of acceptance as a legitimate clinical disorder often requiring treatment. In 1998, Kimberly Young investigated Internet misuse by on-line users who were becoming addicted to it with the first validated instrument to assess Internet addiction (Widyanto and McMurran, 2004; Young, 1998) based on the DSM-IV (American Psychiatric Association, 2000). Albeit from a negative perspective, the Internet addiction phenomenon provides further evidence on the effects of psychotechnologies on cognitive processes and human behavior such as severe emotional, mental, or physiological reactions.

functional structures of which psychotechnologies are composed. Web 2.0 is one of the most extraordinary examples of the user-shaped functional reconfiguration of a psychotechnology; in other words, the needs emerging from a growing experience of interaction have led to the formulation of a new psychotechnology for socialization that allows a new kind of communication, which is more active and participatory than Web 1.0.

3.5   WEB 2.0: FROM A NETWORK SYSTEM TO AN ECOSYSTEM

The web was born thanks to an idea of Tim Berners-Lee, supported by Robert Cailliau, to provide his research team at CERN in Geneva with a platform-independent digital system that would allow the communication and the management of scientific resources (Berners-Lee, 1990a). In a copy of the first web page, Berners-Lee defines, for the first time, the term "World Wide Web" as "a wide-area hypermedia information retrieval initiative aiming to give universal access to a large universe of documents" (Berners-Lee, 1990b). As Berners-Lee said in his proposal, the original objective of the web project was:

> to work toward a universal linked information system, in which generality and portability are more important than fancy graphics techniques and complex extra facilities. The aim would be to allow a place to be found for any information or reference which one felt was important, and a way of finding it afterwards. The result should be sufficiently attractive to use that it the information contained would grow past a critical threshold, so that the usefulness the scheme would in turn encourage its increased use. The passing of this threshold accelerated by allowing large existing databases to be linked together and with new ones. (Berners-Lee, 1989)

The W3 system has been developed to manage information that could be both created by a hypertext language (HTML) and transferred by a HTTP through a system of interconnected computer networks by using a protocol suite (TCP/IP) (Berners-Lee and Cailliau, 1990). In 1991, the web project was made publicly available on the Internet (Wikipedia contributors, 2012e), and the following decade was characterized by the rapid development of the first versions of the current major browsers, such as Internet Explorer (1995), Opera (1996), and Firefox (1998) (Wikipedia contributors, 2012e). Together with the increasing performance of personal computers and the liberalization of the telecommunications market, the web quickly became one of the main channels for sending and receiving information. At the end of the 1990s, about 200 million computers around the world (International Telecommunication Union, 2011) were connected via the Internet. In a very short time, the web became the main channel for sending and receiving information by means of different standards and protocols, and it gradually evolved from a static transmission mode to a dynamic one, toward what is now called the "Semantic Web."

The concept of the Semantic Web has been proposed by World Wide Web Consortium (W3C)—an international community whose mission is to constantly improve web standards and to lead the web to its full potential (W3C, 2012;

http://www.w3.org/Consortium/). As the W3C website says, the main objective of Semantic Web is to provide users with a "web of data" semantically structured:

> In addition to the classic "Web of documents" W3C is helping to build a technology stack to support a "Web of data," the sort of data you find in databases. The ultimate goal of the Web of data is to enable computers to do more useful work and to develop systems that can support trusted interactions over the network. The term "Semantic Web" refers to W3C's vision of the Web of linked data. Semantic Web technologies enable people to create data stores on the Web, build vocabularies, and write rules for handling data. (W3C, 2012; http://www.w3.org/standards/semanticweb/)

Therefore, during recent years, the web has evolved from a data-centered structure to a knowledge-centered one. With a rapid and revolutionary change, society is evolving from the "age of information" toward the "age of knowledge," a new cultural era characterized by the spreading use of ICT and whose economic and social organization is based on knowledge. With the increase in the users' experience of interaction and their needs, the key weakness of the web, that is the impersonal and difficult way of managing the organization of contents, has led the system to a turning point. As Tim O'Reilly points out, the web as it was originally created became overhyped:

> The bursting of the dot-com bubble in the fall of 2001 marked a turning point for the web. Many people concluded that the web was overhyped, when in fact bubbles and consequent shakeouts appear to be a common feature of all technological revolutions. Shakeouts typically mark the point at which an ascendant technology is ready to take its place at center stage. The pretenders are given the bum's rush, the real success stories show their strength, and there begins to be an understanding of what separates one from the other. (2007, p. 17)

In the so-called Web 1.0, a huge amount of information was interconnected through a hierarchical and static model of categorization, in a way which is considerably different from the mental representation of information processes where human knowledge is organized through semantic categorization (Anderson, 1996). In fact, the human mind organizes semantic information through networks of concepts of semantic features, that is, through structures in which concepts are interconnected by associative links (Anderson, 1996; Collins and Quillian, 1972; Rumhelhart et al., 1972). The more knowledge on a specific field is organized and structured by means of semantic networks, the more an individual is able to solve a problem related to that field (Chi et al., 1981; Weiser and Shertz, 1983). The widespread use of the Internet and the increasing expertise of its users have led to a new way of thinking about the web. Web users, who are increasingly skilled, need a web which is even more interactive and accessible for the easy, personalized, and sharable management of information. In 2004, during a conference brainstorming session between O'Reilly Media and MediaLive International, the term "Web 2.0" appears for the first time:

> Dale Dougherty, web pioneer and O'Reilly VP, noted that far from having "crashed," the web was more important than ever, with exciting new applications and sites popping up with surprising regularity. What's more, the companies that had survived the collapse seemed to have some things in common. Could it be that the dot-com collapse marked some kind of turning point for the web, such that a call to action such as "Web 2.0" might make sense? We agreed that it did, and so the Web 2.0 Conference was born. (O'Reilly, 2007, p. 17)

O'Reilly analyzed the phenomenon of Web 2.0 by means of a map (see Figure 3.5) which identifies the elements that constituted the transition to a new web, and gathered the shared ideas that revolve around the core of Web 2.0.

Web 2.0 is a platform for interaction and cooperation services (e.g., Flickr, Gmail, eBay, Wikipedia, BitTorrent) in which the organization of knowledge is based on open protocols and standards and on an indexing system that is both *taxonomic*—organized

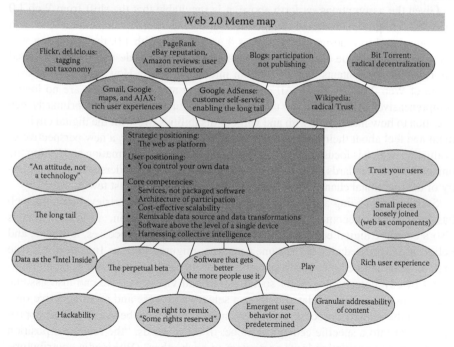

FIGURE 3.5   (See color insert.) Web 2.0 Meme map developed at a brainstorming session during a conference at O'Reilly Media. A meme is "an element of a culture or system of behavior that may be considered to be passed from one individual to another by nongenetic means, especially imitation." (From O'Reilly, T., *Commun. Strategies*, 65 (1st Quarter), 17, 2007; Oxford Dictionaries, "Meme," retrieved September 15, 2012, 2010, from http:// oxforddictionaries.com/definition/meme).

through directories, as with the Web 1.0—and *folksonomic*—organized by means of a collaborative tagging system. In Web 2.0, users directly control and manage both the contents and services, and the qualitative value of their experience determines the success and the survival of the service, leading to what is defined as the phenomenon of the perpetual beta, "in which the product is developed in the open, with new features slipstreamed in on a monthly, weekly, or even daily basis" (O'Reilly, 2007, p. 30), marking the end of the software release cycle. The term "Web 2.0" is then used to indicate a turning point that represents the onset of a cultural revolution. On the basis of the dynamic web (which we can consider as a precursor of Web 2.0), a new way of experiencing interaction through the Internet led from the hypertext being conceived of as a simple network of links between information to a real architecture of participation, in which the content is no longer dependent on its representation. Therefore, Web 2.0 is not a technological invention—it continues to be based on hypertext and TCP/IP and HTTP protocols—but as O'Reilly defines it, it is rather an "attitude" of users (O'Reilly, 2007) or, in other words, the outcome of an interactive, dynamic, and circular process that involves both adaptation and learning processes.

Given the assumptions set forth above, it is inevitable that the shift from Web 1.0 to Web 2.0 requires substantial changes in both user-centered evaluation methods and techniques and web design (see Chapters 4 and 5). For Web 1.0, the evaluation was mainly focused on the accessibility of data in order to provide users with universal information—or contents "for all"—in an interactive space. However, with the evolution of Web 2.0, Design for All and accessibility are measures that are no longer comprehensive. In Web 2.0, the user-centered evaluation and design primarily pay attention to how individuals with and without disabilities live with the digital environment and feel about their interactions with the system. However, a new perspective of evaluation, which is focused more on the personalization of information and less on the universality of standards, is necessary to take account of and understand the complexity of the functional change that has involved the web over the last few years.

Starting from being a simple consultation and information retrieval tool, the web has increasingly become a psychotechnology for socialization, a platform that is also a complex digital ecosystem through which cognitive processes, attitudes, and beliefs are expressed and, at the same time, reconfigured in time. In fact, if it is true that, as demonstrated previously, personality traits can be considered as being influenced by psychotechnologies for socialization and vice versa, we can also assume that this phenomenon is related both to a selective process and to an adaptive one. Through the selective process, some personality traits have been selected as appropriate to fit into a specific ecological niche; in other words, "the relational position of a species or population in its ecosystem to each other" (Wikipedia contributors, 2011); however, the adaptive process leads the human mind to modify its cognitive processes, attitudes, and beliefs. Web 2.0 represents an extraordinary example of how the user–psychotechnology interaction has been responsible for the construction of a new ecosystem where different digital ecological niches have arisen and evolved, as in the case of the social networks of societies where the regime restricts the natural interhuman communication space, such as in the so-called "Arab spring" phenomenon (Marzouki et al., 2012; see also Box 3.4).

BOX 3.4   FACEBOOK CONTRIBUTION TO THE 2011 TUNISIAN REVOLUTION: WHAT CAN CYBERPSYCHOLOGY TEACH US ABOUT THE ARAB SPRING UPRISINGS?

YOUSRI MARZOUKI

The inception of technically powerful social media platforms was already expected to make big changes in our lives but maybe not as expected as to change the history of the Arab world within few weeks. The 2011 Tunisian revolution is a compelling example of this large-scale catalyst effect of social networking media in changing political regimes. This millennium's first revolution have paved the way for a new kind of successful popular uprisings called "leaderless revolutions," which are characterized by the absence of a political figure, party, or organizing capacity. According to many media sources, information sharing via social networking was vital to the success of this revolution, and Facebook was its main vector, as recognized by many observers.

Marzouki et al. (2012) have provided recently an original cyberpsychological account of how Tunisian Internet users perceive the contribution of Facebook to the 2011 Tunisian revolution. The authors hypothesized that a better understanding of Facebook's role may be obtained by assessing the perception of Tunisian Internet users of Facebook contribution to this event. Marzouki et al. (2012) launched their study 5 days after the fall of Ben Ali dictatorship using an online questionnaire where participants were first invited to rate the importance (from 0: *not important at all* to 10: *very important*) of Facebook in the Tunisian revolution and then they had to explain the reason of their rating.

After analyzing a sizeable text corpus of 6640 words from 333 Tunisian internet users' responses using word cloud technique (see Figure 3.6), the authors conducted a cluster analysis based on the Euclidean distance matrix between the 17 most frequent words. The results revealed three main clusters corresponding to what they labeled 1: Facebook political function, 2: Facebook informational function, and 3: Facebook media platform function.

According to Marzouki et al. (2012), this tripartite perception can serve as a proxy to describe the collective state of mind of all users involved in the revolutionary process. This tripartite perception is directly linked to the "collective consciousness" of the participants' cyberspace as shown in the model (see Figure 3.6). Marzouki et al. (2012) consider this "virtual collective consciousness" (VCC) as an updated version of the Durkheimian concept of *collective representation* (Durkheim, 1982) that is also highly comparable to the Žižek's concept of *collective mind* (Gutmair and Flor, 1998) and to "new collective consciousness" used by Boguta (2011) to describe the computational history of the Internet shutdown during the Egyptian revolution.

The acceleration mechanisms of these social movements lead to the crystallization of network interactions into one stance: the VCC. Following up on this idea, I further hypothesize that the dynamic of the Tunisian cyberspace

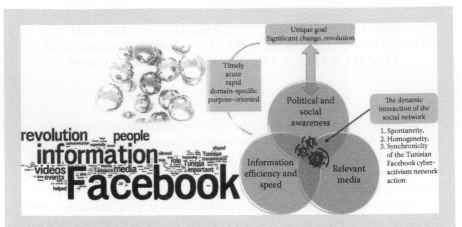

FIGURE 3.6 The word cloud graph based on a text corpus of 6640 words (to the left) and the tentative model describing the dynamic of the Tunisian cyberspace during the uprising (to the right). Note that the model is based on the tripartite perception revealed by the cluster analysis. (Adapted from Marzouki, Y. et al., *Cyberpsychol. Behav. Soc. Netw.*, 15(5), 237, 2012)

reflects the dynamic of its transactive memory (TM). TM is a set of individual memory systems in combination with the communication that takes place between individuals (Wegner, 1986). It represents the group members' ability to benefit from each other's knowledge and expertise being externally and internally encoded. The TM system is defined based on three key components: (1) *Individual expertise* when each member specializes in a particular area based on their relative skills or experiences about the situation, (2) *Knowledge* of each other's informational content, and (3) *Communication* processes between individuals within the network. Overtime members gain responsibility about information encoding and sharing; thus the general knowledge becomes less redundant among individuals.

Although research on TM have been limited to couples, small groups, and organizations, Marzouki et al. study strongly suggests that an effective TM can operate on a very large scale. Indeed, each Tunisian Facebook user had developed a certain knowledge about either acquiring or sharing information related to the uprising. By being involved in the field and filming live action during the uprising, citizen media and journalism are crucial to this part of the TM system. This expertise will help individuals to filter the huge amount of miscellaneous information on Facebook in order to locate what is relevant to the uprising. Ultimately expertise expansion among group members makes the information domain specific, while TM serves to make the group goal achievement efficient (e.g., Brandon and Hollingshead, 2004). Ousting the regime was this goal and Facebook was the TM holder that helped thriving people collective political awareness and ultimately their responsibility toward this goal (see Figure 3.6).

Psychotechnologies for socialization thus constitute complex ecosystems through which a circuit of reciprocal gene–culture coevolution operates. "Gene-culture coevolution is a causal whirlpool in history, where culture is shaped by biological imperatives and genes shift in response to changing cultural opportunities" (Lumsden, 1999). Social networks, mashups, blogs, Wikis, file-sharing repositories, discussion boards, instant messaging, and other web applications are transmission places in which cultures evolve and vary by giving place to new cultural contents that can only survive by means of transmission processes that allow their preservation over time. Twitter, Facebook, and other social networks, which have been created ad hoc to avoid the control of despotic authorities, are becoming alternative militant media (Marzouki et al., 2012; Slimani, 2011) and constitute ecological niches in which a real evolutionary process takes shape by means of new revolutionary cultural systems. People (citizens) who are misfits in their natural (historical) environment become successful individuals able to fit into a new (virtual) ecological niche. Just as an albino crow, shunned by the flock because it is seen as a threat, is saved from certain death by a human who creates a new environment for it, so people living in oppressive regimes find in the (virtual) ecological niches of social networks freedom and the creative expression of their humanity. The new ecological niches created by means of Web 2.0 provide a space for those spontaneous variants that would not normally find expression in a natural environment. Just as some theories argue that genes and culture influence each other's preservation (Lumsden, 1988; Lumsden and Wilson, 1981; Plotkin, 1997), such as double inheritance and other coevolutionary theories, we argue that psychotechnologies for socialization might in time represent places in which the selection of different cultural systems takes place and environments that contribute to both the survival and the evolution of ecological niches.

3.6   CONCLUSION

In this chapter, we have described the role of ICTs in the transmission and modification of human psychological abilities in terms of opportunities for socialization and participation. A new perspective, the psychotechnological one, was introduced to reinterpret the development of ICTs as the result of processes of adaptation that "force users to a cognitive and cultural modification and adaptation" (Miesenberger et al., 2012), and also as the result of learning processes that lead, over time, to a cognitive, cultural, and sometimes structural readaptation of the system. We then described the role of psychotechnologies for socialization as social technologies that emulate, extend, amplify and modify sensory-motor, psychological or cognitive functions of the mind (Federici et al., 2011; Miesenberger et al., 2012), by means of the cognitive and affective processes involved in the formation of attitudes, beliefs, and social activities through media and communication technologies. Finally, we analyzed the phenomenon of Web 2.0 to highlight how the mutual and dynamic relation between a psychotechnology (the web) and its users has led to a mutual functional readaptation and modification.

4 Equalizing the Relationship between Design and Evaluation

4.1 ACTIVE ROLE OF TODAY'S END USER IN THE PERVASIVE INTERACTION WITH PSYCHOTECHNOLOGIES

As discussed in the first chapter, which focuses on the history of human–computer interaction (HCI), the use of devices evolved with the increase of both users' needs and the improvement in the relationship between users and technology. In particular, nowadays, the psychotechnologies for socialization (i.e., the Internet and communication technologies such as computers, mobile devices, and smart technologies) have reached an extensive and pervasive role in our work and lives, allowing users to access and manage information ubiquitously (Ark and Selker, 1999; Saha and Mukherjee, 2003; see also Chapter 3). According to Norbert Streitz, founder of the Smart Future Initiative (see Box 4.1), the use of smart mobile devices is increasingly displacing traditional ways of interacting (e.g., telephones or personal computers) because, in the pervasive interaction contexts, these technologies seem to be disappearing both physically and mentally.

The physical disappearance is the result of "the miniaturization of devices and their integration in other everyday artifacts as, for example, clothes," and the mental disappearance is ascribable to the fact that "the artifacts can still be large but they are not perceived as computers because people discern them as, say, interactive walls or interactive tables" (Streitz and Nixon, 2005, p. 34).

The ubiquitous interaction with psychotechnologies is leading users to become active consumers, that is to say, users that are able to discern the differences among the various technologies and their functioning. In particular, the pervasive presence of devices in everyday contexts allows users to increase their interaction with the psychotechnologies for socialization. Active consumers aim not only to access and use the information, but they also want to develop their own information. In this way, users become developers of ICT content and functions, or in other words, they become active users who should be able to

- Share and promote their information through hypertextual environments, as it happens, in the Web 2.0 environment
- Create structures of information and web interfaces with a minimum knowledge of the mark-up languages, as it happens, with open-source content management systems, e.g., the Joomla (http://www.joomla.org/)

and Wordpress (http://wordpress.org/) projects, thanks to which every kind of user, regardless of the level of their expertise, can create web interfaces by means of a set of tools developed through a collaborative networked process

The progress of both device mobility and software portability, as well as the concurrent interactive possibility of easily manipulating, creating, and sharing information, is strictly related to the increasing use of psychotechnologies for socialization. In 2011, 30.2% of the world's population was using the Internet, with a 480.4% increase in users between 2000 and 2011 (Internet World Stats, 2011). Between 2010 and 2011, 90% of the world's population had access to mobile networks, reaching 5.3 billion people, including the 940 million subscribers to 3G services (ITU, 2010). The International Telecommunication Union (ITU, 2011) reported that data on

---

BOX 4.1   SMART FUTURE INITIATIVE: THE DISAPPEARING COMPUTER AND UBIQUITOUS COMPUTING

SIMONE BORSCI

The Smart Future Initiative (SFI) was founded in January 2009 by Norbert Streitz. The main goal of this initiative is to establish a forum for triggering, developing, and communicating innovative ideas and concepts about smart environments and ambient intelligence in the context of ubiquitous and pervasive computing (see http://www.smart-future.net/1.html). In particular, the SFI group starts from the assumption that the concept of the computer is going to completely disappear within the next years. As Streitz et al. recently stated (2007), the current concept of "the-computer-as-we-know-it" has no place in the information societies of the future:

> It will be replaced by a new generation of technologies, which will move the computing power off the desktop and ultimately integrate it with real world objects and everyday environments. Computing becomes thus an inseparable part of our everyday activities, while simultaneously disappearing into the background. It becomes a ubiquitous utility taking on a role similar to electricity— an enabling but invisible and pervasive medium revealing its functionality on request in an unobtrusive way and supporting people in their everyday lives. (Streitz et al., 2007 p. v)

The key mission of the SFI is to identify the future trends of human artifact interaction, in order to manage by a multidisciplinary approach, the consequences of two kinds of computer disappearance: the physical and the mental (http://www.disappearing-computer.net). Whereas the physical disappearance refers to the "miniaturization of devices and their integration" (Streitz and Nixon, 2005, p. 32) in other everyday technologies, mental disappearance does not pertain to the dimensions or to the visibility of the artifacts, but to the fact that the technologies "are not perceived as computers because people discern them as, say, interactive walls or interactive tables" (Streitz and Nixon, 2005, p. 32). We can say that the physical and the mental disappearance of computers are two key factors of today's increase in the pervasive presence of technology in everyday life. As Mark Weiser, head of the Computer Science Laboratory at the Xerox Palo Alto research center foresaw in 1991, in his analysis of the future scenarios of the twenty-first century technologies, there is a correlation between technology use and technology disappearing due to the fact that the greater the penetration of a technology in human life, the more this technology disappears, gradually becoming part of everyday objects and environments (Mark, 1991).

Today's challenge for HCI professionals (engineers, designers, psychologists, ergonomists, etc.) is to move technology *per se* out of the user's perception, as an isolated component that can be used in an environment, by transforming it into an integrated part of the context that can lead people to ubiquitous computing (Streitz et al., 2007; Streitz and Nixon, 2005). In light of this, when a user perceives, interacts, and experiences technology as part of the environment, the context of use becomes the technology itself, by transforming any physical space in a user-friendly environment in which any kind of people may interact, communicate, manipulate, and modify the context, adapting it to their needs and expectations. As recently clarified by David Armano, executive vice president at Edelman Digital (2012), the future of technology is not the improvement of the mobile, as a technology feature, but the improvement of the mobility that means the improvement of the environment in order to provide ubiquitous information for different kinds of support with different features (e.g., screen sizes). In this sense, mobile refers to the device (i.e., a mobile device), whereas mobility refers to the context that can include and support the device, or not:

> Mobility is radically different from the stationary "desktop" experience. In some cases, mobility is a "lean back" experience like sitting on a commuter train watching a video. In other cases it can be "lean forward"—like shopping for a gift while you take your lunch break at the park. And in many cases, it's "lean free" when your body is in motion, or you're standing in line scanning news headlines or photos from friends while you wait for your turn to be called. (Armano, 2012)

Therefore, today's challenge for the HCI professionals is the design and assessment of adaptable systems in order to integrate technologies and environments, by increasing the users' access and use of information.

In summary, we can propose that the future scenario of the interaction is the disappearance of the computer and the expansion of ubiquitous computing, by the integration of technology in environment. Finally, the SFI aims to identify a comprehensive and multidisciplinary perspective in order to define, manage, and organize this future scenario.

communication-technology use suggest that young people, particularly in school contexts, use the Internet frequently because it offers relevant content in the form of educational material and information, social network services, and other user-created content. At the same time, analysis of World Wide Web use reveals that, each year, the traffic grows with a trend close to 100% (Coffman and Odlyzko, 2002; Odlyzko, 2003).

In the context of pervasive interaction, user behavior has completely changed: today, people use ICT devices in more consistent and richer ways than in the past, revealing more diverse needs and increased expectations of the interaction with the psychotechnologies. For this reason, the designers and the evaluators perceive a growing need to involve the new active and skilled users in the development processes, to design interfaces that fit these new end users, their mental models, and their needs. Therefore, the inclusion of end users in both the design and evaluation processes relates strictly to the aim of releasing products that, by meeting end user expectations, have a high probability of success.

As discussed in Chapter 3, the concept of psychotechnology introduces a new perspective to the analysis of the relationship between designers and evaluators: Although the design of devices and their interfaces mostly concerns the development of the artifact functioning on the basis of a user's model, design assessment mostly concerns the analysis of the designed functions (i.e., the functioning) that are perceived and experienced by users. In fact, what users perceive and use during an interaction is not the functioning of the artifact *per se*, but how the interface works, reacts, and communicates with the users (i.e., the psychotechnological experience). As we shall discuss in the following sections, although the functioning of a device *per se* can be considered the sum of its designed functions, the functioning perceived and experienced by the user during the psychotechnological interaction cannot be reduced to this designed functioning, but as "a *place* for the whole synchronous perception of a meaningful gestalt" (Federici et al., 2011, p. 1179 [italics in original].). In light of this, designers and evaluators should work together iteratively, using a well-planned and integrated methodology that guarantees a successful dialogue between the device and the users, by reaching the aims of Design for All and User Interfaces for All (see Chapter 1).

As Stephanidis (2001) emphasizes, the integration of the designer's and evaluator's work to reach the shared goal of "for all" interaction is the only way to develop context-oriented systems that meet the users' requirements and their adaptable and adaptive interactive behaviors. In line with the goal of interaction for all, the main purpose of the psychotechnological perspective is to create a bridge between designers and evaluators that transforms any designed device into an intrasystemic solution that facilitates and drives the dialogue between users and the interface.

In this chapter, we shall analyze the relationship between the design and the evaluation processes during the product life cycle. Nowadays, in the context of pervasive and ubiquitous interaction, there is a growing need for an integration of aims and communication between designers and evaluators during product development to better answer the new needs of active users and their growing expertise of use. Given this, we shall propose the psychotechnological framework as a new perspective on defining both a new space of communication within the product life cycle and a common shared goal between the designers and the evaluators, that is to say, the development and the release of an intrasystemic solution.

4.2   EQUALIZING THE DESIGN AND THE EVALUATION PROCESSES

As the HCI field developed, different design philosophies have analyzed the relation between design and evaluation (Chapter 1), which moved from the UCD approach to the "User Interfaces for All" approach. Although these design philosophies clearly focus on the limits of the design process by considering the real users and underlining the importance of the evaluation process, they seem to have failed in redefining the relationship between the roles of designer and evaluator. In fact, current design philosophies try to equalize the design and the evaluation processes by proposing that the design process should include the evaluation process. Accordingly, design has priority over evaluation and, as a consequence, evaluation is reduced to a mere confirmatory process for helping designers improve the technology (i.e., by adopting a small usability approach; Chapter 2). In our opinion, this designers' perspective often underestimates the evaluators' role in HCI. In fact, it is quite common that the evaluation, instead of being considered a separate and independent process, is approached only as a supporting process that is integrated in the life cycle to check how the interface works (Robinson and Fitter, 1992). This point of view, which considers the evaluation process as only a "check" of the device functioning, led some researchers to propose different design models, such as the parallel design model, in which the evaluators are totally excluded from the life cycle, while the designers assess their own work (Ball et al., 1994; Buller et al., 2001; Ovaska and Räihä, 1995; Zimmerman et al., 2003).

To equalize the roles of the design and the evaluation processes, it is a necessity to consider them as two opposite and separate points of view on the technology for reaching the same goal (i.e., the success of the device and its interface): While designers develop technologies focusing on a user model, evaluators rethink the same technology from the user point of view by analyzing how the interface's functions interact with the user.

From a psychotechnological perspective, the technological functioning is not the sum of its functions, but is related to how its functions will be perceived and used by users in their context of interaction. Hence, an evaluator should assess both how the technology's functions work relative to the designed functioning and how the user perceives the product functioning.

For instance, when comparing different psychotechnologies for socialization, such as social networks (e.g., Diaspora, Facebook, Google+, LinkedIn, etc.), an evaluator may notice that their interfaces have a similar set of functions, such as the "I like" (Facebook, www.facebook.com) and "G+" (Google+, www.plus.google.com) buttons. From the designer's perspective, these functions are different, because they are components of two distinct interfaces, whereas, from the user point of view, the meaning of these functions (i.e., I appreciate this comment) and the actions for activating them (i.e., by clicking on a button) are the same. By considering both the designer's and user's points of view, in the case of the previous example, an evaluator should measure (1) how each function works, as a component of a specific device, and whether or not it works in line with the designer's expectations (i.e., the functioning *per se*) and (2) the degree of difference perceived by the users in interaction when they use these two functions (i.e., the perceived functioning).

According to our perspective, only the evaluator can discriminate between the device functioning *per se* and the device functioning as perceived by the end user. In fact, only the evaluator can have an external and overall perspective on the interaction, whereas designers and users have a restricted point of view on the interaction. In other words, the designer only focuses on the development of the functioning *per se*, simulating how the user may perceive the interaction, and users only focus on what they perceived, without considering how the functions have been designed.

In sum, when adopting a psychotechnological perspective, the product functioning should be considered as being more than the mere sum of its functions. This concept can be explained easily with different examples—such as the automobile, which was designed not only to be started or propelled by the engine (i.e., its functioning *per se*) but also to be driven by someone (i.e., its perceived functioning), and the television, which was developed not only to be used in its objective functions (the display controls for brightness, contrast, color, etc., i.e., its functioning *per se*) but also to be watched by its users in its perceived functioning—and other examples of technologies used every day include personal computers, mobile phones, video-game consoles, etc.

The evaluation carried out under this perspective is the mean for checking, controlling, modifying, and improving the designed functioning of a device by matching it with its functioning experienced by real users. Therefore, the intrasystemic solution can be achieved only when designers and evaluators share a common perspective—the psychotechnological one—by working in a holistic, iterative way on the following three elements: technology, users, and user interaction.

Whereas the designer works only on the technology by relying on a model of the end-user, the evaluator works on all three elements, by assessing (1) the technology functioning *per se*, (2) how the user perceives the technology functioning, and (3) the dialogue between the user and the technology.

In the following sections, we shall discuss the relationship between the roles of designer and evaluator within the life cycle of a product. Moreover, the concept of technology shall be reread not only in terms of its functioning and adaptability, but also from a psychotechnological viewpoint (Chapter 3), which focuses on developing systems able to foster the user's distributed cognition in pervasive interaction environments.

4.2.1   INTRASYSTEMIC SOLUTION: A NEW PERSPECTIVE ON THE RELATION BETWEEN DESIGN AND EVALUATION

As Steven Krug explained well with his motto "don't make me think" (2000), a user has a good interaction experience only when the interface is "self-evident" (2000, p. 11), i.e., when the user cannot "perceive" the interface. Consequently, designers focus on developing the technological functioning of the system by assuming that the most important component of the interaction is the object itself, i.e., the better the technological system works, the better the user's interaction will be.

Although we agree with Krug's idea that a self-evident interface matches the design "for all" aim, it is important to emphasize that, to create this kind of interface, the designers' improvement of their mental model for designing the product on the basis of a well-simulated end-user is not enough. In fact, as we shall discuss in Chapter 5, designers cannot completely simulate someone else's perspective without relying on their own mental model.

Therefore, we propose that, in order to "...not make me think," the evaluation is a necessary step in which real users are forced to think. In fact, the evaluator represents an external point of view on the interaction, and by observing the user's interaction, he or she can assess the mental model of the users and match it to the designer's mental model; therefore, only the evaluator can measure the distance between the user and the designer. We summarize our position as follows: The only way to allow users to not think during the interaction is to force them to think during the evaluation.

Whereas designers prioritize the development of the technological system by considering the evaluation as a secondary process that improves the product, evaluators, during the life cycle of the product, assume an opposite point of view on the interaction, in which the assessment focuses more on user needs, expectations, and abilities in interaction than on the system functioning.

Considering the designer's and evaluators' points of view, a strong division between the roles of designer and evaluator emerges: The designer usually develops the technological system, whereas the evaluator usually assesses user behavior with the technology (e.g., with user-based analysis) and the technological system reactions to user input (e.g., with model- or expert-based analysis).

The relationship between designers and evaluators is based on the assumption that the design of the object and the assessment of the user in interaction are processes standing at two opposite poles. As discussed earlier, usually when the life cycle prioritizes the design of the technology functioning, these two poles interact and the evaluation is considered a supporting process of the design process. Although in these kinds of life cycles the roles of designer and evaluator are formally separated, the evaluation actually consists in a subordinate process. On the other hand, when the life cycle is not strongly centered on the technological system (i.e., the designer's perspective), the relationship between the two poles is mediated by an iterative shifting of the life cycle focus during the technology's development.

During the evolution of HCI, several approaches to life cycle have been created (for a complete review on lifecycles: Zhang et al., 2005). They differ only in the organization of the moments in which the focus on the interaction is shifted from the object to the subject, or in other words, differing only in the space offered to the evaluation in the life cycle. As Figure 4.1 shows, the shifting is the product of the general goal of the life cycle: When the goal is to improve the technological system, the focus is only on the artifact. User assessment is only a confirmatory test, whereas, when the goal is not only improving the artifact but also adapting it to the user's needs, a greater percentage of life cycle time is dedicated to user testing. Of course, as the UCD suggests, we can focus the entire life cycle on user evaluation by driving the designer's work with the assessment results. Nevertheless, UCD results

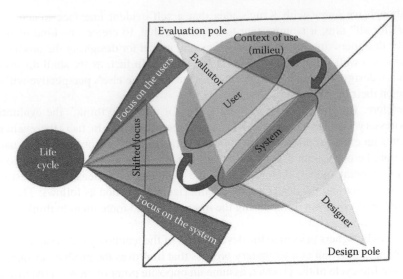

FIGURE 4.1   (See color insert.) The general goal of the life cycle. When the primary goal is to improve the technological system, the focus is only on the artifact. When the goal is both to improve the technological system and adapt it to the user's needs, a greater percentage of life cycle time is dedicated to user testing by shifting the focus during the cycle.

are extremely expensive and are rarely applied in HCI, as Larry L. Constantine, chief scientist of Constantine and Lockwood Ltd., explains:

> The dirty secret that few advocates and practitioners will admit to is that user-centered design in practice is largely trial-and-error design. Stripped of semi-scientific rhetoric and professional self-justification, most user-centered design involves little more than good guessing followed by repeated corrections and adjustments guided by checking with users. (Constantine, 2004, p. 3)

The UCD, focusing the life cycle mainly on one pole of the cycle (in this case, the assessment), creates an unequal relationship between designer and evaluator, in which the evaluation emerges as hierarchically superior to the design. The effect of UCD is the exact opposite of the effect of the life cycle, focused on the product functioning (i.e., designer's perspective). In fact, when the life cycle centers on the user's perceived functioning (i.e., UCD), it may be easy for the user to interact with a product that has been designed according to his or her peculiarities and needs but, at the same time, the technology that has been designed according to this perspective may also result in poor function and design. On the other hand, when the life cycle focuses on the product functioning *per se*, the final product may result in richer functions than a product developed according to UCD. At the same time, however, interaction with its users could be perceived as being much more difficult, given that it was not developed explicitly according to their needs.

   This is not the place to discuss the validity of the different kinds of life cycles; however, it is important to emphasize that the difference among the approaches described above only concerns the shift of focus from the technology to the subject, which is organized during specific steps of the evolution of the technological system and with different kinds of evaluation (e.g., summative evaluation, formative evaluation, or both). Nevertheless, although the shifting of the life cycle focus reduces the orientation to a single pole, it does not solve the main problem: The design and the evaluation continue to be separate processes with a hierarchical relationship. When the focus is mostly on the technological system, the evaluation is subordinated to the design; otherwise, when the focus is mostly on the evaluation, the design is subordinated to the assessment.

We propose that the only solution to really equalizing and integrating design and evaluation in the different life cycles, while creating psychotechnologies (Chapter 3), is to introduce a third pole: the intrasystemic dialogue between the technology and the user (Figure 4.2).

As stated previously, because designer and evaluator exchange information on the technology without a shared aim, design and evaluation should be considered two separated processes. In this kind of exchange, there is not a real matching of different information but only a give-and-take in which designers use evaluators' work only to check the quality of the technological system. Otherwise, when the aim

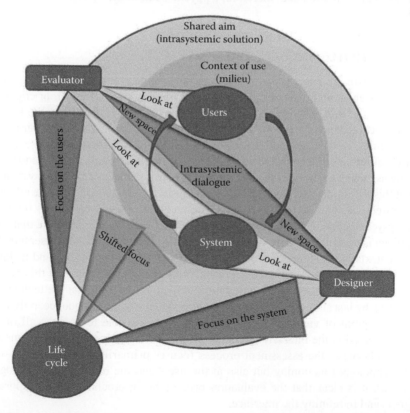

FIGURE 4.2 **(See color insert.)** The new space created by the introduction of a third pole, the intrasystemic dialogue between the technology and the user. When designers and evaluators work together in this space, they share the same aim, equalizing their relationship.

of the design and the evaluation is to develop an intrasystemic solution, regardless of the kind of life cycle applied, designers and evaluators share a common communication space in which the development of the device and its interface functioning (the design process) together with the assessment of user interaction (the assessment process) are two moments both aiming at reaching a common goal, instead of two different aims belonging to separate actors (i.e., the designer of a technology and the evaluator that verifies its functioning). Following this approach, the final goal of the life cycle is to integrate the mental models of the designer and the user through the assessment, to transform a final product into a solution that perfectly meets user needs and accomplishes the standard requirements in an intrasystemic dialogue.

The intrasystemic solution so obtained is the result of the designer's and evaluator's efforts in matching the conceptual model of the system (the device and its interface) and the user's mental model. In this sense, the intrasystemic solution is not the final product *per se*, and not all of the designed products are intrasystemic solutions. In other words, only a technology that is created through both an integrated collaboration and communication between designer and evaluator, and that is assessed and redesigned for reaching the Interface-for-All's aims, can be considered an intrasystemic solution and, therefore, a psychotechnology.

4.3   INTRASYSTEMIC SOLUTION FROM A PSYCHOTECHNOLOGICAL PERSPECTIVE

As discussed in Chapter 3, we define psychotechnology as any technology that emulates, extends, amplifies or modifies sensory-motor, psychological, or cognitive functions of the mind (Federici et al., 2011; Miesenberger et al., 2012). We believe that the psychotechnology is both a medium of systems of symbols—which are organized by rules, restrictions, and knowledge possibilities that force users to a cognitive and cultural modification and adaptation (Miesenberger et al., 2012)—and a way to guide users to a cognitive and cultural readaptation of the environment system. In light of this definition, and considering the analysis carried out so far on the relationship between design(ers) and assess(ors), the analysis of a device and its interface from a psychotechnological point of view should move from the principle that each technology is designed by developers to be used by somebody (i.e., the users) in different contexts of use. Starting from the assumption that between user and technology there is a mutual adaptation, designers cannot capture all aspects of this mutual relationship, because their role focuses primarily on looking only at the technology functioning by just simulating the user's mental model. As a consequence, only from an external point of view (i.e., the evaluation), is it possible to analyze all of the aspects involved in the interaction by matching the designer's and the user's mental models. Otherwise, the assessment process focuses primarily on looking not only at the technology functioning but also at the users and the intrasystemic dialogue. Given this, it is clear that the evaluation process has a crucial role in supporting designers and in refining the interface.

We suggest that designers and evaluators, from their individual observation poles of interaction, should share a common holistic perspective in which the components of the interaction, as entities in an intrasystemic dialogue (i.e., the technology and the users), have a concurrent role in defining the interaction experience. In this way, we propose that a psychotechnological experience emerges as a result of the intrasystemic dialogue between the interface and the users in a specific context of use. As Albert Bandura, professor emeritus of social science in psychology at Stanford University, suggested, by analyzing the emergent properties of the human cognitive processes, the emergent properties of psychotechnologies:

> Differ qualitatively from their constituent elements. To use Bunge's (1977) analogy, the unique emergent properties of water, such as fluidity, viscosity, and transparency are not simply the aggregate properties of its microcomponents of oxygen and hydrogen. Through their interactive effects they are transformed into new phenomena. One must distinguish between the physical basis of thought and its functional properties. Cognitive processes are not only emergent brain activities; they also exert determinative influence. The human mind is generative, creative, proactive, and self-reflective not just reactive. (Bandura, 1999, p. 156)

By extending Bandura's exemplification to the user–technology interaction system, we describe psychotechnology as an emerging phenomenon that is more than the mere sum of the objective components of an artifact. In other words, a psychotechnology cannot be reduced to the device and its interface functioning *per se*. It is the outcome of the dynamic and reciprocal causation among the components of the interaction system—i.e., the technological object and its functioning, the user and his or her subjective experience of the interaction, the environment of use, and the role of this context on the dynamics of the interaction.

In the words of Bunge (1977), designers cannot create "water" (i.e., a new psychotechnology) by knowing only the hydrogen functioning (i.e., the device and its interface). They must also know the chemical bonding between hydrogen and oxygen (in our example, the user's experience in his or her context of interaction with the technology). Nevertheless, although it is easy to simulate the chemical bonding of hydrogen and oxygen (because their relationship is defined by the physical properties of these two "microcomponents" of the water), the interactive bond— i.e., the intrasystemic dialogue between the interface and the users, owing to the generative, creative, proactive, and self-reflective properties of the human mind (Bandura, 1999)—is very difficult to simulate in all its emergent aspects.

In light of this, like chemists, evaluators play a specific role in the product life cycle, because they observe "the water" (the psychotechnology) by defining and measuring both the bond between "the hydrogen" and "the oxygen" (the intrasystemic dialogue) and the emergent properties of their relationship such as the fluidity, viscosity, and transparency of the water (the interaction). The results of the assessment allow designers and evaluators to define a stable bond between the microcomponents of the intrasystemic dialogue, creating in this way a psychotechnology whose emergent properties (i.e., interactions) are a trade-off between the designer's goals and the user's needs and expectations.

Hence, the psychotechnological approach provides designers and evaluators with a shared background that is necessary for analyzing whether or not the life cycle outcome is an intrasystemic solution. By adopting this meta-perspective, practitioners might overcome the limitations of the life cycle process, in which the design and the assessment have different aims. In fact, through this new approach, the outcome of the life cycle is not only the technology as a designed interface, created with different degrees of evaluation and design moments during the cycle, but it is also the technology as an intrasystemic solution. The intrasystemic dialogue, as a third pole of the relationship between designer and evaluator, creates a space during the life cycle which focuses on the relation between the technological functioning *per se* and the functioning perceived by the users. In this space, designers and evaluators collaborate in an equalized exchange for optimizing the adaptation process of both technology to users and users to the technological functioning. Concurrently, because this third pole allows practitioners to focus equally on the objective and the subjective components of the interaction system, designers and evaluators may share a holistic approach, in which:

1. Technology and users are two different interactive systems, one cognitive (user), the other designed (technology) in a specific context of use (milieu and physical environment):
   a. The designed technological system represents the conceptual model of the designers. This conceptual model is the result of a simulation process, in which the simulated end user interacts with the artifact (i.e., conceptual model) in a typified context of use.
   b. The cognitive system (user) belongs to the psychological functions of users' minds, their attitudes, experience, skills, and habits.
2. Both the technological and user systems are integrated entities that play a concurrent role in defining the interaction experience:
   a. Users adapt themselves to the designed technological system in the context of use.
   b. The designed technological system should be developed and assessed in order to be adaptive to the user's needs and expectations and, at the same time, to be easily accessed and used in a specific context by reducing the user's process of adaptation.

Regardless of the kind of life cycle applied to creating a product, when both designer and evaluator endorse a psychotechnological perspective with an equalized relationship, they can consider the mutual adaptation of both the cognitive system to the designed one, and the designed to the cognitive one, to optimize the intrasystemic dialogue of the systems (i.e., the third pole). In this sense, the technology and the user are not considered as two separated entities, the first one developed by the designer and the second one assessed by the evaluator, but as two systems with an adaptive relationship within a specific context of use. Hence, the goal of both designer and evaluator is to work together to construct and optimize this adaptive relationship.

In summary, the psychotechnological perspective and the introduction of a third pole in the relationship between designer and evaluator enlarge the possibility of any kind of life cycle for developing psychotechnologies, which match the end user's needs. In fact, regardless of whether the focus of the life cycle is only on the interface functioning *per se* (i.e., designer's perspective), or it is shifted in different steps from technology to subject (and vice versa) within the life cycle, the psychotechnological perspective supports designers and evaluators in sharing a common goal that is the development of an intrasystemic solution. As a consequence, designers and evaluators establish a space of integration in which their work is equalized and discussed to reach the common goal.

As Figure 4.3 shows, the new space created by the third pole connects designer and evaluator in which the shared goal (i.e., improving the relation between device and its interface and user) is reached only by cooperative work on the information gathered by the user test. In this sense, the modification and the redesign of the technology functioning focuses not only on the system quality, tested within the assessment process, but also on enhancing the intrasystemic dialogue between users and technology. For instance, when testing a graphic interface with a sample of users, the evaluator may identify a graphic element such as a button that, although working

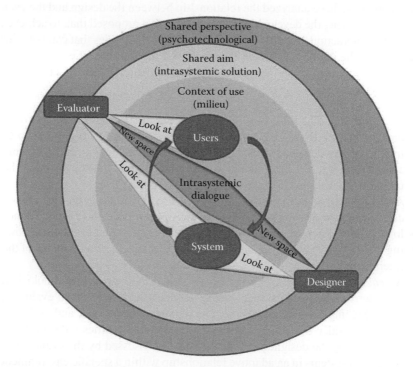

FIGURE 4.3   (See color insert.) The role of the psychotechnological perspective within the life cycle. This perspective, acting as a common theoretical space, strengthens the relationship between designer and evaluator presented in Figure 4.2. Designer and evaluator, in an equalized relationship, share the same goal, namely, enhancing the intrasystemic dialogue between technological system and user in a context of use (milieu and physical environment). In the new space (the psychotechnological one), by discussing the result of the assessment according to the psychotechnological perspective, evaluator and designer reduce the gap between the designed system and the user by focusing on the life cycle in a trade-off between the functioning *per se* and the functioning perceived by the user.

correctly, negatively affects the intrasystemic dialogue by increasing the users' cognitive workload—as in the case in which a user can hardly understand the label of a button or anticipate what will happen when it is clicked. In this case, the designer, in agreement with the evaluator, should work on redesigning the graphic element and its functioning by adapting it to the real user's mental model through a continuous and iterative consultation with the evaluators.

Within a new equalized relationship with designers, evaluators have a growing role, because they act as mediators between the user's and the developer's mental model. Regardless of the kind of design approach used by the designer, to fully accomplish the mediator role, evaluators should assess the intrasystemic dialogue in different steps, using different evaluation techniques. In this sense, the evaluators should approach the interaction assessment by an adaptable process.

4.4   CONCLUSION

In this chapter, we have analyzed the relationship between the design and the evaluation processes during the development of a product. We proposed that, to achieve the main goal of interaction "for all"—releasing psychotechnologies that can both facilitate and drive the dialogue between the users and the interface (i.e., intrasystemic solution)—the relationship between designer and evaluator should be characterized by the following aspects:

- *A shared aim*: The designers' and evaluators' goal should be not only to create a device that has a correct and particular functioning, but also to transform any designed device into a psychotechnology, an intrasystemic solution that can facilitate and drive the adaptive relationship between the user and the technological device.
- *A shared holistic perspective*: The aim to create an intrasystemic solution can be reached only by sharing a common perspective, the psychotechnological one, which acts as a bridge between designer and evaluator, allowing them to focus equally on the objective and subjective components of the interaction.
- *An equalized relationship*: The bridge created by the psychotechnological perspective equalizes the relationship between the designer and evaluator. By embracing the psychotechnological perspective, designer and evaluator do not consider device and user as two separated entities—the first one developed by the designer and the second one assessed by the evaluator—but as two systems in an adaptive relationship within a specific environment of use. Both designer and evaluator should then work together to construct and optimize the adaptive relationship between user and technology, and introduce a new step in the life cycle to discuss the objective and the subjective components that may affect the intrasystemic dialogue.

In light of our discussion, the psychotechnology construct seems to be a powerful framework because it equalizes the relationship between designer and evaluator. This framework opens a new perspective in the field of HCI that overcomes the current limitations emerging in the communication between designers and evaluators during the life cycle of a product, which consequently affect the dialogue between user and product.

In the next chapter, we shall propose an integrated methodology for the interaction evaluation that can be applied in different life cycles and stages of product development. Moving from the psychotechnological perspective, this new integrated methodology supports the equalization between the design and the evaluation process in the product's life cycle, supporting practitioners in the evaluation decision.

5 Why We Need an Integrated Model of Interaction Evaluation

5.1 EVALUATOR'S PERSPECTIVE IN THE PRODUCT LIFE CYCLE

As discussed in the previous chapter, the psychotechnological perspective creates a bridge between designers and evaluators and, in this way, equalizes the relationship between design and assessment processes by focusing on the life cycle on the intrasystemic dialogue between user and technology. In the present chapter, we define an integrated methodology of interaction evaluation (IMIE) that drives the team of evaluators (hereafter, "evaluators," or "evaluator" to refer to a part of the team) to analyze all the emergent aspects of the interaction. This can help designers to redesign the technology so that its functioning is in tune with users' needs and expectations, by following the same designers' main goals and facilitating an intrasystemic dialogue.

The model of interaction we propose only marginally concerns the developers' perspective and their role in the product life cycle, but it mainly aims to take into account all the actors involved in the evaluation process (Figure 5.1), including the users, through whom the evaluators estimate the extent to which a detected barrier is actually preventing their navigation, and the team of evaluators. In turn, the team of evaluators is composed of the following:

- The expert evaluators, who are supposed to detect those barriers that usually prevent the interaction.
- The coordinator of the evaluation (meta-evaluator), who is supposed to integrate the results coming from the "expert-based" tests with the results coming from the "user-based" tests, by performing an evaluation of the evaluation (i.e., a meta-evaluation). For example, the meta-evaluator checks which of the problems detected by the expert evaluators are real problems; that is to say, problems that can also be detected by users.

Figure 5.1 illustrates the functioning of the interaction evaluation process.

Our model of interaction assessment does not aim to provide tools for developing an adaptable system in which the user "should not think" (Krug, 2000) but, through an integrated method of usability assessment, it aims "to let the user think" during the evaluation process. As set out in Chapter 4, we can summarize our position concerning the assessment process as follows: The only way to allow

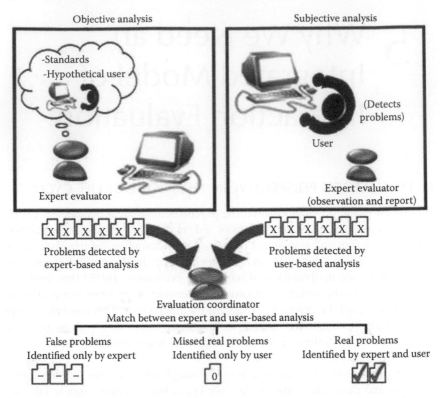

FIGURE 5.1   (See color insert.) The actors involved in the evaluation process are the expert evaluator (in the box at the top left), the user (in the box at the top right), and the evaluation coordinator (meta-evaluator, in the bottom middle). The evaluation coordinator matches the problems detected during the objective analysis with the ones detected during the subjective analysis: the first ones, which come from the analysis carried out by an expert using standards and simulations of hypothetical user's actions; the latter, which come from the analysis carried out by users under observation of an expert. This matching process (shown in the bottom of the figure) identifies three different kinds of problems: (1) false problems, which are detected only by the expert analysis; (2) missed real problems, which are problems identified by the users during the interaction that were not detected by the experts; and (3) real problems, which are problems identified by both the user-based and the expert-based analyses.

users to "do not think" during the interaction is to force users to "do think" during the evaluation. Starting with this assumption, the evaluation process, which we are going to propose, mainly focuses on the inclusion of user's needs and expectations by considering them as a part of the whole psychotechnological system and, in this way, aiming to reduce the users' adaptation to access and use technology. Therefore, since in this model users are called to judge the system they are interacting with, we shall consider the user as a "thinker" within the psychotechnological system.

Our perspective on the human–computer interaction (HCI) evaluation readapts the Krug's concept of a "self-evident" interface (see Krug, 2000) by recovering the "user's thought" as a precious and essential element in developing an affordable and usable system. This kind of evaluation model, based on user-driven evaluation process, can help evaluators analyze the overall interaction by taking into account both the subjective and the objective dimensions that are engaged in the intrasystemic dialogue.

The main goal of the IMIE model is to allow evaluators to detect all the emergent aspects of the interaction process, given that a psychotechnology can only be assessed by the observation of the dynamic and reciprocal causation among the components of the intrasystemic dialogue in the environment of use (see Chapter 4). In this kind of process, the evaluator acts as a mediator between the device and the functioning *per se* of its interface—i.e., the conceptual model of the device, as product of the designers' mental model—and the functioning perceived by the end users—i.e., the user's mental model.

Both the perspective and the model that we intend to propose should be considered as a new synthesis of the HCI field—a synthesis that equalizes, integrates, and distinguishes both the evaluator's and the designer's perspectives on the evaluation process. According to our model, the evaluator should act as the medium of the users' thought (Figure 5.1), by promoting their needs and expectations about the system in an independent, adaptable, and multidimensional evaluation process.

In the next sections, we introduce our model by analyzing two main theoretical issues belonging to the interaction evaluation process: (1) the objectivity and the subjectivity of the measurements and (2) the difference between problems and errors in the intrasystemic dialogue between the designed and the cognitive systems.

5.2   OBJECTIVITY AND SUBJECTIVITY IN INTERACTION: WHEN THE SYSTEM OVERRIDES THE USER

One of the most discussed topics in the HCI literature regards the nature of usability evaluation. This debate points out a dichotomy between objective and subjective measurements: The first ones are considered as quantitative measurement of the user's performance (e.g., task analysis, error analysis, training needs analysis, etc.), whereas the latter ones are considered as a qualitative measurement of an interactive experience (e.g., workload measurement, usability and satisfaction questionnaires, etc.). As John Annett (2002b) claims, this dichotomy is far to be so radical, since subjective measurements can vary according to the "degree of shared meaning" (i.e., the collection of the constructs, tools, and conditions shared by the evaluators). For instance, when two evaluators measure the users' workload during the interaction with two different interfaces, they share the same construct of cognitive workload; a set of measurements, such as the NASA-TLX (Hart and Staveland, 1988); and the administration rules of these measurements. In this case, between the two evaluators, there is a high "degree of shared meaning," and the results of their analysis can be easily compared. Therefore, when the evaluators' community strongly shares a certain set of constructs and subjective measurements (i.e., "meanings"), the evaluators can assign a certain degree of objectiveness to these subjective methods. Although a total agreement rarely happens, when two evaluators analyze the same object in the same conditions and through the same tools, they may also agree to consider their subjective data as an objective "fact":

> In practice, two observers may make their measurements with slightly different instruments, or under slightly different conditions or just at different times. This is normal in science and the process of verification and falsification therefore depends on agreement concerning the *acceptable extent of disagreement* between different observations, known as *experimental error*. (Annett, 2002b, p. 968 [italics in original])

Moreover, given that the evaluator's subjectivity is always involved in the evaluation process, even the most objective measurements have indeed to be considered as influenced by a certain degree of subjectivity (Annett, 2002a,b; Baber, 2002; Drury, 2002; Hancock et al., 2002; Kirakowski, 2002; McKenna, 2002; Stanton and Stammers, 2002). Therefore, although subjectivity seems to be an unavoidable element in the evaluation process, the objectivity of data can only be granted by a shared and reliable form of methodology necessary to individuate the subjective influences emerging in the evaluation process (Annett, 2002b; Michell, 2002). Therefore, subjective measurements have to be considered as an essential part of the evaluation when the dimensions (cognitive workload, degree of stress, motivation, satisfaction, preferences, performance, comfort, and usability) directly related to the user interaction are analyzed by the evaluator (Salvendy, 2002).

In the HCI literature, the distinction between objective and the subjective measurements moves away from the idea that the analyzed technology has to be considered as an "object," which also exists outside the interaction process. Similarly, the user has to be considered as a "subject" who exists independently of his or her interaction with the technology. Therefore, if a subject and an object can exist independently of each other, it should be possible to consider the interaction process as the product of two separate entities, whose proprieties can be separately measured in a reliable way. From this perspective, the properties of the object can be measured by analyzing its accessibility level (i.e., the environmental characteristics of entrance/exit movements), whereas the subject's properties (i.e., the cognitive and physical aspects of the individual differences) can be quantitatively defined by investigating its degree of usability (Federici et al., 2005). Moreover, given that the subject and the object—and the measures of their properties—exist independently of each other, it should be possible to obtain an absolute measure of both accessibility and usability.

By following a distinction between two "subjective–objective" opposite poles, the artifact would be the only component actually measured, while the evaluator's commitment would be solely concerned with the observation of the ability of the system to perform the task for which it has been designed when a specific user utilizes it. Therefore, an absolute objective measure can only describe the interface design (i.e., the objective dimension of the interaction, or, in other words, the technology), whereas an absolute subjective measure can only describe the designed functions of the interface (i.e., all its graphical elements) when it is used by the user, with his or her specific cognitive and physical functioning (i.e., the user's behavior in the system). In both cases, the goal of the evaluation is to analyze the structural and functional dimensions of the technology, whereas what really needs to be evaluated, namely, the intrasystemic interaction between user and psychotechnology, is left out (Federici et al., 2005). This perspective is strictly related to a small usability definition (Kurosu, 2007) and defines both the objective and the subjective dimensions of the interaction only by measuring the functioning of the artifact. As a consequence, the subjective dimension is ultimately defined by objective one: Once the functionality of the artifact is improved, any user (independent of his or her skills and goals) should be more satisfied with the system.

In conclusion, according to this perspective, since the objective measure matches with the number of errors found in the technological functioning, the less number of errors are identified in the object functioning, the better (any) user will evaluate the interaction. This scenario clearly shows why the small usability approach tends to discard the users' involvement in the evaluation process: In fact, by improving the interface, the usability of the system should improve as well, independent of the specific skills and goals of users.

As discussed in Chapter 4, our perspective is far from that the small usability one. In order to take into account all the components of the interaction, we propose that evaluators, as well as designers, should share a new perspective—the psychotechnological one—that goes beyond the above-described dualistic point of view on the interaction system. In fact, a psychotechnology is more than the sum of its objective and subjective components, but it emerges from the relationship between the entire interaction between the objective and the subjective components—the objective components regarding the technological object and its functioning, the subjective components regarding the user and his or her subjective experience of the functioning of technology, the environment of use, and the role of this context on the dynamics of the interaction. In light of this, as we discuss in the next section, the evaluator has to observe the subjective, objective, and contextual components of the interaction in different moments, aiming to measure both the objective and the subjective features of the interaction and, at the same time, also the emergent properties of their relationship, in the form of an intrasystemic dialogue.

5.2.1 BRIDGE BETWEEN OBJECT AND SUBJECT: THE INTEGRATED MODEL OF EVALUATION

As discussed in Chapter 2, accessibility, usability, and user experience (UX) are the three dimensions of the interaction defining the qualitative and quantitative aspects that are necessary to design, judge, assess, measure, and implement both the psychotechnological system and the user's interaction. To assess accessibility, usability, and UX, ISO (see Chapter 2) suggests that the evaluator cannot consider object and subject as two separated entities, since measuring a single dimension of the interaction (e.g., the objective one) is not enough to evaluate the multidimensional properties of the interaction.

In fact, as the "big usability" approach promoted by Kurosu (2007) suggests (see Chapter 2), for analyzing all the different dimensions comprising the interaction, the evaluator should consider the goals that the designed functions of the object are supposed to achieve, along with the analysis of the psychotechnological functioning.

However, given that a product works only in relation to the technological goals for which it has been created, an absolute measure to define the properties of the object will never be possible. For instance, the functioning and the characteristics of a fishing rod will be different whether it is designed for deep sea or for river fishing. The designer can develop these two rods only by simulating the characteristics, required for improving the fisher performances in the specific context of use (sea or river), on the basis of a set of rules and constraints (i.e., guidelines and principles). The rules contain the standard features required for the fishing rods, their possible scenarios of use, and a general representation of the fisher's mental model. The designer can apply these rules to create a fishing rod with a specific set of standard features by simulating at the same time the mental model of the users, e.g., by creating a profile of its hypothetical kind of fishers (i.e., personas) to design a product that shall be accessible for them. Concurrently, after the product has been developed, the evaluator can use these rules for assessing the conformance of the fishing rods to their specific features and to the personas created by the developer, measuring how much the fishing rod will be accessible for fishers by following an objective perspective.

Out of our example, what we aim to underline here is that even the most objective measurement of interaction with a product, such as the conformance analysis, ultimately implies a certain degree of subjectivity. Thus, neither accessibility nor usability can be measured by totally excluding the subjective components of their measures.

As discussed in Chapters 1 and 2, in HCI, there are many different national and international guidelines on accessibility (e.g., WCAG, Section 508) and on the principle of usability (e.g., Bruce Tognazzi, principal at the Nielsen Norman Group for design principles, see http://www.asktog.com/basics/firstPrinciples.html). All these kinds of rules have been created according to a model of possible user that, of course, introduces a subjective dimension into the objective measures of the system. Moreover, the model of possible users is far from stable and immutable. On the contrary, it is historically determined and changes according to the context of use (workplace, home, entertainment, sports, rehabilitation, communication, etc.). In this way, compliance to a standard rule of an evaluation technique has always to be considered as conforming to a certain model of possible user–technology interaction.

As ISO 9241-11 (1998) definition states, the usability dimensions can only be measured in relation to the goals that the user needs to achieve. The mutual relationship between the subjective and the objective dimensions in the interaction system becomes particularly clear when we take into account an evaluation of the users' satisfaction about the interaction with psychotechnology. In such a case, users may be satisfied during a process that leads them to achieve their goals by using the functions provided by the system. In other words, the users' satisfaction depends not only on the achievement of their goals but also on the process of using the psychotechnology that has been experienced when achieving those goals. Even though psychotechnology can induce new goals and needs to users, it is also true that an unsatisfactory evaluation of the interaction with a technology would most likely determine a modification only in the technology and not in the users. Of course, as already described in Chapter 3, a psychotechnological system can emulate, extend, amplify, or modify (Federici et al., 2011; Miesenberger et al., 2012) the users' mind because, during the interaction, users constantly learn specific actions and behaviors and, at the same time, receive feedback from the technological interface. Moreover, the evaluation of a psychotechnological system should not aim to change the user's way of interacting, but just verifying the functionality of the system in relation to the users' needs and goals in a certain historical and environmental contexts. In this way, subjective and objective categories are not to be considered as alternatives; indeed, they need to be understood as different steps of and methodological perspectives for an evaluation process in which a complete objectivity as well as a complete subjectivity limits cases of theoretic interest only. As Federici et al. (2005) state, when objective and subjective elements are referred to accessibility and usability in a user–technology interaction, they cannot be considered as separate entities, but as two different moments that can be included in the continuum of empirical observation:

> Accessibility and usability do not refer to the objective and subjective factors of the user/technology rapport, but rather to a bidirectional way of observing the interaction. In effect, this represents two prospective points from which the one and only observed reality of the user/technology system is drawn. Accessibility of an environment is therefore defined based on how it allows the user to initiate and terminate the operation that completes the machine's task (*functioning construct*) while its usability is based on the user's perception of the user/technology interaction (*user performance*). The functioning construct of a machine is the basis for standard rules, (e.g., *Web Content Accessibility Guidelines 1.0* (W3C-WAI2008)) against which accessibility levels are controlled and assessed. The *user performance* in relation to *functioning construct* of a machine allows us to deduce scales (e.g., efficiency, satisfaction, cognitive load, helpfulness) of usability scores. (Federici et al., 2005, p. 782 [italics in original])

Federici et al. (2005) define this perspective as an "integrated model" of evaluation. This model tries to overcome the objective–subjective dichotomy by defining the interaction process as an intrasystemic dialogue between two main characters— the interface and the user. The evaluation of this dialogue includes different stages during which both the objective and the subjective dimensions of the psychotechnological interaction are taken into account. In this sense, the integrated model of evaluation is able to investigate not only the properties of a single dimension but also the relations that bound the objective part of the interaction to the subjective one (and vice versa). In this context, accessibility and usability are considered as the necessary steps needed for improving the dialogue between the interface and the users (Figure 5.2).

Therefore, we consider the objective- and subjective-oriented evaluation as two necessary horizons/stages of observation that can help evaluators analyze accessibility and usability from the objective and subjective points of view respectively. The outcomes of these two points of observation are necessary to clarify the properties of the intrasystemic relationship between user and technology and, at the same time, can allow evaluators to analyze the emergent properties of the psychotechnological system in its specific context of use.

The evaluator assesses both system and user from two horizons/stages of observation (objective and subjective). At the objective stage, the evaluator uses his or her

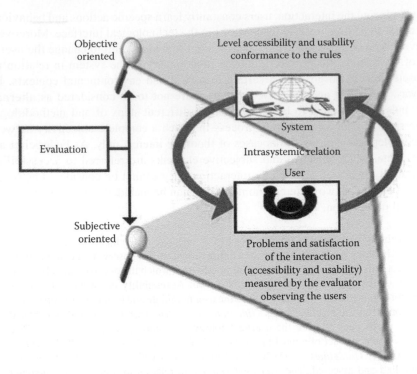

Objective oriented

Level accessibility and usability conformance to the rules

System

Evaluation

Intrasystemic relation

User

Subjective oriented

Problems and satisfaction of the interaction (accessibility and usability) measured by the evaluator observing the users

FIGURE 5.2   (See color insert.) The "integrated model" of evaluation. (From Federici, S. and Borsci, S., Usability evaluation: Models, methods, and applications, in Stone, J. and Blouin, M. (Eds.), *International Encyclopedia of Rehabilitation*, Center for International Rehabilitation Research Information and Exchange (CIRRIE), Buffalo, NY, pp. 1–17, 2010, retrieved from http://cirrie.buffalo.edu/encyclopedia/article.php?id=277&language=en; Federici, S. et al., *Disabil. Rehabil.*, 27(13), 781, 2005)

mental model, by endorsing the accessibility and the usability rules and methods, in order to analyze system's properties. In the subjective stage, the evaluator, by observing the user's interaction, analyzes the interaction problems experienced by the user and his or her level of satisfaction. The outcomes of these two horizons/ stages of observation are used by the evaluator in order to describe, analyze, and report to designers on the intrasystemic relationship between system and user in its context of use.

Moreover, since the focus of the evaluation cannot be merely reduced to either the system or the user, what should be evaluated is the functionality of the intrasystemic dialogue between the user (i.e., the subjective dimension of the interaction) and the interface (i.e., the objective dimension of the interaction) by also considering the context of use. The accessibility and the usability estimations thus need to be understood as the measurements of the users' possibilities of achieving their goals by navigating a given interface within a given psychotechnological environment.

The evaluation of the intrasystemic relation between the user and the psychotechnology includes object-oriented methods as well as subject-oriented ones.

An overall evaluation cannot be achieved merely by the simple addition of results derived from the two different methods.

In this model, when an evaluator observes the system, he or she analyzes what the designers have developed (i.e., the object) from their mental model by simulating the end user's interaction. As we discuss in the next section, the designers' simulation is also driven by accessibility and usability rules and principles. In light of this, when observing the object, the evaluator assesses the conformance of the system functioning—as it is designed by the developers—to the standards of accessibility and to usability principles. On the other hand, when an evaluator observes the end users, he or she analyzes how they experience the interaction with the technology, by measuring the accessibility and usability of the system's functioning as is perceived by the users.

As proposed in Chapter 3, as an external point of view, the evaluator should assess the components of the intrasystemic dialogue by considering that the relationship between user and technology tends to add a certain degree of complexity to these two subcomponents. In light of this, the psychotechnology has to be considered as an emergent phenomenon of the intrasystemic dialogue and, according to the additional attribution phenomena proposed by the Gestalt theory, as being more than the mere sum of its components (Koffka, 1935, p. 176). Therefore, during the assessment process, an evaluator should ever assume that the properties of the sum of the components belonging to the user–technology relationship are different and more complex than the sum of the properties of each of its component. By following an emergentist approach, we can consider that the properties emerging from the user–technology interaction can only be observed within the relation system between the two actors, whereas, if the user and the system are considered in a separate way, it will never be possible to observe the properties of their relations (i.e., the interaction). Theoretically, even though the evaluation process includes multidimensional models of evaluation (which are both subjective and objective), the properties of the observed interaction could also emerge from the results obtained by a single model of evaluation that focuses only on one of the two components. According to this hypothesis, when applying a one-dimensional model, evaluators should be able to analyze the properties of the overall interaction either from an objective or from a subjective perspective (i.e., methodology), in accordance with the dimension that they chose to endorse.

In the integrated model, then, the user–technology relationship (i.e., the intrasystemic dialogue) is the focus of the evaluation, even though this evaluation can be pursued by applying either an object-oriented procedure or a subject-oriented one. Anyway, the possibility to evaluate all the properties of the interaction from a single point of view is to be considered as a theoretical extreme that cannot have a real application. In fact, as previously stated, according to the integrated model, the evaluation of the intrasystemic relation cannot be obtained by a simple addition of the data coming from the objective procedures with the ones coming from the subjective procedures. Therefore, the interactive artifact has to be considered as an objective component of the interaction, but this objective component cannot be evaluated as psychotechnology without considering the user or, at least, a model of possible users.

Since the object cannot be evaluated *per se*, as long as it always falls out of the human experience (Olivetti Belardinelli, 1973), the evaluation process can only take into account what the object allows the user to do. In other words, the object can only be evaluated in relation to the subject and, more specifically, in relation to the meaning that it assumes from the user's point of view (Galimberti, 2002). A technology, in fact, does not have goals; it has only functions. In the same way, in order to evaluate the interaction with the user, the observation should focus on the functions of the object, which represent the technological properties of the psychotechnology. Usually, the functions of technology are designed and implemented by following both specific guidelines and design principles for accessibility and usability; in turn, these general standard lines are based on specific models that try to describe and predict the actions and the goals that a hypothetical user could achieve in the designed interface. Following this perspective, any accessibility or usability error should be considered as being an error in the design or in the implementation of the functions of the object. As Norman (1988) states, an error in the interface is always a "human error" because it depends on an error in the design process. Even when the evaluator detects an error during an objective-oriented analysis, the cause of the error should always be sought in a certain action performed by the designer during the implementation of the interface. During the interaction process, users do not detect an error *per se*; they can only detect those problems that prevent them from performing certain actions in the system. Evaluators, then, observe these kinds of interactive problems during the subjective-oriented analysis.

As Federici and Borsci (2010) suggest, we can distinguish between an error in the interface and a problem occurring during the interaction evaluation as follows:

> Users can only experience problems and not errors: errors are due to bad design or bad implementation of the system, while problems are related to the user's experience of interaction. According to most users, a system does not function when it does not respond properly to their commands. For example, a broken link in the interface would always be experienced by the user as a problem, independent of the fact that the broken link depends on an error in the script (a wrong address or a page that no longer exists) or an error in the pointing procedure of the user (who believes they have clicked the link while actually clicking the background). Even if such errors do exist, they usually remain hidden to the user, who experiences only the "problem" they actually cause. (Federici and Borsci, 2010, p. 5)

In light of this, while an error concerns any kind of barrier appearing in the functionality of the system—even though it is mostly due to a human error occurred during the design process—a problem concerns any difficulty encountered by users during the interaction with the system; whereas a problem in the interaction can be due both to a machine error (e.g., when a link in the interface does not lead to any information) and to an human error (e.g., when a user inserts a wrong password or ID in the field). In the next sections, we explain in depth the difference between errors and problems within the evaluation process.

5.3   PROBLEMS AND ERRORS IN THE EVALUATION

In the interaction design, two main kinds of errors could affect the dialogue between user and system—machine error and the human error (for a complete review on errors, see Norman, 1983, 1988). Machine error refers to an objective error in the programming of (or the code of) the interface. This kind of error can be detected and then corrected by a redesign of the elements of the layout. As the Human Reliability Analysis research field suggests (Swain and Guttmann, 1980), human error is related to the user's actions in the interface and to his or her strategies of problem solving. To solve a human error, the rearrangement of the objective elements of the layout it is not enough, but it is also necessary to rethink all the information architecture that can reduce the possibilities of erroneous behavior.

We do not aim to discuss all the possible kinds of both machine and human errors, but nevertheless we would like to underline that, while the design perspective considers only the "errors," which cause problems that may affect the intrasystemic dialogue, the evaluation perspective focuses only on the "problems" that affect the interaction. Therefore, we should consider that the general goal for the evaluation of the interaction is the identification of a problem, independent of the comprehension of the error causing it.

While many different research fields, such as engineering, ergonomics, and cognitive psychology, have tried to define exactly what an error is and to discriminate between the cause of errors (Norman, 1983), with the aim of improving the design of the system, the international literature about the subjective and objective measurements (see Hvannberg et al., 2007) has never provided a proper definition of "interaction problem." Due to this lack of a unique definition of an interaction problem, there is no clear distinction between problem and error, and the term "problem" seems to be only a label used by the evaluators to indicate an error during the interaction. Nevertheless, in order to assess the interaction by specific kind of methods (such as heuristic analysis, cognitive walkthrough, and task analysis), evaluators usually adopt an empirical classification of usability problems to indicate their severity. As Nielsen claims:

> Severity ratings can be used to allocate the most resources to fix the most serious problems and can also provide a rough estimate of the need for additional usability efforts. If the severity ratings indicate that several disastrous usability problems remain in an interface, it will probably be unadvisable to release it. But one might decide to go ahead with the release of a system with several usability problems if they are all judged as being cosmetic in nature. (1995a)

The severity of a usability problem is a combination of three factors: the frequency with which the problem occurs ("is it common or rare?"), the impact of the problem if it occurs ("will it be easy or difficult for user to overcome?"), and, finally, the persistence of the problem ("is it a one-time problem that users can overcome once they know about it, or will users repeatedly be bothered by the problem?"). Even though severity has several components, it is common to combine all aspects of severity into a single severity rating to achieve an overall assessment of each usability problem to facilitate prioritizing and decision making. Although the evaluators can rate the severity of the problems experienced by users, there is not a distinct theoretical line between problems and errors in the interaction.

As quoted earlier, Federici and Borsci underline that "users can only experience problems and not errors. [...] According to most users, a system does not function when it does not respond properly to their commands" (2010, p. 5). Therefore, a real problem of interaction from the evaluator's point of view can be identified only by a user test. During an evaluation, independent of whether the error that causes the problem is due to a machine or a human error, the problem exists only when a user identifies it: We call these real problems of interaction.

Of course, the machine errors (e.g., errors in the code) exist independent of whether users identify them or not. However, when users cannot experience machine errors, from the evaluators' point of view, they have to be considered as only pertaining to the object (i.e., functioning *per se*) without a direct effect on the intrasystemic dialogue. Therefore, the evaluator can report to the developer that in the interface there are some machine errors that are not experienced by users as a problem. We call these false problems of interaction. Although these kinds of machine errors do not generate real problems, the designer, on the basis of the evaluator's report, should solve them independent of whether they affect (i.e., real problem) or do not affect (i.e., false problems) the interaction. In fact, since users rarely perceive these false problems during the interaction (e.g., link with low visibility, partial unclear labeling, small buttons, etc.), these problems can affect the performance of the technology and the overall UX over time.

Furthermore, during the evaluation process, it could be that some problems unexpectedly affect the user's interaction. This is the case with missed real problems (Hvannberg et al., 2007). In this situation, while evaluators do not detect these problems during their expert analysis, the real user experiences them as well.

Even though we do not want to underestimate the influence of errors in altering the communication flow, we aim to underline that, from the evaluator's point of view, the problems have to be included in a theoretical model that encompasses both human and machine errors as variables in the interactive process for discriminating among real, missed real, and false problems of interaction. This model would not focus on the error *per se*, but it would only consider when and how error influences the communication between user and technology. In fact, it is not up to the evaluation to identify what kind of error may compromise the interaction; this task belongs to the system developers. Considering the problems reported by the evaluator, the developers should identify the kind of errors generating those interaction problems and, then, they should try to fix them by a partial or complete redesigning of the interface.

In summary, we can define a problem as an interruption of the intrasystemic dialogue that is perceived by the user. By moving away from this definition, we can strongly discriminate between errors and problems from the evaluators' point of view as (1) an error concerning the functionality of the system differently or as (2) a problem concerning any difficulty encountered by the user.

1. *Error concerning the functionality of the system (i.e., the design)*. This may be or may not be experienced as a problem by the user. For example, in a website, a link that does not work has to be considered to be a machine error. Nevertheless, it may be that, in a test with a large sample of users,

nobody clicks on the wrong link. In that case, even though the error exists and has to be removed by the designers, the error does not cause an interaction problem (i.e., false problem).

2. *Problem concerning any difficulty encountered by user during the interaction with the system (i.e., the evaluation).* A problem can be classified as
   a. A real problem, which is a problem identified by both the user and the evaluator analysis
   b. A false problem, which is detected only by the evaluator analysis
   c. A missed real problem, which is a problem identified by users during the interaction that is not detected by the evaluator

This distinction between errors and problems, together with the theoretical perspective of the integrated model of evaluation, will allow us to propose and discuss an integrate methodology of evaluation in the next section, in which (1) the role played by designer and evaluator during a product life cycle is clearly defined, marking their perspectives and drawing a clear border between their actions; (2) the evaluation process is strongly linked to a design model; and (3) the objective and subjective measures are integrated in the evaluation process.

5.3.1 PROBLEMS AND ERRORS: FROM THE INTEGRATED MODEL TO THE INTEGRATED METHODOLOGY

The dialogue between the two subsystems (user and technology) comprising the psychotechnological interaction involves two different mental models: the user's mental model, which determines the user's performance, and the mental model that the designer forms according to the conceptual model of the interface, which corresponds to the functioning constructs of the machine. The concept of mental model has been first proposed in the 1940s by the philosopher Kenneth James Williams Craik (1943), and in the 1950s it was introduced to the HCI field by Norman (Norman, 1983; Norman and Draper, 1986). Norman defines a mental model as a system causality conveyance that is created by the user to reason about the system, anticipate its behavior, and explain why it reacts as it does. At the same time, the designers create their own mental model for defining the system functioning (the conceptual model of the system) to simulate how the user will perceive it on the basis of the accessibility and the usability rules and principles. This is an attempt to clarify how the dialogue between user and technology in the interaction process is based on both the users' and the designers' mental models.

In order to be in tune with the psychotechnological perspective—which considers that the evaluation cannot be only focused on the features of technology and the experience of user, but also on their relationship during interaction—the concept of a mental model has to be considered as a key issue in understanding how an evaluator can measure the intrasystemic dialogue.

In fact, the interaction, as previously defined, cannot be understood simply as an objective or a subjective process. Such interaction is actually structured by the distance that separates the mental model of the designer, who creates and implements the interface, and the mental model of the user, who interacts with the interface. In other words, we may say that, being the technology represented by the designer's mental model, and being the user's perception of the functioning of the technology represented by his or her mental model, their relationship can be measured in terms of the distance between these two mental models. In fact, from a theoretical point of view, when the designer's and user's mental models perfectly match (i.e., their distance is equal to zero), the interaction dialogue between user and technology will be effective, efficient, and satisfactory. In this case, we have thus exemplified an ideal psychotechnology, which does not have any problem in interaction with all the emergent properties of the intrasystemic dialogue, which are immediately clear to the end user. Unfortunately, this "perfect" intrasystemic solution is unreachable, unless the designer of the technology is also its end user. In the real world, there is always a distance between a designed functioning technology (the designer's mental model) and the functioning of the product perceived by the end user (the user's mental model). In light of this, this evaluation should be considered as the only means for measuring this distance, and for reducing it, in order to transform a product in terms of psychotechnology.

According to the integrated model of evaluation, the evaluators—on the basis of their assessment expertise; the international standards of accessibility; the principles of usability; and the methods, tools, and techniques of evaluation (i.e., the evaluator mental model)—should not only identify the errors in the interface, but also identify the problems in interaction perceived by the users, in order to define the quality of the intrasystemic dialogue in this way, and the distance between the designer's and user's mental models. In light of this, we can say that the interaction problem can be considered as a unit of measure to assess distance in the intrasystemic dialogue. Of course, when observing the end users' interaction and measuring the distance between the interaction components, the evaluators' ability in identifying the interaction problems depends on their mental model (i.e., their assessment experiences, the tools and techniques they choose to apply for assessing the interaction, and the standards or principles they use as references for observing interaction).

Only the user can detect an interaction problem during the interaction, and this problem can be related either to errors in the architecture of the interaction (object errors) or to errors coming from the users' subjective experience in relation to their goals (subject errors).

During the evaluation process, the evaluator assumes that there will always be a certain distance separating the designer's mental model from the user's one (unless the designer and the user are the same person). Therefore, the evaluator needs to take into account the errors concerning the object (i.e., a machine error that the user does not experience as a problem during the interaction) as well as the problems due to objective or subjective errors identified by the analysis of the user's interaction (i.e., real and missed problems). As Federici et al. (2005) pointed out, in order to integrate subjective and objective elements in a single model of accessibility and usability evaluation, we should consider these elements as different moments belonging to the same continuum of experience. To do so, it is therefore necessary to redefine the rules and the methodology for collecting both the objective and the subjective data. In fact, the integrated model of evaluation does offer a theoretical perspective on the evaluation process that only concerns the evaluators' actions (i.e., the objective- and subjective-oriented evaluation). We can use this model for proposing an adaptable evaluation methodology by connecting the integrated model of evaluation to some of the most common models of designs. We call this model the IMIE.

Since it follows the integrated model (Federici et al., 2005), the IMIE model does not focus just on error prediction but also on the real problems found by users during real interaction with a system. As such, the distinction between the objective and the subjective concerns the point of view from which to observe the interaction, and the distinction between error and problem concerns only the evaluators' perspective and the method applied for describing the interaction.

By using the standard guidelines for assessing accessibility and usability, the evaluators can identify errors in the object, and this identification is needed in order to solve problems in the interaction: Once errors have been detected, the designer can proceed by modifying the object. On the other hand, the problems, which concern only the difficulties that users encounter during the interaction, can be detected by behavioral measurements (e.g., questionnaires, verbal protocols, task analysis, etc.).

During the evaluation process, the evaluator assumes that there will always be a certain distance separating the designer's mental model from the user's (unless the designer and the user are the same). Evaluators can measure this distance by using a multiple set of evaluation techniques and by relying on their experience, skills, and the accessibility and the usability standards and principles that make up their mental model. During the assessment, the evaluator aims to gather both the problems experienced by the users (i.e., real and missed real) and the false problems identified through expert analysis of the system, thus measuring the gap between the real user and the conceptual model of the system.

In conclusion, under the perspective of the integrated model of evaluation, the assessment becomes a process centered on the analysis of the interaction, which should be considered as a whole and not as a mere measurement of the object. Therefore, the evaluation goal should no longer be considered as a way to identify not only errors, but also problems in interaction.

The interaction evaluation process we are proposing reverses the engineering perspective: In our model, in fact, the error (both objective and subjective) is considered to be a part of the problem, and, therefore, aims at identifying problems rather than only the errors that cause them.

5.4   DISCRIMINATION AND MATCHING OF PROBLEMS AND ERRORS: THE INTEGRATED METHODOLOGY OF INTERACTION EVALUATION

In this section, we shall propose the IMIE, an adaptive set of methods, relying on the Federici's model (2005), which can work together with different design processes. According to this model, the evaluation process and the design process should share a common main goal: To release interfaces for all in a pervasive interaction environment that can be used as a tool for distributing the human cognition. Given this, evaluation and design should be considered as parallel processes that define and redefine the interaction features of a technology by analyzing the product functioning and how real users experience the interaction with its interface. By starting from this perspective, which equalizes the design and the evaluation processes, in this section we define the theoretical assumptions and models and the practical process comprising our integrated methodology.

In particular, we describe the IMIE model under the lens of a theoretical perspective on interaction that is focused on

- Discriminating between problems and errors in interaction by (1) defining what an interaction problem is and, at the same time and (2) taking into account the role played by errors in interaction
- Selecting evaluation methods by considering the context and the environment and, at the same time, matching the objective and subjective measures, in order to rethink the technology as an interface for all

While the discrimination between problems and errors is a theoretical issue that can be solved only by identifying a model of HCI that can be applied from the evaluation point of view, the selection and the matching of the methods are practical issues that are linked to the evaluation variables and to the evaluator's decision process.

In the following sections, we present the IMIE model by discussing the decision process of the evaluator in the interaction assessment.

5.4.1 FROM THE CONCEPT OF MENTAL MODEL TO THE INTEGRATED METHODOLOGY OF INTERACTION EVALUATION

To define the components of the IMIE model, we refer to one of the most important models of interface design and, then, to the theoretical perspectives beyond it: the UCD model. As discussed in Chapter 1, the UCD is a model that is able to take into account people's needs and abilities to optimize the interface rather than forcing users to adapt themselves to an interface strictly dependent on the developers' model.

By proposing the UCD model (Norman, 1983, 1988; Norman and Draper, 1986), Norman identifies three elements that could be involved in an interaction, i.e., two mental models and a conceptual model of the system (Figure 5.3). According to the author, there are two mental models involved in the process when the user has an interaction with a system or a technology (image of system): The first one is the designer's model, which describes how a system is designed and implemented; the second one is the user's mental model (how a user thinks the system works), which is build up through the interaction with the interface. In other words, the designer objectifies his mental model in the conceptual model (i.e., the information architecture). The information architecture of the object (i.e., the interface) becomes, then, the only means of communication between the designer's model and the user's model.

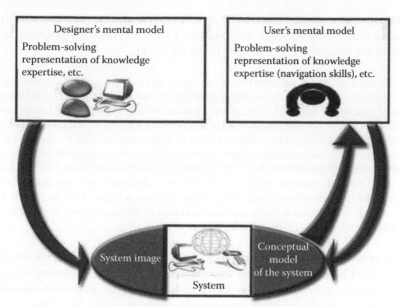

FIGURE 5.3   (See color insert.) The designer's mental model is used by developers to create a technology (i.e., a system) and its functioning (i.e., the system image and its conceptual model visible to the end user) by simulating the user's mental model. The designers can only talk to the user through the "system image." The user, interacting with the technology and its functioning, uses his or her mental model in order to understand how the system works and reacts to the input, thus creating an interpretation of the conceptual model of the system. In light of this, the system image is, like a text, open to interpretation. The users' interpretations depend on their adaptation to the conceptual model of the system. (Adapted from Norman, D.A., *The Psychology of Everyday Things*, Basic Books, New York, 1988.)

The definition and the use of the mental models involved in the interaction process is an open research question. Indeed, in the HCI field, there are many definitions and considerations related to mental models (Craik, 1943; Johnson-Laird, 1989; Legrenzi and Girotto, 1996). As discussed earlier, we endorse the Norman's perspective, which defines the mental models as those models used (1) to reason about a system, (2) to anticipate system behavior, and (3) to explain why a system reacts as it does. During the interaction with a particular technology, a user relies on his or her expertise by applying specific cognitive processes for problem solving and representation of knowledge. According to the Norman's definition (1988), a mental model is a user's cognitive representation of the system and represents the cognitive frame of the system interface. Therefore, a mental model acts as a medium for the user's interaction. In this sense, a higher degree of expertise is therefore related to a more functional, or rather more adaptable, mental model in interaction with the technology.

Nevertheless, although the UCD model defines the specific role played by the image of the system and the user's and developer's models within the interaction system, there is still some confusion concerning the definition of the function that mental models play within the interaction process. In fact, different perspectives consider the different mental proposed by the Norman's model as entities that are other from the system functioning (Gentner and Nielsen, 1996). As Andersen proposes in his analysis of the role played by semiotics in the HCI field,

> the important difference between *the system model* and *the user's model* signifies two interpretations of the same sign-complex produced by two groups that access different parts of it (designer and user). The *system image* is the collection of signs interpreted by the user. The *direct manipulation style* can be defined by the domination of iconic signs based on similarity. The technical notion of a *view* (e.g., in database design) corresponds neatly to the pragmatic notion of *perspective*, the way organizational or geographical position determines the selection and structuring of interpretation. The fact that users normally interpret systems differently than designers do is predicted from the fact that interpretation of signs always happens inside a larger semiotic system. If two semiotic systems are different, the interpretation of the same sign will differ too. (Andersen, 2001, p. 420 [italics in original])

Both the system and the code comprising the physical interface (i.e., the image of system) cannot be simply identified with the mental model of designers, since the image of a system is a product of the designer's mental model. Andersen's idea highlights the role of the distance that separates the user's interpretation of the image of the system and the designer's. However, the system cannot be considered as being simply "a collection of signs interpreted by the user": First, it has been created on the basis of a conceptual model composed of a collection of signs originally organized in an interface, by following the directions coming from the designers' mental models. Therefore, from an evaluation perspective, the distance between the user's and designer's interpretations of the image of the system is also the distance between their two different mental models: These models, in fact, already contain the competences, abilities, and knowledge that are necessary to grant the interpretation of the signs conveyed through the interface. In this sense, the user's mental model integrates also his or her navigation skills, and, in turn, these skills become an important means for the user to widen that same mental model (i.e., more knowledge, more adaptability). At the same time, the designer's mental model should integrate also his or her knowledge of design standards as well as his or her knowledge of the user's possible behavior when interacting with the interface.

For the UCD model, the evaluation process should follow the decision cycle model (DCM) proposed by Huthcins et al. (1985), which considers the interaction as a communication flow. This model describes and separates three main components of the interaction: the designer's mental model, the user's mental model, and the image of systems.

The central idea of the DCM can be described as follows:

> To get something done, you have to start with some notion of what is wanted—the goal that is to be achieved. Then, you have to do something to the world, that is, take action to move yourself or manipulate someone or something. Finally, you check to see that your goal was made. So there are four different things to consider: the goal, what is done to the world, the world itself, and the check of the world. The action itself has two major aspects: doing something and checking. Call these *execution* and *evaluation*. (Norman, 1988, p. 46 [italics in original])

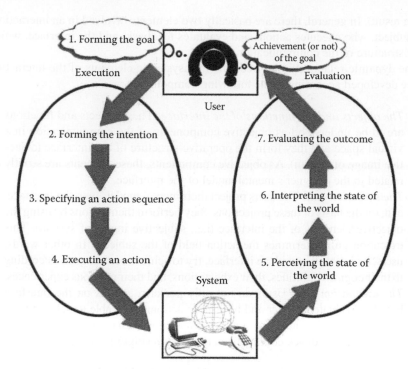

FIGURE 5.4   (See color insert.) Decision cycle model. (Adapted from Hutchins, E.L. et al., *Hum.–Comput. Interact.*, 1(4), 311, 1985)

The DCM is composed of seven steps (Figure 5.4): The first one belongs completely to the individual's subjectivity, while the other six concern the interaction between the individual and the world and are divided into what Norman and colleagues (Hutchins et al., 1985; Norman, 1988) call the "execution gulf" and the "evaluation gulf":

1. *Forming the goal*: Something to be achieved.
   a.   Execution gulf
2. *Forming the intention*: Goals must be transformed into intentions.
3. *Specifying an action sequence*: What is to be done to the world. The precise sequence of operators that must be performed to affect the intention.
4. *Executing an action*: Actually doing something. Putting the action sequence into effect on the world.
   b.   Evaluation gulf
5. *Perceiving the state of the world*: Perceiving what has actually happened.
6. *Interpreting the state of the world*: Trying to make sense of the perceptions available.
7. *Evaluating the outcome*: Comparing what happened with what was wanted.

An important implicit assumption of the DCM (Figure 5.4) is that the interface structure should be accessible for the users interacting with it, both during the execution (i.e., doing something) and during the evaluation phases (i.e., checking the action result). In general, there are basically two elements involved in an interaction: The subject, who executes actions and evaluates feedback, and the interface, which is the structure of the communication channel.

The dynamic relationship between the intrasystemic elements of the interaction can be developed according to the following components:

1. *The objects and the functions of the interface*: These objects and functions are to be understood as objective components of the communication in a virtual space and they form the operative structure of the interface (objective image of system). As objective components, these elements are strictly related to the designer's mental model of the interface.
2. *The execution gulf*: The users project their mental models onto the interface, and, on the basis of these projections, they perform their actions by using the objective elements of the interface (i.e., subjective image of system). This execution gulf determines the action field of the subjects. In other words, users, by interacting with an interface, try to achieve certain goals according to their cognitive abilities, their expectations, and their previous experiences.
3. *The evaluation gulf*: Users do not only perform actions on the interface but also evaluate whether and how these actions were able to achieve their goals. In this moment of the dynamic interaction with the technology, users interpret the feedback coming from the system (Figure 5.5).

Following this model, an interaction problem can be defined as an interruption in the communication flow between the subject and one or more elements of the interface. This interruption can involve both the execution gulf and the evaluation gulf, and it can be caused by a machine error (i.e., an objective error) or a human error (i.e., a subjective error caused by a difficulty for the user in executing their actions in the interface or correctly elaborating the feedback returned by the system) (Figure 5.6).

The evaluation of the UCD is strongly centered on the subjective component of the interaction, and in particular on the user's abilities, and not only on the individuation of the objective failures needed to improve the system by removing the errors. We can identify two fields where interaction problems can arise (Figure 5.6):

1. *Execution*: In this moment of the interaction, a problem can be identified both by a subjective error and by an objective error. A subjective error is mostly due to a lack of user's competence in interacting with the interface, while an objective error is mostly due to a bad design and implementation of the interface components.
2. *Evaluation*: At this moment, a problem in the interaction can be identified both by a user's misinterpretation of the system feedback (i.e., subjective error) and by a lack of output in the system (i.e., an objective error).

5.4.2   Goals of the Integrated Methodology of Interaction Evaluation

Our integrated methodology (Figure 5.8) is based on the idea that the interaction experience (e.g., an exploration of a system) is always linked to the learning skills of

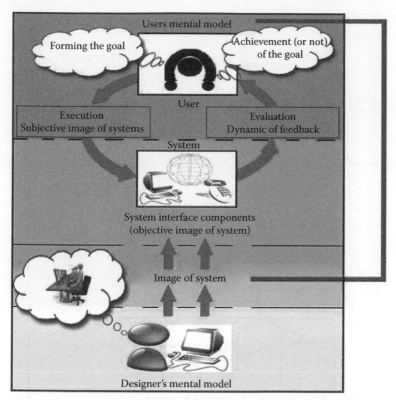

FIGURE 5.5 (See color insert.) Elements comprising the interaction according to the UCD model. The user's mental model is directly involved in the interaction (i.e., execution) and in the evaluation of the system. The designer's mental model, embedded in the image of the system, indirectly affects the interaction because it comprises the objective image of the system and its interface components perceived by the users.

the user and to the learnability of the interface. Presenting their cognitive model of exploratory learning model (i.e., CE+ model), Peter G. Polson and Peter G. Lewis—respectively, professor emeritus of psychology and neuroscience and professor of computer science at the University of Colorado Boulder—claim that "an interface, that must be learnable by exploration must focus on facilitating the problem solving mechanisms" (1990, p. 200). In light of this, the CE+ model allows the designer to both create and evaluate an interface by models related to users' behavior and actions in the interaction. One of the merits of the CE+ model is certainly that it integrates the subjective component of the interaction from two different perspectives:

1. In order to analyze the execution of actions in the interface, the CE+ model considers the users' problem-solving strategies and their exploration abilities as a central information.
2. The CE+ model represents the learnability of the interface—considered as the degree of time spent by a user to perform an action—as the easiness of the interaction.

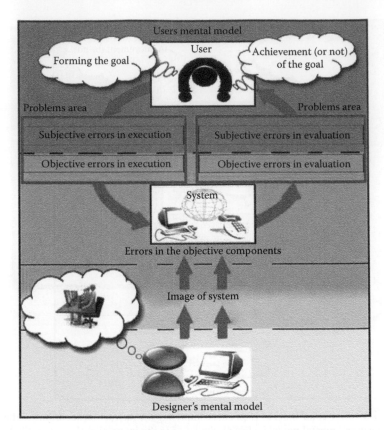

FIGURE 5.6   (See color insert.) Problems in the UCD interaction model: subjective and objective errors in execution and in evaluation can affect the interaction only when the user perceives the error as a problem in relation with the system. The subjective error, as a human error, pertains to the user and can be caused by a wrong action in execution and by a wrong comprehension in evaluation. An objective error, as a machine error, pertains to the system and indirectly to the designers' mental model in developing the system components or in simulating the users in the execution and in the evaluation.

However, although the CE+ model clearly describes the elements of the interaction (i.e., the technology and the user), the ability to integrate these subjective components into the model has an important limit. In fact, the reliability of this model is strictly dependent on users' models rather than on real users (Polson and Lewis, 1990). Therefore, the subjectivity component integrated in the CE+ model follows only standard and predetermined behavior and actions.

We believe that, in order to have a certain degree of reliability and validity, an evaluation model cannot avoid the analysis of real users. A model of interaction evaluation should (1) rely on a standard and shared methodology, (2) avoid becoming dependent on users' models that could be inaccurate (i.e., a usability model should be centered on real user behavior), and (3) strictly relate to a design model.

These three conditions are respected and are followed both by the DCM and by the UCD model. The theoretical perspective that we shall endorse is the one proposed by the UCD model, and, therefore, the model we propose will in turn be based on the DCM model.

Nevertheless, our evaluation model differs from the UCD and DCM models. In fact, the IMIE model, by moving from the distinction between the error and the problem and from the IME's perspective, is strictly focused on those elements in the interaction that determine how good (or bad) the communication flow should be: The identification of the interaction problems and the reduction of the distance between the user's and the designer's mental models are carried out by the mental model of the evaluator. In the following sections, we discuss the two goals of the IMIE model.

5.4.2.1 Identification of the Interaction Problems

As discussed earlier, from an engineering point of view, the evaluation of a system aims mostly to detect the elements in the objective structure of the system that could cause both machine and human errors, whereas the interaction evaluation process that we propose reverses the engineering perspective. In fact, in our model, both objective and subjective errors are considered to be part of the problem, and therefore our model of evaluation aims to identify the problems rather than the errors causing them.

In the IMIE model, we can define an interaction problem as an interruption of the intrasystemic dialogue between user and system. This interruption becomes really significant only when (1) the user perceives it and (2) it is likely to compromise the effectiveness, efficiency, or satisfaction of the interaction (or all three at a time).

This definition of an interaction problem integrates and yet keeps separate both the evaluators' and designers' perspectives. Therefore, the role played by the interaction evaluation (i.e., the identification of problems) is very different from the role played by the design process (i.e., avoiding and fixing errors). In our model, the designer will fix errors retrieved during the evaluation process (i.e., identification of the problems) according to the severity level of the problems identified during the evaluation phase (e.g., the fix needed for the system can range from a simple implementation of an objective error to a total redesign of the interface architecture).

5.4.2.2 Distance between the User and the Designer

From the evaluation point of view, the interaction process not only involves the user's and the designer's mental models, but also that of the evaluator, who plays a significant role since he or she estimates the distance between the first two mental models.

The developer's mental model is composed using his or her preexistent knowledge and competences related to the design process and his or her conceptual model in the image of system. This represents the developer's ideas on (1) the objects that the interface should contain and (2) the functions and the affordances that those objects should have. In this scenario, the elements in the interface (i.e., the objective components of the system) are created on the basis of a developer's subjective perspective, which operates according to its ability to predict the user's actions. From the point of view of the evaluation, such a subjective perspective determines the objective elements that will be evaluated in terms of accessibility and the possibilities of use of those objective elements (i.e., usability). Finally, because the developer's mental model is fundamental in determining the accessibility and the usability of the interface, it also influences the degree of satisfaction perceived by users.

The user's mental model is composed by the user's preexistent knowledge and skills as well as by the effects of his or her subjective interaction with the objective elements and affordances in the interface (i.e., image of system). From the point of view of the evaluation, this subjective perspective determines the user's estimation of the interface properties (i.e., accessibility and usability) and the evaluation of his or her satisfaction of the interaction.

The distance between the designer's and the user's mental model (Figure 5.7) cannot be immediately measured, since the evaluator can observe only the user's interaction with an object created accordingly to the developer's mental model.

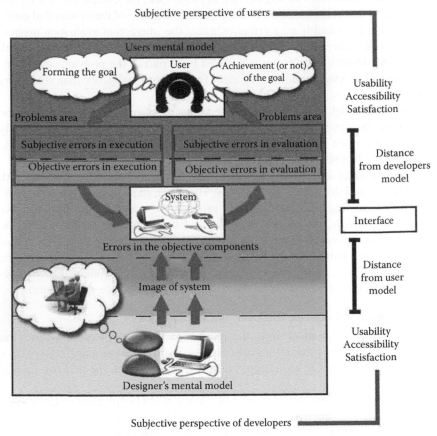

FIGURE 5.7 **(See color insert.)** Subjective and objective errors in execution and evaluation can affect the interaction only when the user perceives errors as a problem in their relationship with the system, as already discussed in Figure 5.6. The user, interacting with the interface, can experience a set of problems of accessibility and usability resulting in a certain degree of satisfaction (i.e., user subjective perspective on interface). When the user's perspective is different from the designer's perspective of the system (i.e., the expected interaction), a gap will exist between the expected interaction and the real one and, as a consequence, a distance between the user's and the designer's mental model can be observed.

The distance between the designer's and the user's mental model opens up two questions:

1. What determines the distance that separates the two mental models (i.e., the designer's mental model considered as how the designer supposes the user will interact with the system and the user's mental model considered as the way the user will actually interact with the system)?
2. Since the user and the designer share the same cognitive, perceptual, and behavioral functions, how is it possible that a product that has been created by following these processes will not fully satisfy the user for which it was created?

The answer to these questions mostly concerns the difficulty that any human being finds when he or she comes to represent and predict someone else's actions and behavior. To fully predict someone else's actions, a designer should be able to completely drop his or her perspective on the system to embrace the user's perspective at once. As we shall show later on, the cognitive processes involved in simulation tasks of the users' performances have been demonstrated to be particularly difficult to perform since the users' simulated interaction styles are expected to be performed during the interaction with the product and can be often different from the real users' style. All these elements allow us to understand how complex the interaction process actually can be, and why the designer's expectations and the user's satisfaction are so often distant from each other.

In order to better understand the concept of distance separating the designer's expectations from the actual users' interaction, we discuss as follows the cognitive process of the two human actors involved in the intrasystemic dialogue (i.e., designer and user) by defining two kind of distances: (1) the distance from the designer to the users and (2) the distance from the user to the designer.

First, we analyze the distance of the designers from the user. As many international studies on the cognitive design have pointed out (Batra and Davis, 1992; Chi et al., 1981; Gugerty and Olson, 1986; Larkin, 1983; Newell and Simon, 1972; Ramaprasad, 1987), the cognitive processes involved in the design process are mostly connected to problem-solving strategies, to the representation of knowledge, and to expertise in complex task environments. Even though these processes have been deeply analyzed, the difficulties due to the "simulation" process have never been properly examined. When designing an interface, the developer simulates how a user would perform in order to achieve his or her goals. Therefore, designers develop the functions of the system according to their idea of a potential user and of a hypothetical interaction. In this way, designers are forced to integrate their design skills with their ability to simulate a user's behavior. Even though a designer is able to represent the typical user's behavior to a certain extent, the application of the standard models, offered by several international guidelines on accessibility and usability, may not be enough to grant the success of a product. Both the accessibility guidelines and the usability principles are tools for guiding designers in simulating the user's needs, expectations, and behaviors. Nevertheless, by respecting all accessibility guidelines and all usability principles, a designer may only guarantee that an interface is somehow accessible and usable in its functioning *per se*; whereas to help the designer in understanding the real user's perception of the product functioning, the evaluator plays a fundamental role because he or she measures both the accessibility and usability experienced by the end user in the context of use.

Therefore, in order to deliver a satisfactory product, the designer needs to possess, to a certain extent, the ability to simulate the possible users' behaviors. However, as previously stated, this ability to simulate someone else's behavior is one of the hardest and most complex cognitive processes that a human being can perform (Decety and Jackson, 2004; Meltzoff and Decety, 2003).

As Gazzaniga points out on his most recent studies, when a person tries to simulate actions and processes that someone else will do, he or she usually strongly relates to his or her previous experiences and competences, whereas it is quite rare to find somebody that is able to completely forget about his or her mental model to assume someone else's perspective (Gazzaniga, 2008, pp. 190–191). In this way, the errors occurring in the simulation process mostly depend on the shared difficulty of a person in not being influenced by his or her own perspective, experiences, and competences. Therefore, from our point of view, a design error in the system (i.e., concerning either an accessibility or a usability issue) should be considered as an error due to the perspective assumed by the designer in his or her simulation of a hypothetical user's behavior. In other words, assuming Norman's point of view (1988), an error in the image of the system depends on the distance separating the designer's and the user's mental models (i.e., distance from developer to user).

The way the user interacts with the system is quite different from the designer's process previously discussed. First, when users interact with the interface, they apply the same cognitive functions used by the designer in the creation of the interface (i.e., problem solving, representation of knowledge, and expertise). Thanks to these shared functions, then, the user may be able to "operate" in the interface (i.e., the interface is understandable and usable). However, while the designer applies these shared cognitive process during his or her simulation of the behavior of an hypothetical user (i.e., in the design of information architecture), the actual user does not need any simulation of the designer's intention: The user's cognitive functions are needed only to perform actions in the interface and he or she does not need to forget about his or her mental model. Therefore, the actions performed by the user in the interface are not based on an "imagined" or "simulated" developer, but the actions are directly experienced.

On one hand, to analyze the designer's mental model, we need to analyze the user's actions that the designer expects to be performed during the interaction with the system (usually, this analysis is performed trough the navigation scenarios).* On the other hand, in order to analyze the user's mental model, we only need to observe what he or she does and how he or she interacts with the system. However, the actions that a user can perform in a system depend on a certain kind of representation, i.e.,

---

* A scenario is a description of the world, in a context and for a purpose, focusing on task interaction. It is intended as a means of communication among stakeholders, and to constrain requirements engineering from one or more viewpoints (usually not complete, not consistent, and not formal) (Jarke et al., 1998, p. 170).

the user's representation of how the system works and functions. Therefore, to a certain extent, even the user simulates something: Indeed, he or she simulates how the system works. Of course, this kind of simulation is very dissimilar to the designer's, since the user does not need to represent and simulate someone else's (the designer) behavior or goals, but only how the system works. In this context, we can figure out a hypothetically perfect coincidence between the user's expectations about system and its real functioning (i.e., system fully satisfies user), even when an image of system does not perfectly express the designer's mental model.

In conclusion, while the designer is forced to simulate the behavior of a hypothetical user, the actual user only needs to simulate the functioning of the system on the basis of his or her previous experiences and competences.

As stated earlier, a second distance affects the interaction: the distance from the user to the developer. This distance usually depends on the fact that humans tend to recognize a certain degree of "humanity" in certain objects, which are considered as entities capable of performing actions on their own:

> The human mind is so generative and so given to animation that we do things such as *map agency* (that is, we project intent) onto almost anything, our pets, our old shoes, our cars, our world. (Gazzaniga, 2008, pp. 1–2 [italics in original])

Consistent with the Gazzaniga's opinion, the user (in execution and feedback) would consider the answers coming from system as the product of an active actor. In general, during the interaction, the user would more easily image that the system possesses a certain degree of intentionality rather than trying to simulate a designer's model. For example, a user may think of an interaction problem and say "this operative system does not work properly" rather than "this operative system was not designed properly." This consideration also helps us to understand why the user can only experience problems and not errors. Errors, in fact, are due to bad design or bad system implementation, whereas problems are related to the UX of interaction. According to most users, indeed, a system does not function when it does not respond properly to their commands. For example, a user will often experience a broken link in the interface as a problem, independent of whether the broken link depends on an error in the script (e.g., wrong address or a page that no longer exists) or on an error in the pointing procedure of the user (e.g., a user who tries to click a link by clicking on the background).

Even if such errors do exist, they usually remain hidden for users, who experience only the "problem" they actually cause. Then, the individual characteristics of each user, and their different attributional styles (Abramson et al., 1978; Heider, 1958), will determine how each user will perceive the problem and its causes. For instance, someone may perceive the problem as depending more on an objective error, whereas someone else could perceive the same problem as depending on a subjective error. For example, in respect of the locus of control (Rotter, 1954, 1966), a user might follow two different paths when trying to identify the cause of the difficulties that he or she is experiencing during the interaction: internal or dispositional way, external or situational way. Regarding the internal or dispositional way, users would tend to ascribe to themselves the causes of the difficulties encountered when they do not feel confident in their competences (i.e., low self-esteem), or when they think they do not possess the appropriate competences for interacting with the system (i.e., low self-efficacy). From the external or situational perspective, users would tend to ascribe to the system the causes of the encountered difficulties when they consider the system not able to meet their competences (i.e., high self-efficacy) or their expectations (i.e., high self-esteem).

Thus, the distance separating the designer and the user in the interaction mostly depends on the different ways of applying their mental model: the designer's simulation of the interaction and the user's interaction with the system. The distance between the simulations and the interactions might be reduced by both of actors of the intrasystemic dialogue by their competences to adapting their mental model to the action required (simulating and interacting): The more competent a designer is in simulating the hypothetical user, the less the distance separating his or her mental model from the actual user's one will be; moreover, the most competent a user is with regard to the system's functioning, the less the distance from the conceptual model of the interface (and therefore with the designer's model) will be.

5.4.2.3   How to Measure the Distance: The Evaluator's Role and Evaluation Model

Both the user's and the designer's mental models are part of the object that an evaluator should measure. Therefore, we cannot use the distance between the designer's and the user's mental models as a measure of expectations of how the system should work (i.e., the designer's perspective), or the experience and the satisfaction perceived by the users in interaction with the system (i.e., the user's perspective). In fact, both these perspectives are only a part of what should be measured. In other words, from an external point of view, the evaluator can observe the interaction between the user and the technology only by using his or her mental model for assessing the components of the intrasystemic dialogue and the emergent properties of their relationship.

Given that the evaluator needs a model to observe and assess the interaction, he or she creates a mental model—on the basis of the available guidelines and evaluation methods for subjective- and objective-oriented observation. When this model reaches maturity, it becomes more and more inclusive along with the know-how necessary for increasing the evaluator (i.e., experience in the assessment).

An evaluator's model created in this way will be able to introduce a new conventional unit of measurement, whose reliability will be granted by the agreement of the international scientific community on the standards, guidelines, methods, and measurements of interaction.

As already stated, the real problems of interaction, which can be identified by a user and observed by an external model (i.e., an evaluator's mental model), can be considered as a unit of interaction assessment. The evaluator, by identifying and matching real, false, and missed interaction problems, can measure the distance between the errors in the functioning of the technology and the problems perceived by the users in the context of use, thus measuring the distance between the designer's and the user's mental models (Figure 5.8).

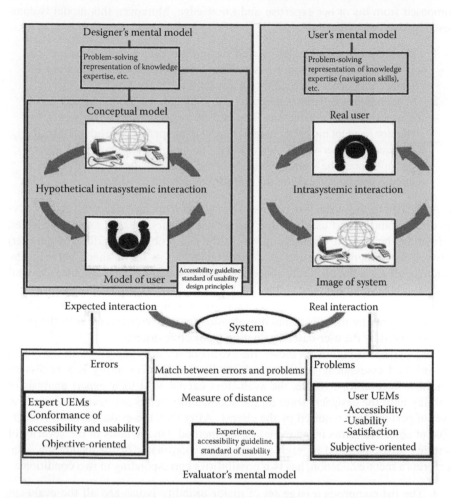

FIGURE 5.8   (See color insert.) The role of the evaluator's mental model from the perspective of the evaluation of problems in the interaction model in the context of the UCD: The designer's mental model is embodied in the system through the conceptual model. The developer designs the system in relation to his or her experience, representation of knowledge, etc. (see the box at the top left: designer's mental model). The designer, taking into account standards and guidelines, images an expected interaction according to the user's model. The real user applies his or her mental model in the interaction with the image of the system (see the box at the top right: user's mental model). The user in "real interaction" experiences problems while the designed system contains errors. The evaluator's mental model is involved in the evaluation, using the usability evaluation methods and the accessibility standards in his or her mental model in order to observe the object and the subject and measuring the distance between the designer's and the user's mental models (see the box at the bottom: evaluator's mental model).

Just like the designer's and the user's mental models, the evaluator's models are composed from his or her expertise and knowledge. Moreover, this model is composed by two other elements:

1. The international accessibility and design guidelines that determine the standards that the evaluator has to take into account when evaluating the interface properties (accessibility and usability).
2. The techniques actually applied by the evaluator for assessing accessibility, usability, and satisfaction. The use of a specific technique forces the evaluator to adapt his or her mental model to the perspective adopted by the technique. In other words, since a specific technique used for the assessment influences the mental model adopted by the evaluator, the evaluation outcome largely depends on the techniques applied.

At the end of the evaluation process, the evaluator should have analyzed the levels of accessibility and usability, the degree of satisfaction, and, as an undirected estimation, the measure of the distance (i.e., the real problems identified by the user) between the designer's and the user's mental model as the distance between the technology functioning (i.e., the conceptual model created by the designer's mental model) and the functioning of real technology perceived by the user. In this way, the evaluator obtains the measure of the interaction distance matching the errors of the object, analyzed by the expert-based evaluation (objective oriented), with the problems observed by the user-based evaluation (subjective oriented).

For instance, as Figure 5.8 shows, the evaluator starts its analysis with the objective-oriented assessment. As discussed in Chapter 2, accessibility is a necessary condition for usability. Hence, the evaluators cannot start their expert analysis of usability until the designers solve all the accessibility errors and reach the aimed-at level of performance required by the clients. After that, the evaluator team collects a list of objective errors by an expert-based method. On the basis of the severity of usability problems rated by each assessor, the coordinator of the evaluation, who performs a meta-evaluation, has two possibilities corresponding to two conditions:

1. The list comprises a large set of major usability issues and all the evaluators (or the majority of them) agreeing that the designers have to solve these errors before processing the users' assessment of the interaction. In this case, the evaluator team generates a partial report on the basis of the objective-oriented analysis (see Figure 5.8) in order to drive the designers to solve errors in the interface functioning. After the redesign phase, the evaluators can run another expert analysis for collecting a new list of errors. Of course, the redesign produces a good result only when in the new list of errors a smaller number and less severe usability problems will occur than in the previous list. Otherwise, a new phase of redesign has to be planned. When all the evaluators agree that the most evident interaction problems (i.e., major) are solved, the user testing is ready to start.
2. The list of errors is composed of minor usability problems, and all the evaluators (or the majority of them) agree that the interface can be assessed by a subjective-oriented analysis (see Figure 5.8). The assessment of the users'

interaction does not concern only the usability issues, but, as discussed in Chapter 2, by following ISO 9241-171 (2008), the assessor in the usability evaluation should also consider accessibility aspects from the users' point of view. The subjective-oriented analysis allows evaluators to collect a list of real problems, corresponding to all the problems experienced and declared by users during the assessment. By comparing the list of errors (i.e., expert-based analysis) and the list of problems (i.e., user-based analysis), the evaluator team can discriminate between real, missed, and false problems, in order to create a complete evaluation report.

The match between errors and problems shows the distance between the interaction imagined by the designer for a hypothetical user and the interaction perceived by the real user. Therefore, the problems perceived by the real users are the units of the interaction distance measurement (Figure 5.8).

To conclude, the consequence of the analysis carried out so far can be summarized in a single assumption: The interaction assessment should follow an integrated methodology, which is able to consider and include all the multidimensional aspects of an interaction.

The IMIE model is a multidimensional process that can be adapted to any kind of design life cycle. It guarantees the equalization of designer and evaluator roles, fostering their communication in order to improve both the designed functioning of the technology and the UX of the interaction. The process is outlined in the following assessment steps:

- *The system evaluation*: The evaluation of the objective aspects of the interface (i.e., accessibility and usability). In this phase (see the box "Errors" in Figure 5.8, on the left of the "Evaluator's mental model"), the evaluator analyses the objective elements of the system. Expert techniques are used to evaluate the interface according to a comparison with some standard design models for both accessibility and usability (WCGA rules, heuristics, etc.). In turn, the data obtained by these techniques will be used as a baseline to be compared with the data collected through the user-based tests. In the objective-oriented observation, the evaluator measures the compliance to the guideline (i.e., WCAG, heuristic lists, and design principles) of the hypothetical interaction designed by the developer (i.e., the image of system). This evaluation not only concerns the identification of errors through a conformance analysis but is also a reconstruction of the designer's mental model from the evaluator's perspective.
- *The subjective evaluation of the interaction*: The evaluation of the subjective aspects of the interface. In this phase (see the box "Problems" in Figure 5.8, on the left of the box "Evaluator's mental model"), the evaluator analyses the elements of the interface as the users experience them during the interaction. User techniques are used to identify the problems perceived by users in real interaction. The data collected can then be matched with the data from the tests carried out by the experts to define the efficacy and

efficiency of the evaluation process. These measures allow the evaluator to observe the distance between the real users' mental model (i.e., the real perceived problems) and the reconstructed designer's mental model (i.e., the objective errors identified by evaluator).

• *The user evaluation of the interaction quality*: In this phase (see the box "Problems" in Figure 5.8, on the left of the box "Evaluator's mental model"), the evaluator assesses the subjective aspects of the interaction. Implicit or explicit measures (i.e., psychometric or biofeedback instruments) are used to collect qualitative and quantitative data and information about the system. These measures allow the evaluator to provide an indirect estimate of the distance between the real user and the hypothetical one (i.e., the user's model) imaged by the designer. Using these kinds of analyses, the evaluator can measure the distance between the two mental models by also taking the user's individual differences (directly or indirectly, depending on the instruments) in terms of skills, preferences, and attitudes, which otherwise would be excluded from the evaluation, into account.

It should now be clear enough that a single evaluation technique does not comprise all the dimensions of the evaluated interaction, even if it is performed either by an expert or by a user. In order to obtain a fully exhaustive evaluation, it is necessary to compose an IMIE.

5.5   HOW TO USE THE INTEGRATED METHODOLOGY: THE DECISION PROCESS CARRIED OUT BY THE EVALUATOR

The IMIE model is a multidimensional process that can be adapted to any kind of design life cycle. As an external point of view on interaction, the professionals involved in the assessment (such as psychologists, ergonomists, and experts in human factors) can analyze all the aspects of the intrasystemic dialogue between user and interface while collaborating with the designer, in order to transform the product into an intrasystemic solution (i.e., a psychotechnology). By applying the IMIE model, the evaluator can work out how to collaborate with designer during the product life cycle, by deciding on two main aspects of the assessment:

1. When and where a certain evaluation step has to be carried out. For instance, the process for assessing a prototype (i.e., formative assessment process) requires an expensive investment, because such an assessment is comprised of a multiple set of steps in which each evaluation step is followed by a redesign step, in an iterative collaboration between designer and evaluator, for forming and refining an interface and the overall aspects of the interaction. Otherwise, the assessment of a product (already released or close to be release in the market) would require a minimal set of evaluation steps (i.e., summative assessment), in which the assessment is completed

only when all the aspects of the interaction (from accessibility to UX) have been evaluated (for a complete review on formative and summative evaluation, see Hartson and Hix, 1989).

2. Which kind of evaluation techniques are the most efficient and effective, and which kind and how many users the evaluator has to test in order to gather reliable results can be assessed (Borsci et al., 2011; Nielsen and Landauer, 1993). The efficiency and the effectiveness of the IMIEI depend strictly on the selected evaluation methods. As Borsci et al. (2012a) suggest, the efficiency of an evaluation method can be estimated by considering all the costs of the evaluation for reaching the aim, while its effectiveness can be estimated by considering how many real problems are identified during the assessment.

The IMIE model (Figure 5.8) clarifies the role of the evaluator and his or her goal (i.e., the measure of the distance between the designers and the users), driving the evaluator in taking into account all the variables that may affect the intrasystemic dialogue. Nevertheless, the evaluator, in order to define his or her collaboration with the designers and the evaluation techniques for the assessment, has to consider at least three main variables that affect the efficiency and the effectiveness of the assessment process: (1) the contextual variables, (2) the internal variables, and (3) the behavioral variables.

By considering these three variables, the evaluator adapts the IMIE model to the design process and selects the evaluation methods by creating a counterbalance between the cost of the evaluation techniques (efficiency) and the number of the real problems that have been identified (effectiveness). While, theoretically, any evaluator aims to select the assessment methods that produce a minimal impact on the budget (high efficiency) and allow him or her to find the maximum number of identified problems (high effectiveness), in fact the evaluator cannot select the final methodology without considering several variables affecting the assessment: First, the design process by which the product under assessment is created and the kind of technology under assessment (the contextual variables); second, what the evaluator experiences in the assessment, and the advantages and limits of the different evaluation methods (the internal variables); finally, the number of subjects needed for both the experts' and the users' assessment, and the number of real, missed, and false problems identified in the overall interaction assessment (the behavioral variables).

- *The contextual variables.* We can define as contextual all variables that affect the decision of the evaluator in selecting a specific set of methods for assessing the interaction (Figure 5.9). In the application of the IMIE model, an evaluator should consider two kinds of contextual variables: the relationship between design and evaluation process and the features of technology under assessment. An evaluator has to consider the decision process of the designers and their mental models in order to define how to adapt an evaluation methodology to the design process. For example, for a practitioner, it is different to adapt or select the evaluation methodology, in a formative context, according to whether the designers adopt (1) a cooperative and

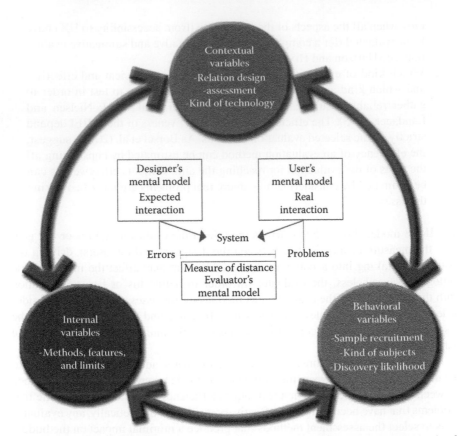

FIGURE 5.9 **(See color insert.)** By considering the contextual, internal, and behavioral variables, the evaluators can adapt the IMIE model to the design process. The contextual variables concern the relation between design and evaluation process, and the kind of technology under assessment. The internal variables concern the limits, the advantages, and the features of the selected evaluation methods. The behavioral variables concern the sample recruitment, the kind of subjects involved in the assessment, and the sample discovery likelihood.

participatory design or (2) a goal-oriented design (see for a complete review, Cooper et al., 2007; Greenbaum and Kyng, 1994; Schuler and Namioka, 1993). In the first case, the stakeholders' involvement in the design requires both a design and redesign process, in which the evaluation methods are included in the design phases. In the second case, at first, the evaluator has to collaborate with the developers during the design of the prototype, in order to build up the user's model together with them and he or she has to test the interface with the real end users in order to suggest how to improve the product to match a specific kind of user model. Finally, the evalua-tor has to select the evaluation methods that, in a way that needs to be compatible with the design process, can minimize the cost (efficiency) by concurrently identifying a large number of real problems (effectiveness). The second contextual variables regard the features of technology under assessment. When an evaluator has to assess a specific kind of technology, he or she selects a specific set of evaluation tools for testing the interaction, by considering the features and the different possible uses of the technology. Nevertheless, the context of use in which the evaluator should test the interaction could be very different on the basis of the kind of technology that is under assessment. For instance, the methods selected by an evaluator for testing a web interface and an assistive technology may be similar, but the evaluation of an assistive technology requires that the evaluator takes into account not only the interaction between the user and the technology but also the environmental interaction among users, technology, and environment (Borsci et al., 2012b). In light of the kind of technology, an evaluator should consider during the assessment a different number of interaction variables, thus defining the time and the costs of the evaluation (efficiency of the assessment).

- *The internal evaluation variables.* We can define all the variables that are related to the limits of the methods and tools applied in the experts' and the users' methods as being "internal" (Figure 5.9). For example, in order to conduct an expert evaluation, Sears (1997) suggests that a coordinator of the evaluation can use the classic cognitive walkthrough method if the experts involved have great experience of evaluation (e.g., more than 2 years), whereas, when the experts have a low level of expertise, it may be more useful to apply an heuristic cognitive walkthrough. At the same time, in order to evaluate the users' levels of satisfaction, a practitioner could use different standardized questionnaires that may require a different minimum number of users for obtaining reliable data. The internal limits of tools and methods are variables that an evaluator has to consider in selecting the steps and the methods that make up the integrated methodology. The internal variables affect both the efficiency and the effectiveness of the assessment. In fact, the selection of the evaluation methods defines the costs and, potentially, how many false, missed, and real problems that experts gather at the end of the assessment. For example, an evaluator can use heuristic analysis for assessing a website instead of a cognitive walkthrough (Lewis et al., 1990) because using heuristic analysis reduces the overall costs (Nielsen and Molich, 1990). Nevertheless, according to the experience of the evaluators that make up the team and on the basis of the details of the evaluation they aim to obtain, the evaluators can select different kind of heuristic lists, such as the one provided by Nielsen (1995c) that comprises 10 points, or the one provided by Tognazzi (2005) that comprises 16 points. The evaluators' final choice will depend on internal evaluation variables that will affect the efficiency and effectiveness of the assessment.
- *The behavioral variables in the evaluation.* We can define all the variables related to the behavior of a sample of users in discovering interaction problems as behavioral (Figure 5.9). The number of subjects needed for the assessment affects the cost of the evaluation process. Usually, following the five-user assumption (Nielsen and Landauer, 1993; Turner et al., 2006; Virzi, 1990, 1992), a sample of five users, such as a sample of five experts, is enough for discovering more than the 80% of the problems. Nevertheless,

as we discuss in Chapter 6, this is only an ideal assumption. The evaluator can only check the problem discovery behavior of a sample, but there are no magic numbers that an evaluator can use for forecasting how many subjects he or she has to involve in the assessment. As the IMIE model proposes, analysis by experts allows evaluators to collect a set of problems that could affect the interaction, even though only the user testing can discriminate among real, missed, and false problems. In light of this, the selection of the users is one of the most important steps of the evaluation. In Chapter 6, we discuss the selection and the recruitment of the users with and without disability and how to estimate the users' behavior, in order to discover real interaction problems which affect the level of assessment reliability. Usually, practitioners apply the estimation models of users' behavior to define how many subjects should be used for evaluating an interface (Borsci et al., 2011; Lewis, 1994, 2006; Nielsen and Landauer, 1993; Turner et al., 2006; Virzi, 1992). In Chapter 7, we propose a grounded procedure that can drive practitioners to define the most useful number of users for the assessment on the basis of sample discovery likelihood.

5.6   CONCLUSION

In this chapter, we proposed an integrated methodology, the IMIE model, which can be used by an evaluator to assess the interaction in any design life cycle. This model drives evaluators in a step-by-step process of assessment that, together with the measurement of accessibility, usability, and UX, leads the evaluators to measure the distance between the designers' and the users' mental models. In light of this, the IMIE model results in a multidimensional model in which the evaluator has a specific role: the external observation of the interaction components and their relationship. As discussed in Chapter 4, this evaluator role is equalized with the designer one. In fact, by adopting the IMIE model, the evaluator is not reduced only to being a "verifier" of the designer's product. At the same time, the evaluator is not a users' advocate who, by questioning all the technology, features as the basis of the user's needs, thus forcing designers to rethink their work, as happens in the UCD. Starting from the common goal of releasing an intrasystemic solution shared by the evaluator and the designer, for the IMIE model, the main aim of the evaluation is to transform the designed artifact in a psychotechnology. The evaluators work separately in an iterative dialogue with the designers for improving both the functioning of the technology *per se* and the functioning perceived by the users, in order to reduce the distance between the designer's and the user's mental models. Therefore, to achieve the intrasystemic solution, the evaluator works in the opposite way to the designer: While the designer aims at creating an invisible interface about which the user does not need to think, the evaluator creates conditions in which the user has to think about the interface (i.e., the evaluation test) in order to transform the technology into a form of psychotechnology, about which the user does not have to think.

The IMIE model represents the application, from the evaluator's point of view, of a psychotechnological perspective, in which the interaction emerges as a whole that cannot be measured only as the sum of the components of the intrasystemic dialogue.

In light of this, the interaction can be assessed only by a multidimensional process in which the evaluator analyzes its components (i.e., technology functioning *per se* and the functioning perceived by the user), and the distance between the designer's and the user's mental model can be seen as a measure of the intrasystemic dialogue, which is defined by the interaction problems experienced by the end user.

By applying the IMIE model, the dialogue between the evaluator and the designer is defined by two main aspects: (1) when and where a certain evaluation step has to be carried out and (2) which kind of evaluation techniques are the most efficient and effective, and which kind and how many users the evaluator has to test in order to gather reliable results. In order to define the aspects of the assessment in the life cycle, the evaluator, in agreement with the designer, has to consider three main variables that can affect the assessment outcomes: (1) contextual variables, (2) internal variables, and (3) behavioral variables.

In the following chapters, we analyze the identification of the assessment variables that represent the main way for adapting the IMIE model to the life cycle and to the features of the product that is under evaluation. In Chapter 6, by discussing the role of disabled users in the interaction assessment, we talk about the different aspects of the behavioral variables that an evaluator has to consider in the IMIE model, underlining how the inclusion of disabled users in a sample cohort can improve the reliability of the assessment outcomes. Furthermore, in Chapter 7, we see how to perform an interaction evaluation by considering all the assessment variables, describing the methods and their limits (i.e., contextual and internal variables), and proposing a specific procedure for managing the behavioral variables. Finally, in Chapter 8, we present a list of evaluation techniques by considering their adaptability to the disabled users' evaluation.

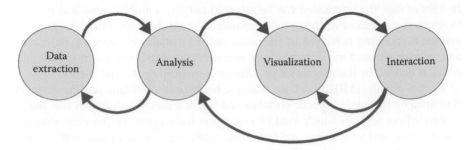

FIGURE 1.1 Conceptual design tasks for the functional layer.

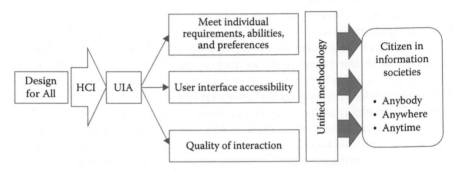

FIGURE 1.2 Conceptual application of the UIA aim in the design process.

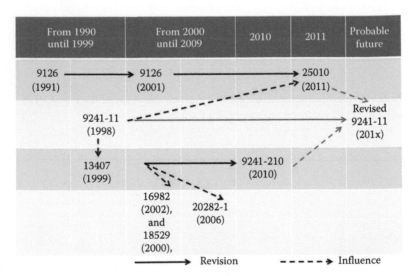

FIGURE 2.3 The usability standards relationship from the 1990s until today, and the possible future revision of ISO 9241-11 to create a unified standard of usability.

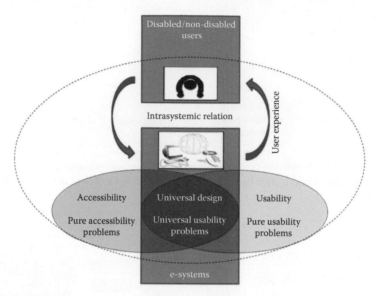

FIGURE 2.4 The intrasystemic relationship between users and technology.

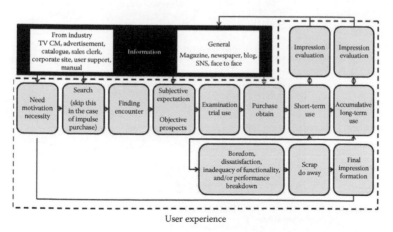

FIGURE 2.6 Overall stages of the UX.

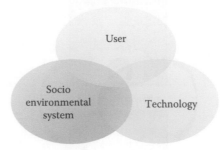

FIGURE 3.3 Reciprocal triadic causation between the components of the user–technology interaction.

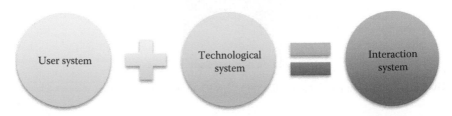

FIGURE 3.4 Dyadic perspective of interaction between a subjective component and an objective one.

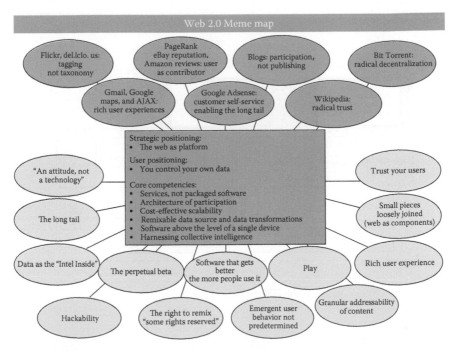

FIGURE 3.5 Web 2.0 Meme map developed at a brainstorming session during a conference at O'Reilly Media.

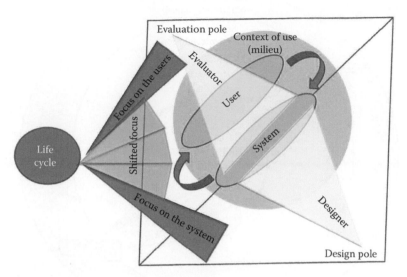

FIGURE 4.1 The general goal of the life cycle.

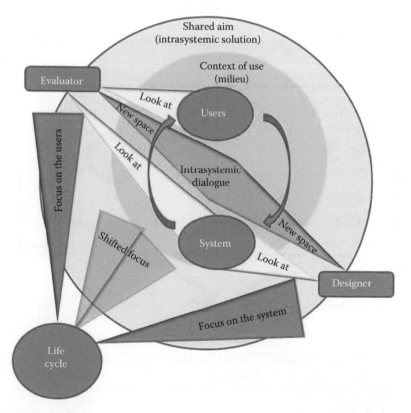

FIGURE 4.2 The new space created by the introduction of a third pole, the intrasystemic dialogue between the technology and the user.

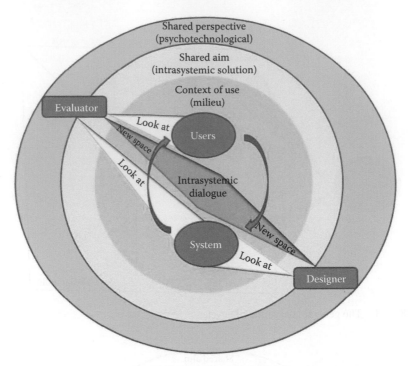

FIGURE 4.3 The role of the psychotechnological perspective within the life cycle.

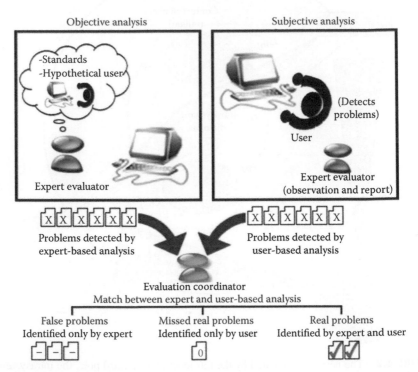

FIGURE 5.1 The actors involved in the evaluation process are the expert evaluator (in the box at the top left), the user (in the box at the top right), and the evaluation coordinator (meta-evaluator, in the bottom middle).

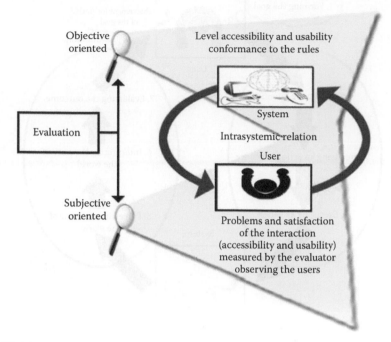

FIGURE 5.2 The "integrated model" of evaluation.

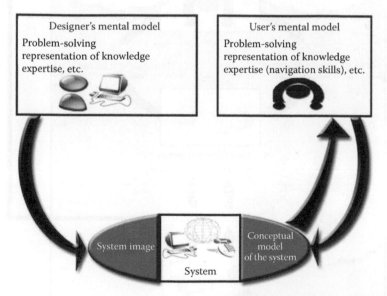

FIGURE 5.3 The designer's mental model is used by developers to create a technology (i.e., a system) and its functioning (i.e., the system image and its conceptual model visible to the end user) by simulating the user's mental model.

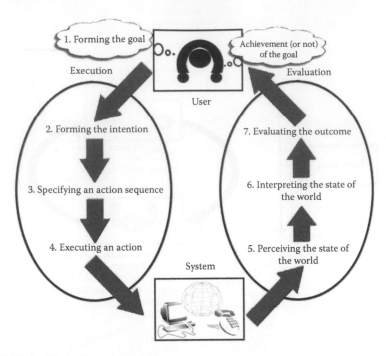

FIGURE 5.4 Decision cycle model.

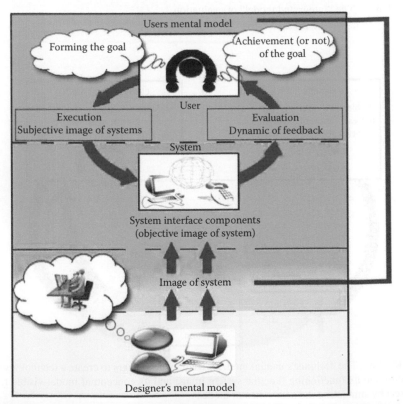

FIGURE 5.5 Elements comprising the interaction according to the UCD model.

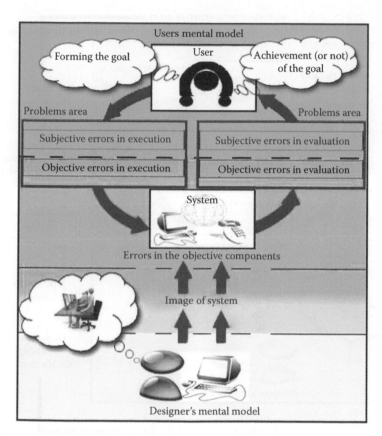

FIGURE 5.6 Problems in the UCD interaction model.

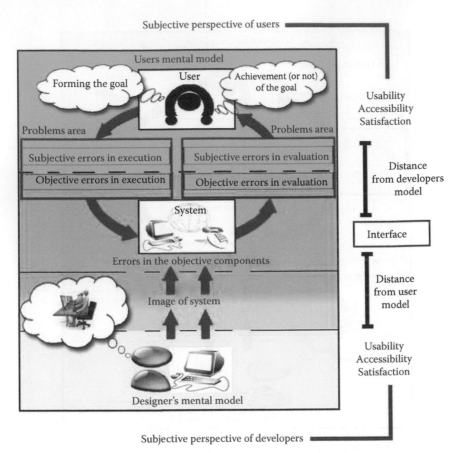

FIGURE 5.7 Subjective and objective errors in execution and evaluation can affect the interaction only when the user perceives errors as a problem in their relationship with the system, as already discussed in Figure 5.6.

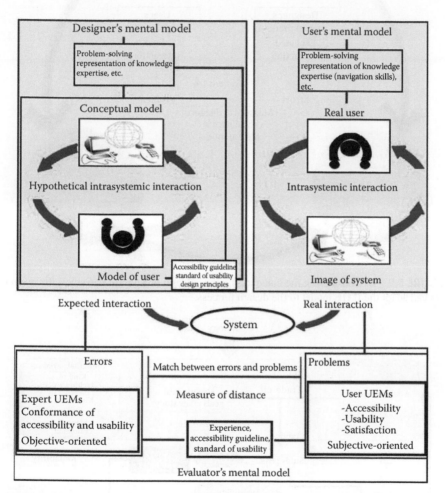

FIGURE 5.8 The role of the evaluator's mental model from the perspective of the evaluation of problems in the interaction model in the context of the UCD.

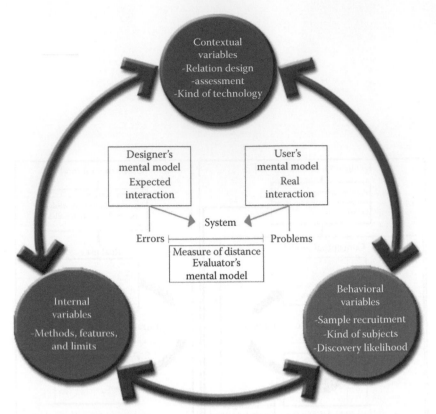

FIGURE 5.9 By considering the contextual, internal, and behavioral variables, the evaluators can adapt the IMIE model to the design process.

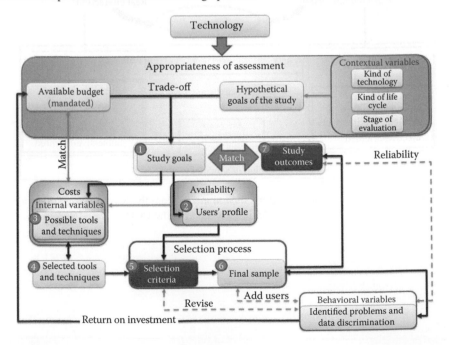

FIGURE 6.1 User testing decision flow.

Method class	Method type	Meaning	Safety	Reliability, compatibility, durability, sustainability, cost	Effectiveness	Efficiency	Satisfaction	Pleasure, joy, etc.
UX								
			Quality				**Kansei**	
					Usability			
(1) Qualitative and subjective measurements for the interaction analysis	Interview	X	X	X			X	X
	Observation	X	X		X		X	X
	Diary	X	X	X			X	X
	Satisfaction questionnaire	X	X	X			X	X
	Psychometric questionnaire	X					X	X
	Eye-tracker		X		X	X		
	Biofeedback analysis		X				X	X
(2) Usability testing and analysis of a real interaction	Concurrent think-aloud				X	X		
	Retrospective think-aloud				X		X	
	Remote testing				X	X		
(3) Inspection and simulation methods of expected interaction	Heuristic list				X	X		
	Cognitive walkthrough				X	X		
	Task analysis				X	X		

FIGURE 7.4 Synoptic representation of the most common evaluation techniques and measures of the UX and usability divided into three groups of methods.

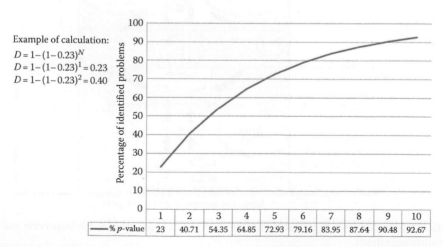

Example of calculation:

$$D = 1 - (1 - 0.23)^N$$
$$D = 1 - (1 - 0.23)^1 = 0.23$$
$$D = 1 - (1 - 0.23)^2 = 0.40$$

	1	2	3	4	5	6	7	8	9	10
% p-value	23	40.71	54.35	64.85	72.93	79.16	83.95	87.64	90.48	92.67

FIGURE 7.5 Example of the error distribution formula application on the base of the return on investment model, in which the sample's discovery likelihood is estimated by the raw p-value of the cohort.

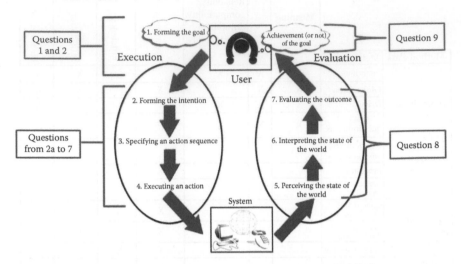

FIGURE 8.2 Adapted representation of the decision cycle model of Hutchins et al. (1985), integrated with the nine questions of the original CW inspection.

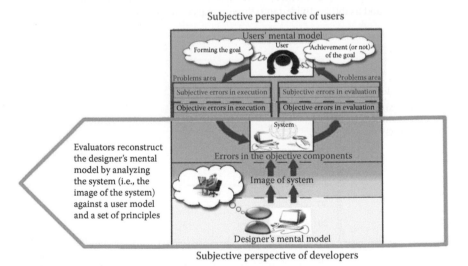

FIGURE 8.3 Synoptic representation of the interaction observed through inspection and simulation methods.

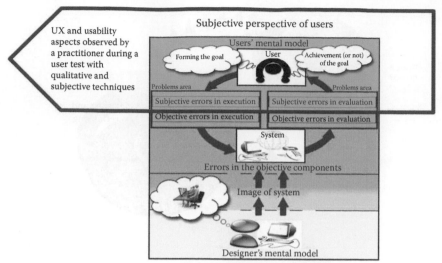

FIGURE 8.4 Synoptic representation of the interaction observed by qualitative and subjective methods.

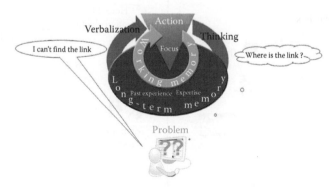

FIGURE 8.6 The users pay attention to the action while they are forced to verbalize their thoughts.

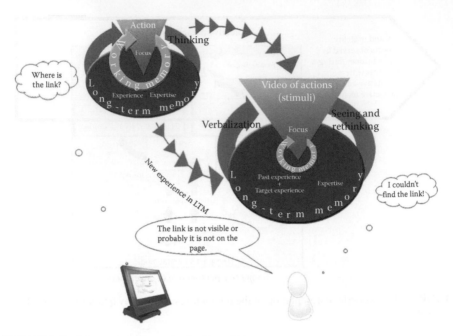

FIGURE 8.7 Memory processes in the Retro-TA.

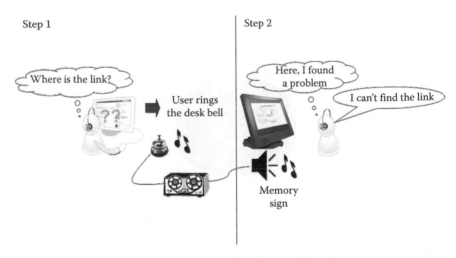

FIGURE 8.8 Evaluation process of partial concurrent thinking aloud.

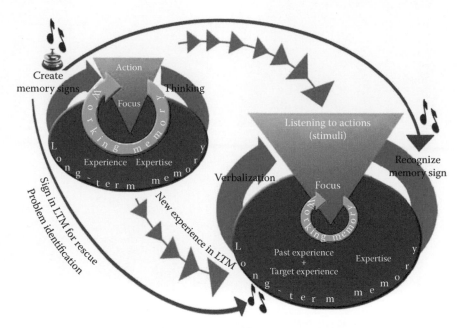

FIGURE 8.9 The memory processes in the PCTA.

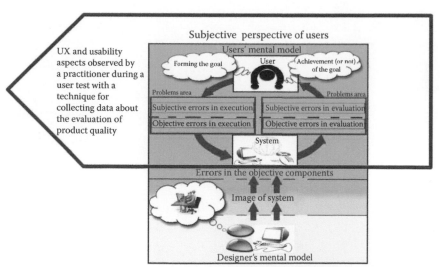

FIGURE 8.10 Synoptic representation of the interaction observed through methods of evaluating the product quality (user evaluation of quality).

6 Why Understanding Disabled Users' Experience Matters

6.1 DISABLED USERS' EXPERIENCE

As we discussed in Chapter 1, the accessibility of artifacts is a well-debated issue in human–computer interaction (HCI). In particular, researchers and practitioners have remarked strongly on the ethical aspects of the "right of access" for all users (Roulstone, 2010), concurrently supporting the diffusion of the international rules and guidelines for assessing and verifying the accessibility of technological products (e.g., Section 508, WCAG). Nevertheless, while accessibility is a well-discussed topic, the role of disabled users and the advantages of their involvement in the interaction evaluation are often undervalued as a secondary issue.

In fact, disabled users are mostly only involved in the evaluation to analyze the accessibility of the technological products and for comparing their interactive behavior with a baseline of users without disability (see Bohman and Anderson, 2005; Fairweather and Trewin, 2010; Feng et al., 2008, 2010). In this sense, usually disabled users play only a functional role (e.g., when people with disability are involved as users with special needs for defining and testing the features of a product) in the development and assessment of a given technology and are only involved in some phases of both the design (e.g., for defining the device and its interface main features) and the evaluation of accessibility in order to respect the international rules and accessibility guidelines. Moreover, disabled users are still excluded from the possibility of full participation in the overall interaction design and assessment. Indeed, professionals rarely involve disabled users along the product life cycle, from the initial definitions of the prototype features to its overall assessment (i.e., accessibility, usability, and user experience [UX]), until the final evaluation of the released product.

As Bob Regan, senior product manager for education and government at Macromedia, notes (2004), in analyzing the relationship between accessibility and design, currently designers approach accessibility only as a technical issue by considering the design of accessible interfaces as a restriction on their creativity. In this designer's perspective, accessibility is considered only as a feature of the device (and its interface) for accomplishing a need of a particular kind of users. Concurrently, in line with this designer's perspective, disabled users are often involved by evaluators as specialists in the assessment of accessibility, whereas practitioners rarely select disabled users for assessing the UX, since they are, generally, considered as a group outside the target market of the product.

Implicitly, a large number of designers and evaluators consider disabled users as people with divergent and special kinds of needs. In fact, for designers, accessibility is a technical issue that concerns only disabled users and, on the other hand, for the evaluators only disabled users may assess accessibility.

We can say that, although today there is a shared agreement, as we discussed in Chapter 2, on the fact that accessibility is a dimension of the interaction instead of a feature of the interface, developers are usually perceived as being forced to design standard and uncreative interfaces, simply in order to allow the interaction of this "little" percentage of end users (see Harper and Bechhofer, 2007; Harper et al., 2006; Jay et al., 2007; Regan, 2004). The functioning of these uncreatively designed interfaces has then to be assessed by these "users with specialness" only for testing and checking the conformance of the interface's functioning to the standard rules. As Pradipta Biswas and Pat Langdon, researchers at the Engineering Department of Cambridge University, recently reported

> existing design practices often isolate elderly or disabled users by considering them as users with special needs and do not consider their problems during the design phase. (Biswas and Langdon, 2011, p. 73)

Evidence that this perspective is still largely endorsed by HCI professionals (i.e., designers and evaluators) comes from the first World Web Accessibility Audit, which the United Nations commissioned in 2006 to the Nomesa agency. The study, as Nomesa's website reports,* evaluated 100 websites from 20 different countries across 5 sectors of industry (media, finance, travel, politics, and retail) and showed that only three websites passed the basic accessibility checkpoints (i.e., Level A) outlined in WCAG1.0, and not a single site passed all checkpoints.

What we are going to propose is that the development of an accessible interface and, moreover, the inclusion of disabled users in the evaluation cohort for the interface assessment (i.e., by composing a mixed sample of end users with different characteristics of individual functioning) is not only a necessary step for guaranteeing the right of access, but also an investment for developers and evaluators. In fact, the main aim of designers when they realize any product is that it achieves success in the market. Nevertheless, the only way to manage an aleatory variable, such as the success of the product, is to reduce the uncertainty in the design decision making. As we discussed in Chapter 4, only through the assessment of real users and communication with the evaluator can designers have a reasonable level of confidence that the product might satisfy the end users. In particular, as we are going to discuss in this chapter, the reliability of the assessment data and the end user cohort representativeness of the entire population are key factors for creating a psychotechnology that matches end users' expectations and needs. In light of this, the involvement of disabled users in the evaluation cohort is today an investment in increasing the assessment reliability and in capturing different kinds of users' needs and expectations in order to implement the technology features and improve the intrasystemic dialogue between user and interface.

---

* http://www.nomensa.com/blog/2007/practical-plans-for-accessible-architectures/

Finally, we must highlight another aspect that supports the necessity today for disabled users' involvement in all the phases of the product life cycle—the market of technology. In fact, the undervaluation by HCI professionals of interaction accessibility shows a serious lack of forecasting the future market of technology. Indeed, as demographic data of 2007 show (UN, 2007), the elderly (over 60) in the world are already suggesting more than young people (under 15) that accessibility is a key factor for e-inclusion in the information societies. Moreover, the trends of demographic data show that disabled and elderly users are going to comprise a large part of the consumers of future markets, in which, for instance, elderly users will be equal to 20% of the world population (WHO and World Bank 2011; see also Box 6.1). Accessibility, in the next 10 years, will be the main factor for the success of technology, and assessment by a mixed sample of users with different ranges of abilities will be the only way to understand and meet consumers' needs.

In this chapter, we are going to propose that the way in which accessibility is approached and managed by designers and evaluators determines, as in the case of the usability and the UX, the final intrasystemic dialogue between user and technology, and that disabled users' involvement in the evaluation of the overall interaction is an investment that professionals should make in order to capture and meet all the real users' needs, thereby increasing the possibility of a product's success in the market.

6.1.1 BIG ACCESSIBILITY APPROACH

In Chapter 2, we extensively described the distinction between the two concepts of "small" and "big" usability, primarily concerning two different ways to involve end users, including disabled ones, in the designing and evaluation processes (Kurosu, 2007). In the same way, we apply this distinction to the accessibility construct, dividing it into small and big approaches.

We consider as being affected by a small accessibility approach all the technologies that have been created and evaluated, respectively, by designers and evaluators on the basis of the prejudice that disabled users in interaction are persons with "special needs" of access. This small accessibility approach is characterized by two main shortcomings:

1. It considers the interaction by focusing on "users' special needs" rather than on a range of human functioning. In fact, when a disabled person interacts with a product, he or she should not be considered as a "special" user, but as an end user with his or her attitudes, needs, skills, and functioning. Indeed, as a universal model of human functioning and disability, "disability is not a human attribute that demarks one portion of humanity from another (as gender does, and race sometimes does); it is an infinitely various but universal feature of the human condition" (Bickenbach et al., 1999, p. 1182). Therefore, disability is not to be considered as just a special need, regarding a minority group of users, but as a way of human functioning (WHO, 2001)—"disability is a matter of more or less, not yes or no" (WHO and World Bank, 2011, p. 5). As a consequence, a disabled user in interaction should not be considered as a special user with a special need, but as a user who finds more or less accessible barriers in the system (see Box 6.1).

BOX 6.1   HOW MANY PEOPLE WITH A DISABILITY ARE THERE IN THE WORLD?

STEFANO FEDERICI AND FABIO MELONI

The question of how many people are there in the world with a disability is a difficult one to answer. Although several global surveys and national population censuses have provided reliable estimates about the demographic prevalence of people with disability, the data nevertheless do not coincide with one another, leaving a broad range of variance to be reconciled. Estimates vary even within a given sample population. The Irish population census of 2006, for instance, found that 9.3% of the population (393,785 individuals) reported the presence of a disability. Later in 2006, the Irish Central Statistics Office's National Disability Survey (NDS), using a broader definition of disability, identified an additional 8.1% of the population as "false negatives"—people with a disability which had gone undeclared—thereby increasing the number of disabled individuals in Ireland to 18.5% of the population (749,100 individuals) (Central Statistics Office, 2008). Even when a comparison is drawn with other European countries that share the same or a similar health care system, the answer to our question remains elusive. In 2005, an Italian sample survey found that 4.7% of the Italian population (about 2,600,000 individuals) have declared to have some form of disability (ISTAT, 2007). This figure has actually declined as compared to the figure recorded in previous years. According to the Italian sample survey, persons with disabilities are defined as those individuals who, excluding conditions related to temporary limitations, have said they are not capable of performing typical activities of daily life, even taking into account the possible use of medical devices such as prostheses, walking sticks, glasses, etc.

The need for reliable estimates of the global prevalence of disability has led the World Health Organization (WHO) and the World Bank, working jointly, to produce the first ever *World Report on Disability* (2011). The report was based on two primary data sources: the WHO *World Health Survey* of 2002–2004 (Üstün et al., 2003b; WHO, 2002–2004), which includes data from 59 countries, and the WHO *Global Burden of Disease* study, updated in 2004 (WHO, 2008). The first comprises the largest multinational health and disability survey ever to use a single set of questions and consistent methods to collect comparable health data from across multiple countries; the second is an overall assessment of the health of the world's population which provides exhaustive estimates of premature mortality, disability, and loss of health from different diseases, injuries, and risk factors, drawing on available WHO data sources and on information provided by Member States. The *World Health Survey* and *Global Burden of Disease* study, however, as they are "based on very different measurement approaches and assumptions, give global prevalence estimates among the adult population of 15.6% and 19.4% respectively" (WHO and World Bank, 2011, p. 29).

There are three main reasons that contribute to the difficulties in accurately measuring the prevalence of disabilities through censuses and that combine to render the data ambiguous and nonunique. These are (1) the universality of disability, (2) the definitional paradox of disability, and (3) the contextual factors affecting the self-perception of disability.

The *universality of disability*. Since the 1980s, starting with Irving Zola's (1989, 1993) universal model of disability and continuing through to the biopsychosocial model of disability adopted by the WHO as a universal framework for classifying (2001) and for collecting disability data (WHO and World Bank, 2011), disability has come to be defined not as something which is to be experienced only by minority groups—due to bias, prejudice, segregation, or discrimination—as a fixed and dichotomous entity that "demarks one portion of humanity from another (as gender does, and race sometimes does)" (Bickenbach et al., 1999, p. 1182). Only in a purely theoretical construct, one might find in an individual either a full disability or a full ability. Disability is instead properly understood as a fluid and continuous experience that any human being has to tackle over the course of their life: "it is an infinitely various but universal feature of the human condition" (Bickenbach et al., 1999, p. 1182). Disability is a type of individual's functioning in which the term "impairment" is not adequately descriptive.

> Disability is not a set of immutable characteristics that define a person over another nor is it predictable by a medical diagnosis since it is not a direct consequence of disease, but it is, instead, a multidimensional process that lasts a lifetime and involves the physical, psychic, and social spheres of the individual. (Federici et al., 2012a, pp. 27–28)

Given this broad meaning of disability (universality) and its strict relation to human functioning (the biopsychosocial model), any classification of an individual as having a disability is a question of a threshold of severity that any survey might arbitrarily state. The universality of disability is therefore the first reason that makes it difficult in measuring disability.

The *definitional paradox*. A major problem encountered by experts in disability measurement is closely related to the complex definition of disability (Üstün et al., 2003a). In the *International Classification of Functioning, Disability and Health* (ICF), in fact, disability arises out of activity limitations and participation restrictions, which are determined by the interaction between the functioning of body functions and structures and the conditions set by the contextual factors (see also Box 3.1)

> Since only one or two of these dimensions of disability are reflected in measures in any given survey [...], the data will only capture a portion of the population, those who exhibit the specific aspects of disability the questions represent. (Altman and Gulley, 2009, p. 544)

The "definitional paradox" (Madans and Altman, 2006) surrounding disability is derived from the operational nature of the disability concept, according to which any theoretical definition implies aporia while any operational meaning is determined by the purpose of research. Madans and Altman have stated that "there is no single operational definition of disability (multiple sets of questions, linked to the different purposes of measurement, may be needed)," and consequently, that "different operational definitions lead to different estimates" (2006). In a complex model such as this,

> each domain represents a different area of measurement and each category or element of classification within each domain represents a different area of operationalization of the broader domain concept. To generate a meaningful general prevalence measure one must determine which component best reflects the information needed to address the purpose of the data collection. (Mont, 2007, p. 4)

Put simply, the selection of the purpose motivating the data collection determines which definition is to be used. Since disability is a complex, multidimensional experience, the numbers of people with disability and their circumstances (paradoxically) vary both across (e.g., between the *World Health Survey* and the *Global Burden of Disease* study) and within countries (e.g., the earlier instance of the Irish population census as compared to the NDS) influenced by these different approaches to the measuring of disability.

The *contextual factors*. People with the same impairment can perceive very different types and degrees of social participation restrictions and activity limitations depending on context (WHO and World Bank, 2011). According to the ICF

> contextual factors represent the complete background of an individual's life and living. They include two components: Environmental Factors and Personal Factors— which may have an impact on the individual with a health condition and that individual's health and health-related states. (WHO, 2001, p. 22)

Two women, one of whom lives in Stockholm and the other in Kabul, both of whom lost the use of their legs due to a spinal cord injury and are thus reliant on a wheelchair for mobility, would experience their individual functioning and disability in very different ways. The condition of the streets, the availability and accessibility of public transportation, the housing spaces available, and the sociocultural status of and the attitudes toward women would all conspire to make each woman's actions in her current environment drastically different from one another, even though both have the same individual abilities to execute the same actions. In addition to these socioenvironmental factors, which make it so difficult to census disability around the world, one must consider personal factors such as those relating to perceptions of the morbidity of a disease, as well. As the Nobel Prize-winning economist Amartya Sen has stated (1998, 2002), there is a conceptual contrast between health perception versus observation. Tension often exists between internal or subjective views of health and health-related conditions, based on the individual's own perceptions, and external or objective views of that same individual's health status based on the observations of doctors or professionals. In Sen's research into differences in the self-perception of own pathological conditions (also understood as morbidity; Sen, 1998, 2002), North Americans were found to have a morbidity score 10 times higher than that perceived by the people of Bihar, one of the poorest Indian states. According to these results, we should infer that the health conditions of the people of Bihar are better than those of North Americans (Federici and Olivetti Belardinelli, 2006). Therefore, the contextual factors, the third reason affecting the self-perception of disability, are considered to have a strong impact in the way that a same health condition is perceived as disabling.

How many people with a disability are there in the world? Among the adult population, the figure is estimated between 15.6% and 19.4% of the global population. Since "global aging has a major influence on disability trends" (WHO and World Bank, 2011, p. 34) and "one third [2 billion] of the population is forecast to be 60 years and older in 2050" (WHO, 2011, p. vii)—which would be "more than double the number of children in developed countries" (UN, 2007, p. 8)—seriously considering the accessibility of products, services, environments, or facilities is not just a matter of human rights but is an issue of numbers and marketing, as well.

2. It approaches accessibility as a world apart, an optional feature of the interface, instead of a main component of the interaction. In light of this, the access is something that pertains to the technology, without any link to the UX of the interaction.

As we have already discussed in Chapter 2, and underlined in Chapters 4 and 5, the assessment of accessibility does not consist in a test for granting access to people with special needs, but rather it is a necessary step of any kind of interaction evaluation for improving the intrasystemic dialogue between a psychotechnology and any typology of user. Moreover, disabled users, as well as users without disabilities, must be involved by evaluators in an overall assessment of the interaction (i.e., measuring accessibility, usability, and UX).

Therefore, the assessment of accessibility cannot be reduced to an analysis of conformance to the rules, because it is part of a multistep process in which accessibility, usability, and UX are measured by different techniques involving experts' and mixed users' samples (i.e., with and without disability).

The main advantage of this multistep process is that the overall interaction data collected in the assessment, by the evaluator, can be discussed with the designers for concurrently deciding how to modify the product's features and how to optimize the intrasystemic dialogue, in line with the real needs and expectations analyzed by a mixed sample of users. In particular, the involvement of the disabled users in the evaluation cohort, by extending the population of interaction behaviors tested by the evaluator, increases the reliability of the data and generalization of the outcomes, thus providing designers with concrete and reliable evidence for making their decisions.

For this reason, a different perspective—which we call here the "big" accessibility one—has to be taken into account. This approach, in contrast to the "small" accessibility one, endorses the psychotechnological perspective (see Chapter 3) by considering accessibility (as well as usability and UX) as one of the main elements of the intrasystemic dialogue, instead of a feature of the interface. In light of this, the assessment must pertain not only to the features of the product and the needs of the users but also to the measure of the distance between the device and its interface functioning *per se*, and the functioning perceived by the users in the environment of use. This measure can only be obtained by assessing (1) the technology and its functioning *per se*, i.e., accessibility and usability of the product; (2) the interaction as the functioning perceived by the users, i.e., accessibility, usability perceived by the users, and their interaction experience with the product; and (3) the users, i.e., their satisfaction, workload, needs, expectations, attitudes, and skills. Hence, in accordance with the *International Classification of Functioning, Disability and Health* (ICF; WHO, 2001) perspective, we should consider any user, with and without disabilities, as a bearer of a special need consistently with his or her own individual functioning performed in a specific environment of interaction with a psychotechnology (see Box 3.1). As Federici et al. recently pointed out

> it is impossible from this perspective to isolate disability from the functioning of an individual and vice versa, or rather hypothesize one without the other, not only at the level of social organization but also at the level of a single individual. Disability implies functioning and vice versa. (Federici et al., 2012b, p. 12)

For our purposes, we can apply this perspective to the assessment of the interaction with a psychotechnology since the disability has to be considered as a way of functioning among the infinite possibilities of the human functioning that an evaluator has consider when selecting a sample of users which represents, in a reliable way, the overall population of users. Hence, disabled users cannot be involved in the assessment only for analyzing the accessibility of a system, but they have to take an active part in the overall assessment of the psychotechnological interaction. We can consider this approach, under the lens of the ICF's biopsychosocial model, as the big accessibility one. Accessibility is not a "special need" that has to be measured by users with specialness; accessibility is a necessary condition for the interaction between people and psychotechnologies that has to be measured in all its aspects (i.e., objective and subjective) by a sample of users that can represent well the whole possible variety of human functioning (i.e., a mixed sample of users with and without disabilities).

Accessibility, together with usability and UX, are properties of the interaction, and each designer can develop an interface by finding design solutions that can support the users' access, use, and interaction experience without, at the same time, giving up their own creativity. Of course, a final designed solution, which aims to achieve the goal of the Interface For All (Stephanidis, 2001), is a trade-off between both the imagination and the creativity of designers, and the real expectations, attitudes, and needs of users. This trade-off can only be made possible by means of a redesign process that is based on the measure of the distance between the mental model of the designers and the users.

As we discussed in Chapter 5, only an integrated assessment (i.e., the IMIE) composed of experts' and users' analyses can identify and measure this distance. In particular, by aiming to obtain a reliable and generalizable set of data on the overall interaction, evaluators must select a sample of users that can represent as much as possible the end user of a psychotechnology. In line with the IMIE, the exclusion of disability from the sample selection criteria has to be considered a severe mistake: evaluators who do not test a mixed cohort of users (with and without disability) cannot actually guarantee the assessment's reliability, since they may not observe a representative sample of human functioning.

In this chapter, we shall discuss user testing and the procedure for the selection of the assessment sample, showing that the involvement of disabled users is one of the most important resources for the improvement of the simulation process of designers and for the development and the assessment of psychotechnologies.

In order to explain both the role of disabled users in the evaluation and the benefit of creating a mixed sample of users, in the following sections we shall discuss two main issues involved in the design and evaluation decision processes, which are strongly related to the exclusion or inclusion of disabled users in the assessment. In particular, we will describe

1. The simulation processes, i.e., all the processes, driven empirically or through specific models and techniques, for designing and evaluating the interaction relying on a specific model of user
2. Sample selecting rules for the user testing, i.e., all the rules that an evaluator has to consider during the assessment decision process in order to increase the representativeness and the reliability of the evaluation data

6.2 MODELING USERS' INTERACTION BEHAVIOR: THE SIMULATION PROCESS

As we discussed in Chapter 5, the evaluation process is the means for reducing the distance between the interaction of real users with a psychotechnology (i.e., the perceived functioning) and the technology functioning designed by the developers, through a simulation of the possible users' mental models (i.e., the functioning *per se*). As we have already underlined (see Chapter 5), the simulation of human functioning is one of the hardest cognitive processes that a human being can perform that increases its complexity the greater the distance between the simulator mental model and the object of the simulation. The risks of a developer designing an inaccessible psychotechnology become greater as his or her human functioning diverges from the users' functioning. Diversity in functioning/disability, age, culture, gender, etc. increases the distance between the developer's mental model and that of the user, increasing the developer's difficulty in simulating users' actions.

To help designers, manufacturers, and decision makers, many specific simulation techniques and approaches have been created in HCI, such as the human processor models (Card et al., 1986). We can consider simulation models as techniques used in different fields for reducing a system's complexity in a step-by-step process by means of algorithms (Winsberg, 2003, p. 107).

The simulation in HCI is a necessary step for both designers and evaluators:

- Designers have to image the impact of the features and functioning of the psychotechnology in the real world by simulating the behavior, attitudes, habits, and reactions of the possible users (i.e., users' mental models).
- Evaluators have to define a list of selection rules (such as age, expertise, etc.) on the basis of the expected (simulated) end user of the psychotechnology, in order to decide how to assess the product with a sample of users and compare the interaction experienced by real users with the expected interaction designed by the developers.

Designers and evaluators can apply two different kinds of simulation techniques and tools:

1. *Empirical simulation driven by guidelines and principles*: Empirical models composed of lists of rules and principles or scripts, such as, for example, design principles, heuristic lists, and accessibility guidelines. These empirical simulation models rely on a specific model of general end user and, as a consequence, their reliability is based on the degree of agreement with their rules by the national and international community for representing the different skills, abilities, attitudes, and habits of a large population. We can list as empirical models:
   a. *Accessibility standards*, such as WCAG 2.0 and US section 508, which are used for designing systems that, in their functioning, can be accessed by users with different kinds of disabilities and by means of different kinds of assistive technologies (e.g., screen reader), and also for assessing accessibility conformance.
   b. *Design principles and heuristic lists*, which are used as rules (or checklists) in order to analyze and rethink the usability of a system from an end user's perspective, such as Nielsen's heuristics, Tognazzi's principles of interaction design, Shneiderman's golden rules of interface design, and Gerhardt–Powals' principles (for a complete review, see Dix et al., 2004; Gerhardt-Powals, 1996; Hvannberg et al., 2007; Nielsen and Mack, 1994). On the one hand, designers rely on these empirical simulation models during the life cycle to develop a product that matches a model of user (embedded in the rules) and to address the largest possible population of real users. On the other hand, the evaluators rely on those empirical simulation models to assess a device and its interface functioning *per se*.

2. *Predictive simulation driven by estimation models*: Models aimed at representing the human performance during the experience of the interaction with a psychotechnology, by focusing on the subject perception and elaboration of external stimuli. We can divide these models into at least two subgroups:

a. *The human processor models* (Card et al., 1986), which are generally applied for developing and analyzing the performance of a "simulated" user, based on the measure of how long he or she will take to perform a certain task in the system. These models are mostly used for defining a user's standard behavior created by a set of rules and scripts, in order to compare the real users' interaction performances with a baseline. The most famous human processor models are the Goals, Operators, Methods, and Selection rules model (GOMS; see Chapter 1, Box 1.3) and the keystroke-level model (KLM) (for a complete review, see John and Kieras, 1996a). Recently, a new application of this kind of model has been found in the novice-expert model (NEM) (Urokohara et al., 2000), which provides a quantitative measure of the efficiency and effectiveness of an interaction with a system by calculating a performance index obtained by the mean of the times required by a group of novices to achieve a task divided by the mean of the times required by an expert group to achieve the same task.

b. *Estimation models of discovery likelihood.* We can list as predictive simulation all the models applied in the user testing for estimating the outcome reliability. Those models are used for estimating an index that represents the likelihood of discovering interaction problems for each subject of a sample (for a complete review, see Lewis, 1994, 2000, 2001, 2006; Nielsen, 2000; Nielsen and Landauer, 1993; Turner et al., 2006; Urokohara et al., 2000; Virzi, 1990, 1992). We shall briefly present these models in Section 6.3.2., which discusses the representativeness of the sample.

Both the empirical and the predictive simulation models can be used, on the one hand, for supporting developers in the interface design, and, on the other hand, for driving evaluators in the assessment of the product. Nevertheless, even if a simulation can represent the behavior of a certain population of users with a certain degree of validity and accuracy, this kind of process can never replace the information gathered by the analysis of the real users' behavior. The application of the simulation models remains only a support tool that can be applied by a designer or an evaluator for optimizing a system or for harmonizing the expected interaction between a simulated user and technology during the preliminary phase of a product life cycle.

In summary, our thesis is that the simulation has to be seen as a limited resource in which the infinite variability of the human being is reduced to a set of stereotyped users' behaviors. Finally, the use of the simulation processes can support an exhaustive measure of the interaction gathered by real users' evaluations (i.e., the user testing) without replacing it. In light of this, the selection criteria of the sample of users and the representativeness of the data gathered by the real user assessment characterize the quality of the evaluation process. In fact, the selected sample of users determines the measure of the distance (i.e., the interaction problems) between the mental model of designer and the real user.

6.3 DECISION PROCESS FOR USER TESTING: SAMPLE SELECTION AND REPRESENTATIVENESS OF DATA

The involvement and the selection of users, together with the composition of the sample and its representativeness of the overall end user population, is a very hot topic in HCI evaluation studies.

As Thomas S. Tullis and William Albert, respectively, senior vice-president and director of user insight at Fidelity Investments, indicate, one among the most common criticisms of the evaluation studies is that a selected sample does not necessarily represent a larger population of users or the target audience of the product (Tullis and Albert, 2008). The authors suggest that selecting participants for assessing the interaction is a trade-off among different factors, such as "cost, availability, appropriateness, and study goals" (Tullis and Albert, 2008, p. 16).

Starting with Tullis and Albert's considerations, we aim to analyze the relationship between those factors affecting the selection of the users and the evaluation variables affecting the selection of the evaluation techniques (previously discussed in Chapter 5; see Figure 5.9), that is to say: (1) the contextual evaluation variables linked to the relation between the design and evaluation process and the kind of technology under evaluation; (2) the internal evaluation variables due to the limits of the techniques and tools applied in the experts' and users' evaluation; and (3) the behavioral variables related to the sample behavior in the interaction (e.g., number of problems discovered).

Figure 5.1 shows all the factors and variables that an evaluator has to consider for defining a user test. The decision flow starts with an analysis of the appropriateness of the assessment, in which the evaluator defines, in agreement with the designers, the study goals (Figure 6.1, point 1) by a trade-off between the hypothetical goals of the assessment and the available budget.

Usually, the budget is imposed on the evaluator by the customer (who commissions the assessment), while the hypothetical goals are defined according to the following three contextual variables:

1. The kind of interface under assessment and its features. For instance, the interaction and the environmental variables that an evaluator has to consider when he or she assesses a game for a touch screen mobile phone are different from those affecting the evaluation of the same game in the version for computer or for console
2. The developmental stage of the product under assessment (i.e., formative or summative)
3. The kind of life cycle and the relation between the designers and the evaluators

The final goals of the study drive evaluators to define the users' profile (Figure 6.1, point 2), and all the possible techniques and tools employed for the assessment

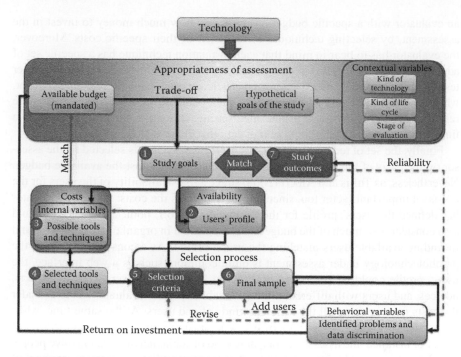

FIGURE 6.1 (See color insert.) User testing decision flow. By starting from the technology and the appropriateness of the assessment, and considering the overall cost against the budget, the evaluator defines (1) the study goals, (2) the users' profile, (3) the possible evaluation techniques, (4) the final techniques and tools, and (5) the selection criteria. On the basis of these criteria, the final sample (point 6) is involved in the assessment and the final outcomes (point 7) are matched with the study goals. During the assessment, the evaluator can improve the reliability of the study by monitoring the users' behavior in discovering problems (behavioral variables) in order to add more users to the sample (in line with the users' profile), or by revising the sample selection criteria for including other kinds of users in the sample. At the same time, at the end of the assessment, the evaluator can use the gathered data to analyze the evaluation return on investment.

(Figure 6.1, point 3). The techniques and tools for the assessment (Figure 6.1, point 4) are selected by considering the overall costs of the assessment against the budget.

The costs of the assessment are generally defined by considering the cost and the kind of analysis of the possible evaluation techniques (i.e., the internal variables), estimating the number of subjects needed for the analysis (users or experts), the time required for data collection and analysis, and the costs for a coordinator (Bias and Mayhew, 2005). In light of this, the costs and the selected evaluation technique (Figure 6.1, point 4) are in a mutual relationship in which the costs against the budget influence the choice of technique, and the technique's internal variables affect costs. For instance, it is a quite common assumption that a heuristic analysis carried out by experts is cheaper than a cognitive walkthrough, as a remote user testing is cheaper than a thinking-aloud analysis (Bias and Mayhew, 2005). As a consequence, an evaluator with a specific budget has to decide how much money to invest in the assessment, by selecting techniques on the basis of their specific costs. Moreover, the evaluator has to bear in mind that each evaluation technique has a specific set of advantages and limits (i.e., internal variables); e.g., an evaluator using a remote user testing obtains data on effectiveness and efficiency in an uncontrolled environment, while with a thinking-aloud analysis, the data obtained by a practitioner are more reliable since the users are in a controlled setting. Of course, the evaluator selects a final set of techniques in order to obtain data that achieve study goals.

Finally, the set of techniques and tools for the assessment is selected by the assessor on the basis of the goals of the study and the costs against the available budget. Nevertheless, as Tullis and Albert (2008) suggest, the availability of the users for the test is an important factor too, since it directly affects the costs: When an evaluator has defined the users' profile for the testing (Figure 6.1, point 2), he or she should also consider how much of the budget will be invested in organizing the analysis and in finding available users matching the users' profile. As a consequence, when the psychotechnology under assessment is quite common, such as a web interface, the users' profile could be composed of different kinds of end users, such as experts, novices, and users with different kinds of disabilities. The evaluator has to consider the costs for recruiting all the different kinds of end users. At the same time, when the product is a new one or an innovative one, it can require a very specific kind of user. For instance, the assessment of a new kind of social network can involve people less than 25 years old with a certain level of Internet addiction; or the assessment of a new kind of game can involve users that spend more than 3 h per day on gaming activities. In these cases, the evaluator may find it very difficult to recruit users that are available for composing the sample and, as a consequence, the overall evaluation costs increase.

In summary, the evaluator defines the evaluation techniques (Figure 6.1, point 4) by considering the overall costs of the assessment (i.e., availability and internal variables) against the budget and the goals of the study. Thus, the evaluator can define the selection criteria (Figure 6.1, point 5), which are a direct product of the selected techniques (Figure 6.1, point 4) and the users' profile (Figure 6.1, point 2). These selection criteria are used for composing the final sample (Figure 6.1, point 6), thus determining the final outcomes of the users' assessment (Figure 6.1, point 7). In fact, on the basis of the selection criteria, the evaluator defines which kinds of users have to be tested, and how to discriminate their data in order to achieve the study goals and to generalize the assessment outcomes. As we shall discuss in the following sections, user testing and, consequently, the generalization of the assessment data may be affected by the behavioral variables of the evaluation (i.e., the ability of users to identify interaction problems). During the assessment, the evaluator can monitor users' behavior in discovering problems by applying specific estimation models for analyzing the representativeness of the sample composed by the end user population. Through this analysis, the evaluator can check and revise the selection criteria (Figure 6.1, point 5) and add new users to the evaluation cohort (Figure 6.1, point 6) when the sample does not represent the overall population in a reliable way. In light of this, the core step of this decision flow is the selection process because it defines the quality of the final outcomes (Figure 6.1, point 7).

At the end of the process, the final outcomes (Figure 6.1, point 7) are matched with the study goals (Figure 6.1, point 1), and the individual likelihoods of encountering a problem (i.e., behavioral variables) can be used by a practitioner for checking how much of the budget has really been invested in achieving the study goals and how much of it has been wasted on unreliable tests (i.e., the return on investment [ROI]).

In conclusion, the selection has to be considered as the core process of the user testing decision flow, since it determines the behavior of the final sample. The users' profile, the possible discrimination of the data, and the generalizability of the outcomes are the three main keys to obtain reliable and useful data from the users' testing (Tullis and Albert, 2008). We shall describe and discuss these components in the following section.

6.3.1 THREE KEYS FOR MONITORING PARTICIPANTS' SELECTION PROCESS

According to Tullis and Albert (2008), an evaluator has to answer three key questions when he or she is going to create a sample:

- *Question 1: Do participants represent the target audience of the product?* In other words, is the users' profile complete and have the selection criteria been respected during the users' selection? Tullis and Albert answer this question with the following example: "If you're designing a new medical application for doctors to use in their practices, try to get practicing physicians as your participants. In some situations, however, you may have to settle for participants who are only close approximations of the target users. In those cases, be aware of the limitations of the data you collect. Many of the statistics you will calculate assume that the sample data reflects the larger population" (Tullis and Albert, 2008, p. 16).
- *Question 2: How can participants' data be separated and analyzed in distinct groups?* In other words, can users' data be managed and compared in line with the study goals? Tullis and Albert (2008) suggest that a practitioner can analyze the data of the participants separately by dividing the sample by participants' demographic data (e.g., gender, age, status, etc.), their kind of interaction with the product (e.g., use of particular functionality or features), their level of expertise (i.e., novice, intermediate, expert), and their frequency of use (e.g., number of web visits or interactions per month).
- *Question 3: Can I generalize the data gathered?* In other words, do the gathered users' data represent the overall population of users? Tullis and Albert (2008) suggest that, in order to gather data that represent the overall user population, a practitioner has to organize a sampling strategy, such as, for example, a randomization strategy, which guarantees the reliability of the assessment.

Although we totally agree with Tullis and Albert (2008) when they suggest that practitioners should select participants from within the target audience of the technology, we have to underline that in an interaction test it is not always clear who should be the end user of a technology. For instance, by following the example proposed by the authors, and described earlier in point 1, the target audience of a medical device can be seen as the specialist that has to use it, but, at the same time, we can also list the medical staff that have to manage it and the patients that will undergo the treatment as possible end users. With other technologies, such as for newspaper websites, the virtual population of end users cannot be identified just by considering the users' age or status or their frequency of use; it is also necessary to take into consideration the possibility that end users may be elderly and/or disabled users. Of course, for certain kinds of technology, it might be easier to define a user's profile. For instance, the end users for a hearing aid might be identified as a certain percentage of deaf users, with the specific characteristics usually identified by a market analysis. Nevertheless, in this case, there are also a lot of questions to which an evaluator has to respond: Is there a cutoff for selecting and excluding subjects? In which contexts of use must a practitioner test the interaction with the product?

Considering these questions, we can say that the target market of a product can be used as a reference point for composing the evaluation cohort, but it is not enough for defining a complete users' profile. When practitioners aim to analyze how a product works with the most probable buyers and/or users, the users' profile will coincide with the user model defined by marketing analyses. As the director of Frontend.com, Frank Long (2009), claims, these kinds of users' models, known as "personas," are

> fictional user archetypes based on user research. Through a process of analysis and refinement, the data from user interviews is distilled into one or multiple fictitious characters. Each character is developed in realistic detail, and how that character wants to interact with the design is described as task scenarios. (Long, 2009, p. 1)

Although the use of the personas allows designers to simulate users' requirements by strongly focusing the design on the users' characteristics, the simulation is a useful tool that cannot, however, replace the real users' interaction analysis, as we discussed earlier. Evaluators well know that the "expected" users, or personas, rarely coincide with the real end users of the psychotechnology in the real world.

Let us exemplify our discussion with a brief assessment case:

An evaluator has to assess a hearing aid designed to be as hidden as possible from other people and esthetically accepted by consumers. In order to create a users' profile, the evaluator asks the designers what kind of personas are being used for developing the product. The developers report that the product has been designed following a list of personas, with different functioning and personal characteristics, created on the basis of the following market target: people from 15 to 40 years old, with a certain degree X of deafness.

We aim here to underline that the evaluator can assess the product by selecting a group of participants from within the target market, obtaining, in this way, reliable data. However, there are also good reasons for including other "divergent" participants within the sample, such as, e.g.: (1) consumers between 41 and 80 years old, who could be interested in buying the product and (2) caregivers, who have to manage and store the product for end users with other impairments associated with deafness. Continuing with the previous assessment case example:

The evaluator, according to the recommendations of the U.S. Food and Drug Administration guidelines for medical device development (2011), has to validate the device—i.e., analyze the usability and safety of the product in line with ISO/IEC 62366 (2007)—by testing at least 15 participants per possible major group of users (i.e., specialists, doctors, patients, etc.) or with the major group of users with distinctly different characteristics (e.g., use responsibilities, age ranges, skill sets, or experience levels). In our case, the evaluator decides to create 2 groups of 15 users each: the first group is composed of users that match the target, whereas the second group is composed of users with different characteristics, such as a different age from the target (i.e., outside of the target). These 30 subjects allow the practitioner to gather data about interaction problems that can affect the users' experience of the aids, considering a large set of possible behaviors and needs that are in line with the marketing target and outside the target. In this way, the practitioner can include in the evaluation report: (1) how to meet the real users' needs and how to solve specific problems that can affect the interaction of users, in and outside the target and (2) how to adapt the aid to a broad range of consumers' needs, attitudes, habits, and skills, thus increasing the possibility of technological success.

In summary, to answer the question about when participants represent the target audience of the product, the evaluators should consider the goals of their study by focusing the assessment on testing a representative set of possible interaction behavior in line with the budget. The users' profiling is a key factor of the sample selection and the personas taken into account for designing a reliable starting point product usable by profiling users. However, a complete interaction evaluation aims to analyze as much as possible all the possible divergent behaviors of interaction with a psychotechnology, by running a sort of "stress test" of the product. In light of this, the evaluator has to include in the sample not only participants that fit to a certain degree the "expected" end users, but also other typologies of virtual consumers in different contexts of use.

Finally, turning to the last two questions proposed by Tullis and Albert (2008), after the sample composition, a practitioner also has to consider how to discriminate between the different participants to analyze data (see Question 2 mentioned earlier) and how to generalize the evaluation outcomes (see Question 3 mentioned earlier).

In the interaction evaluation studies, the separation of data is mainly focused on discriminating the participants' expertise in the use of the technology, measured by the time spent in interaction and by the frequency of use, and the differences within users' interaction styles (Howard et al., 2001; Mendelson and Papacharissi, 2004; Turkle, 1995; Weiser, 2001). In particular, expertise is generally considered one of the most important factors that can affect the interaction experience with a psychotechnology; however, some other factors may also play a role in the assessment: age and gender, spatial memory and reasoning abilities, learning style, and cultural background (Nielsen, 1993). In light of this, we can claim that the discrimination of the participants' data mostly depends on what the evaluators are looking at.

Finally, practitioners, in agreement with designers, and respecting the budget and the features of the product under assessment, have to identify how to discriminate the data of the users' assessment by considering different factors, such as their age, their expertise, their disability, etc. Furthermore, as we shall discuss in the next section, a key factor for deciding how the participant data can be used for redesigning a psychotechnology is the degree of reliability of the evaluation outcomes.

6.3.2 REPRESENTATIVENESS OF THE SAMPLE

Recently, Borsci et al. (2012a) defined the representativeness of the sample in the interaction evaluation as the degree to which errors or problems identified by a sample represent the problems that can be identified by all the virtual users of a specific product. As Tullis and Albert (2008) suggest, while sample randomization is a necessary step for any kind of evaluation process, for the specific purpose of the interaction assessment the randomization procedure is not enough for guaranteeing the reliability of the data gathered. In fact, in the interaction evaluation, the sample representativeness not only concerns the personal characteristics of the users involved in the test but also the degree to which the possible interactive behaviors of the entire population is represented by the selected sample. By testing a sample, practitioners aim to identify a certain percentage of UX problems. Therefore, the participants' ability to discover problems represents the efficiency and the effectiveness of the evaluation.

During the evolution of HCI, many different models have been created for estimating the problem discovery likelihood, such as the ROI model, the Good–Turing (GT) procedure, the bootstrap discovery behavior (BDB) model, and the logit-zero truncate model (for a complete review, see Borsci et al., 2012a). By considering different parameters, these models are used for increasing the accuracy of the p-value estimation (i.e., the average percentage of errors discovered by one user). The p-value is used in the following error distribution formula to estimate the percentage of problems identified by the users during an interaction:

$$D = 1 - (1 - p)^N \tag{6.1}$$

where
   D is the percentage of problems discovered by the sample
   N is the number of subjects

When the p-value is equal to or greater than 0.3 (i.e., the standard), the sample has a high ability in discovering problems. Sometimes this topic is discussed as a five-user assumption and is presented as follows: "How many users are needed for obtaining a certain number (e.g., between 80% and 85%) of the interaction problems in a user testing?" According to Borsci et al. (2012a), it depends on the behavior of the sample. In fact, there is no minimum number of users that can assure a practitioner that a sample reaches $p \geq 0.3$. For instance, if in a sample that is composed of six users all the subjects identify the same five problems, the p-value is certainly over 0.3, because all the problems are evident and have a high impact on the interaction. So, by considering the homogenous behavior of the sample, the practitioner can report to the designers' team that they must solve these problems before reevaluating the prototype. Otherwise, if the behavior of these six users is not homogenous (as represented in Table 6.1), the practitioner has to apply the estimation models, calculating

TABLE 6.1

A Hypothetical Sample of Six Users That Has Identified Five Problems of Interaction

Subjects	Problem 1	Problem 2	Problem 3	Problem 4	Problem 5	p-Value
1	1	0	0	0	0	0.2
2	0	1	0	0	0	0.2
3	0	0	0	0	0	0
4	0	0	0	0	0	0
5	0	0	1	1	1	0.6
6	1	0	1	0	0	0.4
					Raw p	0.23

Note: The subjective behavior in discovering problems is considered as a binary issue, in which "0" corresponds to a problem/error not found by a subject and "1" corresponds to a problem/error found by a subject. The evaluator uses this table for estimating the raw p-value of the sample.

the p-value in order to analyze the representativeness of the sample. In Table 6.1, the raw p-value is equal to 0.23; this value is usually applied for calculating the ROI. In this case, the model indicates that at least two other subjects are needed for reaching the 80%–85% of the interface problems, albeit we have to consider that in literature many studies (Borsci et al., 2011, 2012a; Caulton, 2001; Faulkner, 2003; Lewis, 1994; Schmettow, 2008, 2012; Spool and Schroeder, 2001; Woolrych and Cockton, 2001) underline that the ROI model overestimates the discovery likelihood.

We shall discuss the models for estimating the index p and their limits in Chapter 7, by proposing a grounded procedure (GP). This technique, for organizing and managing the sample representativeness, uses the average p-value empirically obtained by the application of the different estimation models in order to avoid the overestimation of the classic raw p applied in the ROI model. In this section, we intend to underline that, when selecting a sample, a practitioner must aim to collect the larger set of subjective behaviors, in order to enlarge the representativeness of the sample to the entire population of end users. According to this framework, the involvement of disabled users in mixed samples is a resource for the evaluators, since a sample with different personal characteristics in functioning and disability enrich sample representativeness measuring divergent interaction behaviors. In fact, by discovering and experiencing divergent problems of users with different personal functioning and disabilities, the probability of a sample fitting the behavior of a larger population is extended.

6.4 SIMULATION AND SELECTION OF DISABLED USERS FOR COMPOSING MIXED SAMPLES

We have previously clarified that, in the design and the evaluation processes of a psychotechnology, disability is not to be considered as a special need to take into account for respecting the guidelines or the national laws, but one of the possible ways of human functioning and, at the same time, a resource for the assessment of the overall interaction experience.

By moving from the "hypothetical end user" imagined by designers, practitioners have to select users that are "in and outside" the target market of the product under evaluation, by embedding in the sample users with different levels of individual functioning and disability—i.e., with cognitive, physical, and sensory impairment and nondisabled—skills, attitudes, and degree of expertise in the use of the technology under evaluation. These mixed samples (i.e., in or outside the target) are not selected by aiming to fit the "simulated end users" but, conversely, for representing as much as possible the virtual population of the users' interaction behaviors. In this framework, disability becomes a selection criterion that can be used together with the frequency, the expertise in use, and the predisposition to use for composing a sample.

In contrast to the other subjective variables, disability and disabled users' interaction are very hard for designers to simulate and anticipate. As previously discussed in Chapter 5, since the cognitive simulation of a psychotechnological interaction is a process in which someone (i.e., the designer) has to take the perspective of someone else, through a lot of imaginative effort, a question arises: How can someone realistically simulate something that he or she can hardly imagine, as in the case of a disabled user's interaction simulated by a nondisabled practitioner or vice versa? Related to this question is the advice given by Shawn Lawton Henry—leader at the W3C for the promotion of web accessibility for people with disabilities—to both designers and evaluators for taking into account the perspective of disabled users

> don't make assumptions about people or their disabilities. Don't assume you know what someone wants, what he feels, or what is best for him. If you have a question about what to do, how to do it, what language or terminology to use, or what assistance to offer, ask him. That person should be your first and best resource. (Henry, 2007, p. 21)

In other words, by endorsing the well-known motto of the disabled users' associations, "Nothing about us, without us" (Charlton, 1998), we can readapt the same motto by extending it to the interaction context as "nothing is for all, without us" (Borsci et al., 2012a).

In summary, we can suggest two steps for including a realistic disabled perspective in the product life cycle:

1. Designers should involve disabled users during the design as stakeholders, in order to analyze their needs and expectations, thus enlarging the features of the prototype and its functioning *per se* and the model of the users simulated by the designers (i.e., the personas).
2. After the release of the prototype, evaluators should perform an evaluation with a mixed sample of users in an iterative cycle, until the release of the final product.

One of the risks in promoting the disabled users' assessment as a resource for the evaluation consists in the possibility that practitioners, directly or indirectly, could assume that for testing disabled users, for example, blind people, and solving their interaction problems, it is enough to report that the interface has a good level of accessibility and usability for all the blind users. We have to clarify that a practitioner should not confuse a person with his or her own disability. For instance, testing an interface with a sample of 25-year-old users does not mean that the interface will be accessible and usable for all users of the same age; and testing an interface with a sample of blind users does not mean that the product will be accessible and usable for all blind users. As Henry underlines,

> people with disabilities have different preferences. Just because one person with a disability prefers something one way doesn't mean that another person with the same disability also prefers it that way. (2007, p. 21)

We aim to underline that the generalization of the evaluation data gathered does not depend only on the kind of subjects making up the sample but also on their discovery likelihood (i.e., the sample representativeness). In fact, disability is an important resource for extending the possibility of the sample representativeness in a test and retest cycle, whereas the generalization of the evaluation outcomes mostly depends on the quality and on the quantity of the problems identified by the users' sample. In light of this, it is not enough to test the interaction with a sample of disabled users (e.g., blind) to report that the interface is accessible and usable for all blind users, but the practitioner must also analyze the discovery behavior of the cohort, in order to measure the sample's representativeness of the overall population, to indicate to the designers, with a certain level of confidence, how the intrasystemic dialogue works with all the possible blind users.

6.5 TESTING DISABLED USERS

In the previous chapter, we discussed at length the selection of the users and in particular how a practitioner has to involve disabled and nondisabled users equally in each step of the assessment process, from the recruitment of subjects until the final product evaluation. However, it is still necessary to analyze how to test and compare disabled users' data with those of users without disability.

Due to the nature of the disability of the users involved in the evaluation sample, practitioners have to select the evaluation techniques, bearing in mind that, at the end of the assessment, it will be necessary to manage all users' data gathered as a comparable data. While, for example, we can test users with physical disabilities by means of a concurrent thinking aloud, thus providing data that are comparable to users without disability, this technique may be a non-natural way of interaction for persons with other kinds of disabilities, such as blind people, and it could therefore affect their evaluation. Moreover, people with intellectual or cognitive disabilities may have speech or reading problems (e.g., aphasic and dyslexic users), or a low degree of attention, quickly reaching a cognitive overload in multitasking actions (e.g., Down's syndrome users).

Usually, studies on disabled users' interaction are mostly focused on understanding how disabled users interact instead of investigating how to involve users in the evaluation of psychotechnological interaction (see Bohman and Anderson, 2005; Fairweather and Trewin, 2010; Feng et al., 2008, 2010). This shortcoming opens a research space in HCI on different possible ways to test disabled users' psychotechnological interaction, by respecting their functioning and equalizing the data gathered from these users with those obtained from users without disability. Currently, specific tools such as eye-trackers (see Chapter 8), involving users in a silent evaluation, are often used for testing users with different typologies of disability. However, the limit of this kind of evaluation is that the users cannot directly identify or verbalize the problems they are experiencing during the psychotechnological interaction. At the same time, as Federici et al. have shown (Federici et al., 2010a,b), it is possible to create methods adapted to the users' functioning, as for blind users with partial concurrent thinking aloud (see Chapter 8).

The development of the methods used to evaluate the psychotechnological interaction of disabled users is one of the most interesting future fields for HCI. Since in current societies psychotechnologies are becoming every day more pervasive, the challenge of including disabled users in the evaluation, in order to reach the Interface For All aim, is today a crucial issue. This pervasive presence concerns not only the personal use of psychotechnologies for socialization (see Chapter 3), such as the Internet and mobile phones, but also the use of technologies for education, work, health, and home environments, which increases more and more every day. The increasing presence of technologies in everyday life contexts without a concurrent increase of their accessibility, usability, and UX of the interaction—which are necessary conditions to transform the systems into psychotechnological intrasystemic solutions—enlarges the social and environmental exclusion instead of leveling the human possibilities.

6.6   CONCLUSION

In this chapter, we proposed a big accessibility approach for HCI design and assessment in which accessibility is not a "special need" that has to be measured by users with specialness. We suggested, in tune with our psychotechnological perspective, that the involvement of disabled users in interaction design and assessment is a necessary condition for measuring the interaction between people and psychotechnologies in all its aspects (i.e., objective and subjective), by representing the whole possible variety of human functioning (i.e., a mixed sample of users with and without disability). In light of this, disability in the HCI field must be considered as a way of functioning among the infinite possibilities of human functioning that an evaluator has to consider when selecting a sample of users. In our big accessibility perspective, disabled users are an important resource for assessing and improving the intrasystemic relationship between user and technology. As we discussed earlier, the evaluator can only obtain reliable and generalizable data, with a certain level of representativeness of the overall population, by investing the budget in selecting users with different functioning in order to test the interface with mixed samples. In fact, for helping designers to make decisions during the product life cycle, evaluators should discuss with developers on the basis of reliable data that can represent as much as possible the overall population of end users.

In conclusion, we propose that pervasive psychotechnologies can match the aim of inclusive societies only by fulfilling the "Interface For All" aim. This goal can be reached only by involving disabled users in both the assessment and design process in order to develop psychotechnologies that are able to reduce the problems that affect the intrasystemic dialogue between any kind of user and a given technology.

7 How You Can Set Up and Perform an Interaction Evaluation *Rules and Methods*

7.1 WHAT IS THE EVALUATION PROCESS?

In Chapters 5 and 6, we described our IMIE model and the variables a practitioner must consider in assessing the intrasystemic dialogue between users and technology. In light of the previous discussion, this chapter aims to present a means by which to set up and manage an integrated evaluation process (i.e., IMIE). In particular, as we underlined in Chapter 2, a complete evaluation process should include measures and techniques for assessing the three dimensions of the interaction—accessibility, usability, and the user experience (UX). These three dimensions are organized in a hierarchical manner, so that nothing can be considered "usable" if it is not already accessible and, at the same time, we cannot arrive at a realistic measure of UX without measuring and solving first the accessibility and subsequently the usability problems. As was noted in Chapter 6, although the accessibility assessment plays a part in the evaluation process as well, our focus in this handbook is on depicting a complete procedure that may be used by evaluators in order to assess usability and the UX. To achieve this goal, we shall analyze the rules and methods of these two dimensions of the interaction.

Bearing in mind that the assessment of UX includes, but is not exhaustively measured by means of, the usability assessment, we must first clarify exactly what we mean in attempting to "evaluate" the interaction if we are to fully explain how to apply the usability and UX assessment techniques. Due to its empirical nature, evaluation of the interaction is in fact often considered by lay people and by professionals not directly involved in the assessment process as a simple collection of users' elicited criticisms about an interface or a product use cycle. This kind of a folk psychological approach can result in wrong ideas as to what an evaluation process is and its value.

The set of beliefs and interpretations people use in everyday contexts in order to predict and explain behaviors play an important role in daily life (Malle and Knobe, 1997; Wellman, 1990). This kind of "common knowledge among us" (Lewis, 1999, p. 258) constitutes an important framework within which we attempt to fit ourselves to the real context through a process of assessment and adaptation. Nevertheless, we cannot confuse the processes behind the evaluation of the interaction and those we apply in everyday life. In fact, in our life, to criticize or elicit judgment can be considered either a direct or indirect assessment, while an interaction assessment is a rigorous and well-structured process of evaluation in which, together with the user's verbalizations concerning the interaction problems, a practitioner gathers a set of objective measures via specific techniques and tools.

Some evaluators may have experienced a gap between their expertise and approach and the expertise and approaches of other professionals (i.e., designers, clients, marketing experts, etc.), which in turn might lead them to assume that an evaluation is a collection of criticisms about a product. We may claim, for instance, that a strong commonsense approach is behind the idea that the UCD is a trial-and-error design process that is "followed by repeated corrections and adjustments guided by checking with users" (Constantine, 2004, p. 3), instead of a rigorous process of design and evaluation. At the same time, this approach can be identified in the broadly shared belief among lay people that a discounted analysis is better than nothing in attempting to improve a product, because "any data is data" (Nielsen, 1994b), and so an evaluator can organize an evaluation by gathering suggestions and impressions about the use of a product from a group of three or five randomly selected users.

In order to clarify the distance between the commonsense approach and a psychotechnological evaluation process, in the next sections we shall describe the difference between subjective criticisms and everyday judgments, as well as describing a well-structured process of assessment. We shall then describe how an evaluation process differs from an evaluation technique, in part by underscoring the fact that, while a technique is composed of measurements and criteria applied by professionals in order to perform an assessment, an evaluation process is composed of a set of techniques. Finally, we shall describe how practitioners can control users' goal achievement during an evaluation test. On the basis of this analysis, we shall introduce and discuss the evaluation of UX and the usability.

7.1.1 Significance of Evaluation: From Commonsense to Evaluation Criteria

The acts of evaluating and judging are psychological processes that shape the ways in which human beings behave and interact with the world in their daily lives. We do not intend to enter into a discussion about the cognitive processes and the psychological and sociological factors behind human decision making; in order to understand why the act of evaluating something cannot be reduced to a collection of the users' judgments, however, we have to exemplify the difference between everyday criticisms and judgments and the critiques and comments elicited from users as they assess a product. On the basis of our perceptions and previous experiences, for instance, we are able to predict whether an event is about to occur—e.g., it is going to rain—and, as a consequence, we may either make a decision related to our prediction—e.g., we go out with an umbrella—or analyze a contextual situation as informed by our judgments, such as (1) "I'm out and it is raining, unfortunately I do not have an umbrella" (judgment), so (2) "I have to run until I find some cover" (decision), and (3) "in order to avoid becoming ill" (reason on the basis of previous experience). Such decision processes are based on our natural tendency to assess and judge events and to apply these judgments in assessing objects and their use in context. When we interact with different technologies, we are accustomed to expressing criticisms and complains such as "The button on this smartphone is too small," "the procedure to set up the recording of a TV program takes too many steps," and "the 'EXIT' button is not easy to find on the screen." Such criticisms represent users' actual perceptions of an interaction. In sum, criticisms are simply the act of pointing out the inadequacies and defects of the design and they will always be present. On the other hand, an evaluation is a structured process that deals with the information about the inadequacies and defects as perceived by users engaged in an intrasystemic dialogue in order to send back to the design team feedback about the product pertaining to its effectiveness, efficiency, and ability to satisfy users' expectations.

In our daily lives, we are not able to determine *a priori* other people's goals, but we can guess at and anticipate peoples' intentions before the action on the basis of our cognitive structures and processes, as in the case of brain activity that involves mirror neurons (Buccino et al., 2001; di Pellegrino et al., 1992; Rizzolatti and Arbib, 1998). At the same time, in assessing other people's actions and their processes of goal achievement, we may infer their intentions *ex post*, on the basis of their final achievement, by concurrently assessing the efficiency and effectiveness of their actions in achieving the said goal.

As opposed to real life, during an interactive evaluation process, evaluators must know *a priori* the goals of the users and the steps they must take in order to achieve those goals. In light of this, the observing of the interaction in real-use contexts is a useful means of obtaining data about the use of a product and the UX, but it is not enough for a UX or a usability evaluation. In fact, together with ethological approaches, evaluators must associate other techniques that involve users in a more controlled environment by using a range of different techniques (i.e., the IMIE model).

Although gathering users' judgments and observing their interactions can be enough for an evaluation in the commonsense approach, in the human–computer interaction (HCI), the assessment is considered to be a complex process based on a mixed set of measures and criteria.

Although the distinction between gathering user criticism and assessing the interaction is clear for evaluators, this is often less clear for both designers and users. From the designer's point of view, given that the evaluation report could be perceived as a collection of criticisms, it is sometimes difficult for the design team to "neutrally" accept the feedback for a variety of reasons, including the following:

1. *A management problem*: Only a limited period of time is available before the release of the product or service, and no time is left for product assessments or redesigns. The evaluation report, therefore, can be perceived as a barrier to the market release of the product.
2. *A miscommunication between the designers and evaluators*: Designers may feel insulted and become unpleasant when exposed to negative feedback as reported by evaluators. The evaluation report, therefore, can be perceived as an aggressive set of judgments of the designers' skills and their professional role.

3. *An underestimation of the evaluation process*: Designers do not have the time or simply do not want to read the evaluation report. The evaluation is perceived only as a means of checking the most complex design processes. The assessment is therefore seen only as a minimal step that cannot improve the real performance of the technology or product.

As has been discussed earlier, in Chapter 4, the gap between designers and evaluators in relation to the management of the (re)design and (re)evaluation phases can be bridged only by adopting a psychotechnological perspective in which the relationship between designers and evaluators is equalized by the creation of a new communication space focused on the intrasystemic dialogue that occurs between users and technology. It is important that designers cooperate with evaluators in order to achieve the highest possible level of usability; this can be facilitated by their understanding that the evaluation is not a set of user complaints, but rather a set of useful feedbacks meant to help them improve the intrasystemic dialogue and ensure the success of the technology on the market. A simple strategy to create this communication space would be to involve designers in a collaborative atmosphere by inviting them to the evaluation site and letting them observe the interactions of actual users with the product they have designed.

The participants' perception and comprehension of the assessment's aims are also important. Independent of the evaluation technique applied for the analysis, practitioners, therefore, inform participants that their skills are not under assessment, because the goal of the evaluation is not to assess either the users or the technology, but the dialogue between the two. It is important that participants genuinely understand that practitioners are not looking for their complaints about the product or for affirmation of the quality of the designers' work. It is therefore very important that practitioners provide participants with as much detail as possible about the interface under assessment, the evaluation procedure, the resultant measurements, and the tools they will use to gather data. At the same time, an evaluator should remark to the users both before and after the assessment that the primary aim of the test is to understand their actual perceptions of the interaction and their reactions to the problems they might have experienced in using the product. Finally, it is important that practitioners remark upon the distance from a commonsense notion of evaluation by explaining that an evaluation process is based on specific measures and criteria (i.e., evaluation techniques) and that the users' judgments about the product are only one aspect of the overall assessment process.

7.1.2 EVALUATION IN TERMS OF MEASUREMENTS AND CRITERIA

The measurement process plays a fundamental role in any evaluation process designed to provide a practitioner with a criterion and a unit of measure by which to assess an interaction as efficient or inefficient, effective or ineffective, satisfactory or unsatisfactory, and, moreover, by which to categorize the product under consideration, as good or bad, adequate or inadequate, or acceptable or unacceptable. In line with the overall aim of the evaluation and the budget, the evaluation technique selected by practitioners should provide evaluators with a specific set

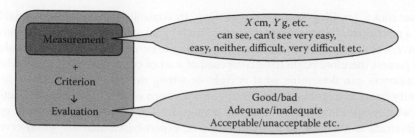

FIGURE 7.1 Each evaluation process is composed of methods and techniques designed to obtain quantitative or qualitative units of measure (i.e., measurements) and methods and technique to use in interpreting such units (i.e., criteria).

of measurements composed of either or both a quantitative unit (e.g., centimeters, grams, etc.) and a qualitative unit (e.g., the user's elicitation, "I can see" or "I cannot see," or the ratings of a sale as "very easy, easy, neither, difficult, or very difficult"; see Chapter 6, Figure 6.1 for more information about the selecting of techniques in user testing). Moreover, the selected technique must provide a criterion by which the evaluators will be able to gather and interpret quantitative or qualitative units for assessing the interaction. In other words, the evaluation technique is a combination of the criterion and the measurement, as shown in Figure 7.1.

As discussed in Chapter 5 (Section 5.2), the evaluation process has a threshold by which we can judge and classify the aspects of the interaction under assessment. The evaluators can interpret the data on the basis of the technique selected for the assessment, because the evaluation technique will determine the measurements and the criteria applied in analyzing the quality traits of the interaction. Last, according to the psychotechnological approach, in order to obtain an overall assessment of the UX, practitioners should not use only single and separate techniques but instead a set of integrated techniques that compose an IMIE—i.e., a process of integrated measurements and criteria. In Chapter 5, we identified three main kinds of analysis a practitioner should use to create an IMIE:

- Expert-based analysis, which concerns elements of the system's features and functioning, such as the expected effectiveness and efficiency of use as simulated by professionals using specific tools (e.g., heuristic lists, cognitive walkthroughs, etc.)
- User-based analysis, which concerns the measuring of the effectiveness and efficiency of the system the user interacts with, gathered through techniques such as thinking aloud
- Analysis of users' perceptions of the quality of the intrasystemic dialogue as gathered by explicit or implicit measures, such as psychometric tools, questionnaires, biofeedback, etc.

In order to apply all of these kinds of analysis during the assessment, any evaluator should define and control for both the users' tasks and all of the steps users must complete when interacting with the system in order to achieve their goals (e.g., mouse clicks, scrolling, searching, etc.). Only by controlling for these two variables can a practitioner determine the process of users' goal achievement and, as a consequence, which part of the product users are going to perceive and assess. An evaluation process therefore ought to be composed of a set of controlled analyses, in which practitioners can determine what is right or wrong during the users' interaction, identify errors and problems, and distinguish between what is efficient and effective and what is not. Finally, the evaluators' management of the users' processes of goal achievement is a key factor in simulating (i.e., expert-based analysis) or observing (i.e., user-based analysis) the potential problems experienced by users through the measurement of the deviation from the correct set of steps in terms of time, number of clicks, etc.

7.1.3 PROCESS OF GOAL ACHIEVEMENT AND ITS ASSESSMENT

As discussed earlier, during the assessment of the interaction, the evaluators cannot hypothesize the end users' intentions, especially when the practitioner's aim is to test the effectiveness and efficiency of the interaction. Conversely, evaluators should control for the variables that affect the interaction by providing goals to the participants either directly or indirectly (e.g., scenarios). In this sense, while some techniques contained within an evaluation process can be used to obtain qualitative information, practitioners will use other techniques to measure users' deviations from the correct pathway toward goal achievement. As Kurosu (2012a) has suggested, we can graphically represent the process of goal achievement (Figure 7.2) by imagining a distance between the initial state of the user (i.e., when a user starts the task) and the goal state in a conceptual space (i.e., when a user thinks he or she has achieved the goal of the task). In order to bridge the gap between the initial and the goal states, users try to achieve the goal by interacting with the product while relying on their motivation, previous expertise, and understanding of the scenario.

Users will sometimes fail to achieve the goal, as shown by the dotted line in Figure 7.2; in other scenarios, they will reach the goal but only via a long and winding

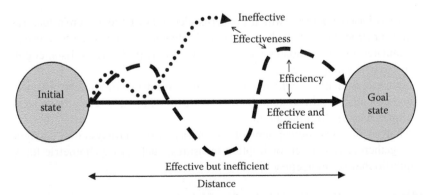

FIGURE 7.2 The goal-achievement process. The distance between the initial and goal states can be described as a gap bridged by an efficient and effective path (straight line), by a not effective path (dotted line), or by a not efficient path (dashed line).

path, and by experiencing interaction problems, as represented by the dashed line in Figure 7.2. The difference between the dashed line and the dotted line in Figure 7.2 lies in the effectiveness of the interaction—the dashed line represents those cases in which a user reaches the goal state but experiences some problems in doing so, while the dotted line represents those cases in which the users encounter problems during the interaction that lead them to fall short of the goal. On the other hand, the straight line represented in Figure 7.2 represents those cases in which users have no problems in achieving the goal (i.e., they adopt an approach with a high level of effectiveness and efficiency). The difference between the straight line and the dashed line is the efficiency experienced by users in reaching the goal—because the straight line is shorter (i.e., it requires less time or fewer steps to complete—while the difference between the dotted line and the straight line is the effectiveness of the process of goal achievement.

In conclusion, practitioners can measure the interaction in a reliable way through evaluation techniques (i.e., measurements and criteria) only by defining the goal and controlling the path the user will pursue in attempting to achieve it. This is the main difference between the evaluation process as applied by professionals and the commonsense understanding of what constitutes an assessment: the controlling for variables and the reduction of subjectivity. On the basis of this distinction, in the next sections, we will discuss the UX and the usability evaluation processes.

7.2 UX AND USABILITY: THE IMPORTANCE OF THE USER'S LONG- AND SHORT-TERM USE OF A PRODUCT

As Chapter 2 underscored, usability professionals worked toward improvement as the sole goal of usability until the end of twentieth century, with the concept of UX having emerged at the turn of the century. The UX concept understands the measure of quality in use and covers a wider area than does usability alone. As was discussed in Chapter 5, practitioners can apply different sets of evaluation techniques based on their overall aims and budget restrictions in order to assess UX and usability. Nevertheless, to assess the complexity of the interaction and to measure the distance between the expected interaction (i.e., the designer's mental model) and the user's interaction (i.e., the user's mental model), practitioners ought to use all of the applied techniques within an integrated framework.

It is now clear that, while usability concerns the interaction analysis carried out by users with a minimal level of experience with the product, UX analysis can be considered to be a follow-up assessment. The evaluators can gather data about the UX only once users have gained a certain level of expertise, in terms of time having used the product. Whether a practitioner gathers data about the assessment of a car, for instance, by engaging a sample of purchasers intending to buy that model or immediately after having purchased that model, the data collected will regard the usability of the car. On the other hand, were the assessment to be performed 3 or 6 months after the purchase, the data would focus on the UX. For certain systems, such as cash machines, ticket machines, or other walk-up-and-use systems, it is rare that users will acquire long-term experience of use (i.e., UX); in such cases, the short-term experience (usability) may be considered the same as the long-term experience. In these cases, practitioners can gather data about both the usability and the UX independent of the time spent by users in the use of the product. For most products, however, users will use them for several months or years, as happens with smartphones, personal computers, cars, etc. During this long-term period of use, users will experience different unexpected events during their interaction. As such, and in order to monitor the long-term experience, evaluators should select only those users that have acquired a certain level of expertise in the use of a given product. In the following sections, we shall describe in detail the UX assessment process and, as part of this, the usability evaluation of a product.

7.2.1 DYNAMIC PROCESS OF THE USER EXPERIENCE

Kurosu (2012b) recently proposed three aspects that may lead an evaluator to pursue a UX evaluation process. These aspects, summarized in Figure 7.3, are the meaning of the product, its quality, and its *Kansei* aspects (from the Japanese word *Kansei*, meaning "emotional" or "affective").

The meaning of the product (meaningfulness) represents how well the product fulfills the needs or requirements of its users, independent of its aesthetics and usability features. It is important for an evaluator to consider and assess, in a qualitative

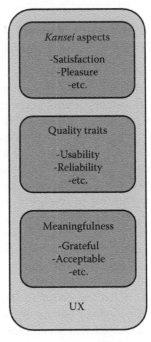

FIGURE 7.3 The three main aspects of UX interaction—the *Kansei* aspects, the quality traits, and the meaningfulness of the product. (From Kurosu, M., Three dimensions of artefact design—Meaning, quality and Kansei, paper presented at the *Human Interface Symposium 2012*, Fukuoka City, Japan, 2012b.)

manner, the users' motivations for using the product, and how these motivations can influence users' evaluations of the interaction (see for a review on UX, Hassenzahl and Tractinsky, 2006). Nevertheless, it is not easy for a person to state directly whether a given product is meaningful or not. A practitioner therefore can conduct qualitative observations of users' interactions in their use context in order to measure the frequency of product use and the user's dependency on the product. In some cases, for example, within social networks, heavy and extensive use can engender a pathological relationship with the technology, such as Internet addiction (Widyanto and McMurran, 2004), and measurement of the meaningfulness may be replaced by specific psychometric measures, such as the Internet addiction test (Young, 1998). In most such cases, however, the meaningful analysis—and especially analysis undertaken during the product's formative cycle—will act as a direct assessment of how much the users' needs are or have been taken into account by the designers. In fact, when a product provides little meaning to the user, it is usually a clue that the product has been generated by a design process that lacked an appropriate analysis of the market and of user requirements.

The quality traits and the *Kansei* aspects (Nagamachi, 1995; Xu et al., 2011) are similar to the notions of the practical and the hedonic attributes of the interaction as proposed by Hassenzahl (2005), and concern the analysis of the quality in use. In order to capture these aspects during assessment, the evaluator has to assess the usability and all of the quality traits of the interface. The most familiar quality trait for professionals is the usability, or the quality in use; an evaluator who aims to assess the UX, however, also ought to consider other qualitative aspects that may affect the interaction, such as the reliability in use, the safety, the cost, the compatibility, the durability, and the sustainability (Mirza et al., 2012). A well-structured usability evaluation will typically cover different aspects of the quality of the interaction. A practitioner might assess a website, for instance, by focusing on the usability aspects while minimizing measurements of the safety and the reliability, whereas reliability and safety become very important factors when the product to be assessed can affect or damage its users, as is the case with, for instance, medical devices. In such cases, the evaluator must collect information and data about the level of safety and reliability users experienced both during the individual interaction (usability) and over time (UX).

Finally, the *Kansei*, or the hedonic aspects (Hassenzahl, 2005), regard the measurement of users' satisfaction, happiness, joy, and pleasure in use. Such factors are typically assessed by evaluators through interviews, questionnaires, or specific psychometrics tools.

As was discussed in Chapter 2, each user, in the course of the evolution of his or her use experience, passes through different stages (see Chapter 2, Figure 2.6). The measurement of the UX in this sense is a dynamic process—in aiming to assess the UX, practitioners should measure the three aspects discussed earlier over the course of the development of the users' experience with the product.

In summation, in order to capture the users' overall experiences evaluators have to consider modifications to the intrasystemic dialogue between the subject and the product that might occur at each step. In order to determine the overall UX as perceived by users, evaluators can make a comparison between the short-term use (usability) and the long-term use (UX); this can be done only at the end of the UX process, by analyzing the data gathered through the integrated set of techniques (the IMIE model).

7.3   BRIEF OVERVIEW OF THE TECHNIQUES FOR ASSESSING UX AND USABILITY

During the evolution of the HCI, a huge corpus of techniques designed to measure interactions were created by practitioners. For reasons of space, it is not possible to provide an exhaustive description of all such practices in this section; there are ample resources that explain the evaluation techniques in detail available on the Internet (e.g., http://www.usabilitybok.org/methods, http://www.usabilitynet.org). This section attempts to depict how some of the most extensively applied evaluation techniques can be used by practitioners to assess both the UX and usability.

One of the most complete taxonomy of the usability evaluation methods was provided in the 2001 by Melody Y. Ivory and Marti A. Hearts—researchers at the University of California. They proposed to classify the usability methods on the basis of four main characteristics (Ivory and Hearst, 2001):

1. In five-method class, the type of evaluation conducted by the evaluator is described:
   a. The testing class, in which an evaluator observes the users interaction in order to identify the interaction problems
   b. The inspection class, in which an evaluator analyzes the interface by means of criteria or heuristics in order to identify potential interaction problems
   c. The inquiry class, in which the users provide feedback on an interface via interviews, surveys, and the like
   d. Analytical modeling class, in which an evaluator tries to predict by models the users' interaction
   e. Simulation class, in which an evaluator simulates by model the users' interaction
2. Method type, in which the evaluator selects a specific evaluation technique through possible classes such as thinking-aloud protocol, the GOMS model, etc.
3. Four automation types. The evaluator can choose among different levels of automatic data recruitment on the basis of the selected method:
   a. None automatic type, in which all the data are gathered manually by the evaluators
   b. Capture type, in which an evaluator uses a software for recording the data (e.g., log data, screen recorder, etc.)
   c. Analysis type, in which an evaluator uses a software that records and identifies potential problems of users' interaction (e.g., eye-tracker software)

    d. Critique type, in which an evaluator uses a software that analyzes on the basis of a model or a set of criteria the interface in order to suggest how to improve the product (e.g., automatic tools for the web usability analysis)

4. Four effort levels. The effort concerns the endeavor required to the evaluator in order to apply the selected method during the assessment:

    a. Minimal effort for the evaluator. It happens when there is a high degree of automation of the data recruitment

    b. Model development for applying the evaluation type. The effort of the evaluator is due to the development of a user model and in applying this model for simulating or predicting the interaction

    c. Informal use of evaluation type, in which the evaluator involves users in free navigation and use of the product

    d. Formal use of the evaluation type, in which the evaluator involves users in scenario analysis of the product

This deep taxonomy provides a useful way for discriminating among the techniques. However, some limits can be identified in the organization proposed by Ivory and Hearts (2001). First, this taxonomy concerns only the usability, and second, it can be used by evaluators in order to describe one technique without help practitioners in mix different kinds of techniques for composing an integrated evaluation process. Finally, the Ivory and Hearts (2001) mostly analyze only the evaluator effort for gathering and recording the data (effort level), without considering the effort for analyzing and interpreting the gathered data.

By moving from these limits, we aim to propose a reorganization of the first two level of the Ivory and Hearts taxonomy (i.e., the class and the type of the methods), without any intent to propose a deep and exhaustive taxonomy, but for depicting how some of the most used evaluation techniques can be used by practitioners for assessing both UX and usability.

In tune with this goal, we propose an innovative holistic representation of the UX and usability in relation to three main groups of evaluation methods (Figure 7.4):

- *Qualitative and subjective measurements for the interaction analysis*: In this group, we list all of the techniques in which the evaluator will have to involve users in order to collect qualitative information about the interaction (e.g., interviews, observations, etc.), or in order to measure aspects such as satisfaction, workload, stress, and visual foci through direct testing of users with specific instruments (e.g., questionnaires, eye-tracking, biofeedback tools, etc.).
- *Usability testing and analysis of real interaction*: In this group, we list the user-based techniques in which practitioners engage a sample of users in product interaction in order to test the effectiveness and efficiency of the intrasystemic dialogue by gathering specific data such as the percentage of users able to achieve the prescribed goals, the percentage of users able to successfully complete a task, the average accuracy of completed tasks, the time to complete a task, the tasks completed per unit of time, the cost of performing the tasks, etc. (for a complete list of measures, see ISO9241-11, 1998).

- *Inspection and simulation methods of expected interaction*: In this group, we list the expert-based techniques in which a sample of experts analyze the product in order to simulate the expected interactions of a real user in terms of effectiveness and efficiency—i.e., heuristic analysis, cognitive walkthroughs, and task analyses.

Practitioners can use Figure 7.4 as an indication for selecting the best set of techniques for measuring the UX or the usability from among the set of most common practices and based on the goals of their evaluation. There are also other reliable and widely used evaluative techniques that could be included in the table, such as card sorting (Nielsen, 1995a), which could be inserted in the first group, or formal usability inspection (Gunn, 1995), or the GOMS analysis (see Chapter 1, Box 1.3), which could be included in the last group. Our primary interest here, however, is only to provide a holistic representation of the relationship between the UX and usability and how the evaluation techniques can be used to measure these two dimensions of the interaction.

Method class	Method type	UX						Kansei
		Quality			Usability			Pleasure, joy, etc.
		Meaning	Safety	Reliability, compatibility, durability, sustainability, cost	Effectiveness	Efficiency	Satisfaction	
(1) Qualitative and subjective measurements for the interaction analysis	Interview	X	X	X			X	X
	Observation	X	X		X		X	X
	Diary	X	X	X			X	X
	Satisfaction questionnaire	X	X	X			X	X
	Psychometric questionnaire	X					X	X
	Eye-tracker		X		X	X		
	Biofeedback analysis		X				X	X
(2) Usability testing and analysis of a real interaction	Concurrent think-aloud				X	X		
	Retrospective think-aloud				X		X	
	Remote testing				X	X		
(3) Inspection and simulation methods of expected interaction	Heuristic list				X	X		
	Cognitive walkthrough				X	X		
	Task analysis				X	X		

FIGURE 7.4   (See color insert.) Synoptic representation of the most common evaluation techniques and measures of the UX and usability divided into three groups of methods: (1) qualitative and subjective measurements for the interaction analysis, (2) usability testing and analysis of a real interaction, and (3) inspection and simulation methods of expected interaction.

Figure 7.4 highlights the fact that evaluators cannot use just one method to obtain a complete assessment of the interaction. Practitioners who intend to assess usability have to integrate expert-based and user-based techniques as well as qualitative measures. We discuss in the following section the evaluation techniques presented in Figure 7.4; we first must consider, however, how an evaluator can manage the data gathered through the various evaluation techniques (i.e., the effort level for interpreting the gathered data) and how he or she can most accurately estimate the reliability of the evaluation process. We shall focus in particular on the question of how a practitioner can show someone (i.e., a designer, a client, an authority, etc.) that the integrated set of evaluation techniques (i.e., the evaluation process) as applied for the assessment is effective and efficient. We shall answer this question in the following section.

7.4 EFFECTIVENESS AND EFFICIENCY OF THE EVALUATION PROCESS AND THE MANAGEMENT OF THE GATHERED DATA

As was discussed earlier, in Chapter 6, the techniques selected for the evaluation and to assess the representativeness of the participants constitute two key factors in ensuring the overall reliability of the data gathered by practitioners. We can identify two principles that ought to guide practitioners seeking to apply an efficient and effective evaluation process:

1. *Respect the rules of the techniques*: The extent to which practitioners respect the rules of the technique they have decided to apply is important in guaranteeing that the evaluation will be replicable and the outcome will be reliable.
2. *Manage the data properly to discover all of the real problems*: The manner in which the data gathered from both users and experts are managed by the evaluators is an important factor in estimating the representativeness of the evaluation cohort, the number of problems identified, and for determining the generalizability of the results.

The first principle is quite obvious—in fact, the reliability of any evaluative technique is based on a certain set of procedures and constraints the evaluator must respect in order to achieve his or her evaluation goal.

Conversely, the second principle is less evident. Evaluators often focus on obtaining data, while they consider the management of the results to be a secondary issue. As Borsci et al. (2012a) have claimed, practitioners cannot assume an evaluation process is reliable because it is composed of reliable techniques and measures (e.g., the time spent by users to achieve a goal or how many tasks were failed or achieved by users); they also must control for how many real interaction problems were identified during the analysis (the effectiveness of the process) and the sum of all costs associated with the evaluation, understood as the time devoted to and money spent for the analysis (the efficiency of the process). Moreover, together with efforts to identify interaction problems, a practitioner should also consider the costs and benefits of all of the qualitative analyses applied to gather specific information about users' perceptions, workloads, satisfaction, pleasure, etc. The procedures applied by professionals to manage the data therefore are a key factor to controlling the effectiveness and efficiency of an evaluation process in terms of the information gathered about the product and the costs of doing so within a budget.

There are different kinds of data management procedures that professionals typically apply. We can divide these into two main groups: data management through software and manual data management.

The management of data carried out by evaluators using software is applied when attempting to organize and analyze a huge dataset drawn from evaluation tests done with hi-tech devices, such as biofeedback or eye-trackers. This is done mostly because such devices have specific software packages for the collection, organization, and analysis of a large set of physical data (e.g., heart rate, saccadic movements, etc.). At the same time, practitioners may use specific computer applications to manage the data generated via satisfaction questionnaires and various psychometric tools.

The adoption of data management software is useful in assessing physical or subjective reactions (e.g., fixation points, workload, etc.); currently, there is no software, however, that can help evaluators discriminate during a test—for instance, when a user or expert identifies an interaction problem—and then analyze the effectiveness and the efficiency of the interaction. In order to make such discrimination possible, evaluators have to apply a manual means of data management.

Manual data management is used when professionals want to systematically analyze a qualitative dataset. In such instances, professionals apply either exploratory and descriptive analyses or specific approaches such as the grounded-theory approach (GTA), a well-known sociological method, for achieving a bottom-up analysis of data (Glaser and Strauss, 1967). At the same time, manual data management is often used by practitioners to extrapolate the number of problems discovered by a sample of users or experts during an evaluation test. In such instances, professionals analyze the data collected by various techniques such as usability testing or inspection analyses by applying specific algorithms (i.e., estimation models) in order to estimate the discovery likelihood within a sample, indicated in literature by the value p (Lewis, 1994, 2006; Nielsen, 2000; Nielsen and Landauer, 1993; Schmettow, 2012; Turner et al., 2006; Virzi, 1990, 1992). As we discussed in Chapter 6 (Section 6.3.2), by estimating the p-value and applying it in an error distribution formula (Chapter 6, Equation 6.1), practitioners can then calculate how many problems have been discovered during the assessment and estimate the most effective sample size that will allow them to identify a certain percentage of problems in the product. Finally, evaluators can use these data concerning the evaluation process (i.e., the number of problems and the sample size) together with data about the time and resources allocated to the assessment to obtain specific information about the efficiency and effectiveness of the evaluation process.

In summary, in order to estimate the effectiveness and efficiency of the overall evaluation process, practitioners must consider (1) how much information they have gathered about the interaction using different instruments (e.g., eye-trackers, questionnaires, interviews, etc.); (2) how many problems have been identified by an evaluation cohort; and (3) the costs in terms of time and resources allocated to the gathering of these data.

The use of hi-tech instruments and software and, moreover, the assessment of interactions by qualitative techniques, are essential to addressing the different aspects of the UX assessment (i.e., meaningfulness, qualitative traits, and *Kansei*). The qualitative analyses therefore can be seen as a fixed cost, part of any evaluation process that aims to cover all aspects of the UX (for a review about the measures and the costs, see Law et al., 2012; Sauro and Lewis, 2012). An evaluator carrying out a one-technique assessment will incur fewer expenses than an evaluator performing an integrated set of evaluation techniques; moreover, any time a practitioner follows up a round of analysis by performing a new test with another tool or instrument to expand upon the body of data collected, he or she will affect the efficiency of the overall evaluation process (i.e., more time and money will have to be invested for the collection of the additional information). Conversely, this added investment of time and money will typically increase the effectiveness of the assessment (e.g., more information about the interaction will be available). The composition of an IMIE therefore will always represent a counterbalance between the costs and aims of the assessment on the one hand and the efficiency and effectiveness of the evaluation process on the other.

Many evaluators prefer to use and rely upon specific devices for the assessment— e.g., log-analysis software, eye-tracking, and biofeedback systems—instead of applying more qualitative procedures that require long analytical processes, such as GTA, because the former assessments are more efficient in terms of time. Nevertheless, when practitioners aim to collect a deep dataset in the wild, or to inspect specific aspects of the interaction (e.g., the *Kansei*), they are forced to use a qualitative technique in their IMIE. In such cases, GTA is often considered the most important systematic approach of analysis that can lead evaluators to make reliable inferences about the UX from the qualitative data gathered (Muller and Kogan, 2010).

At the same time, analysis of the sample's p-value against cost is considered by many researchers (Borsci et al., 2011, 2012a; Lewis, 1994, 2006; Schmettow, 2012; Turner et al., 2006) to be the main procedure for distinguishing between an efficient and effective evaluation process and a bad investment in the assessment.

In the following section, we shall discuss the manual management of qualitative data, analyze the strengths of the GTA, and present a pragmatic of management in order to determine the number of problems discovered within a sample (i.e., the p-value), a process referred to as grounded procedure (GP).

7.4.1 MANAGEMENT OF THE QUALITATIVE DATA: AN OVERVIEW OF THE GROUNDED-THEORY APPROACH

As discussed earlier, collecting qualitative data is important for obtaining a clear picture of the intrasystemic dialogue. To manage such data in a manner that allows the drawing of inferences about the UX requires that evaluators apply a range of statistical analyses (e.g., exploratory and descriptive). Among the different approaches to the analysis of qualitative data, GTA—created in 1967 by Barney G. Glaser and Anselm L. Strauss, sociologists at the University of California—is the most often applied data management process in the HCI.

Michael Muller and Sandra Kogan (2010)—researchers at the IBM Watson Research Center of Cambridge—reported on an extensive set of international articles published from the 1990s through to the present day that have applied GTA in the study of a range of interaction topics, such as software engineering, software testing, quality processes, etc. This wide range of applications is due to the fact that GTA, by avoiding the use of hypotheses, is in tune with the goal of the qualitative analyzing of the interaction itself (e.g., interviews, observation, etc.), a process in which a practitioner does not aim to prove or falsify a hypothesis, but only to gather information from users about different aspects of their interaction and use experience. We aim to present here a brief picture of GTA's strengths, with no attempt to exhaustively explain its rigorous process of qualitative data codification and interpretation.

As Muller and Kogan (2010) have suggested, in order to apply GTA, an evaluator must first undergo a certain training period in order to learn the basic notions of the method and its procedure. The procedure is usually represented as follows (Charmaz, 2000, 2006):

1. *Coding of the data*: The data are transcribed and codified in different categories (i.e., axial coding) in order to identify core data (i.e., selective coding)
2. *Memo writing*: The first description of the most evident relationship among the data, and the drawing of first inferences
3. *Process analysis*: The detailed analysis of all data to create a framework or theory within which to examine the emerging relationships among the data. This is usually associated with a holistic representation, such as a diagram, which may aid the researchers in this and subsequent analyses

By avoiding premature conclusions concerning the object under assessment, this long data management process ends with the drawing of a category relationship diagram (Muller and Kogan, 2010), which is useful both in exploring an event or an object without a governing theory or hypothesis and in constructing a theory through a process of abduction driven through the discovered relationships among the elements under assessment.

In conclusion, GTA is a bottom-up methodology through which practitioners can extrapolate important aspects about the relationship between the users and the product from the data at hand.

In the next section, we describe a new procedure for data management that uses GTA as a bottom-up approach created by the researchers of the MATCH program—a 10-year project focused on the design and assessment of medical devices and funded by the UK Engineering and Physical Sciences Research Council Grants. This procedure aims to extrapolate information about the sample discovery likelihood (i.e., the *p*-value) by using the data to have emerged from the evaluation to (1) make specific decisions about the assessment, (2) estimate the effectiveness and efficiency of an evaluation process, and (3) compare the results of different evaluation processes (Borsci et al., 2013).

7.5 GROUNDED PROCEDURE FOR THE MANAGEMENT OF DATA AND TO DETERMINE THE NUMBER OF PROBLEMS DISCOVERED BY A SAMPLE

As discussed in Chapter 6 (Section 6.3), GP is a pragmatic data management process that can be used by evaluators to analyze the sample's behavior in order to discover interaction problems. In line with recent HCI literature (Borsci et al., 2011, 2012a; Lewis, 2006; Schmettow, 2008, 2012), GP assumes that there is no predetermined sample size that can guarantee that an evaluation cohort will discover a high percentage of problems because the p-value depends on the ability of each participant to perceive and identify problems during the interaction. As Schmettow (2012) has noted, a sample of neither 5 nor 50 participants therefore is able to guarantee a practitioner an efficient and effective evaluation. In any analysis of the p-value, an evaluator in fact cannot calculate the D-value (i.e., how many problems are been discovered by a sample) solely by the error distribution formula (see Chapter 6, Equation 6.1).

GP attempts to overcome the one-size-fits-all solutions, such as the well-known idea that five users are sufficient to allow for the discovery of 80%–85% of all problems present, by proposing a dynamic control of the sample's behavior according to J. R. Lewis's idea that

> practitioners can obtain accurate sample size estimates for problem-discovery goals ranging from 70% to 95% by making an initial estimate of the required sample size after running two participants, then adjusting the estimate after obtaining data from another two participants. (Lewis, 2001, p. 474)

As Borsci et al. (2013) have proposed, this procedure is based on three main assumptions:

1. An evaluation is a counterbalanced process. In light of the aims and the available budget, evaluators can reduce the variability of divergent UXs (i.e., the range of possible interaction behaviors) by typifying the kinds of users that are involved in the assessment, the tasks and the goals of the interaction, and the use environment.
2. Reductions in variability lead practitioners to select specific evaluation techniques, thereby affecting the resultant data (Tullis and Albert, 2008).
3. Monitoring the p-value (i.e., the sample discovery likelihood) beyond the first four or five users allows practitioners to obtain reliable information about the data gathered in order to determine whether the problems discovered via the sample have a certain level of representativeness of a larger population of end users (i.e., the reliability and quality of the test).

Applying GP during the data collection process allows practitioners to assume a specific p-value standard (e.g., $p = 0.30$, if the aim is to achieve the identification of

80%–85% of all problems), and thus to use this value to compare the *p*-value of the tested sample to the standard in order to inform the following two decisions:

- *If the sample fits the standard*, the practitioner reports the results to the client and determines whether the product should be redesigned or released.
- *If the sample does not fit the standard,* the practitioner adds more users to the sample and re-tests the *p*-value in a cyclical manner until the predetermined percentage of problems (D_{th}) has been achieved.

GP is an information-seeking process that works dynamically during data collection to drive practitioners to obtain reliable evidence for deciding whether it is necessary to add users to a sample or whether they can conclude the evaluation because they have obtained sufficient information. The practitioners can make these decisions after completing each of the following three steps:

1. *Monitoring the problems*: A table of problems is constructed to facilitate analysis of the number of problems discovered, the number of users that have identified each problem (i.e., the weight), and the average *p*-value of the sample
2. *Refining the p-value*: A range of models are applied, after which the number of users required is reviewed in light of the emerging *p*-value
3. *Making a decision based on the sample's behavior*: The *p*-value is applied in Equation 6.1 (Chapter 6) and, based on the results, the evaluator can make a decision while considering the available budget and the aims of the evaluation.

In the following sections, we discuss these three steps of GP in order to show how a practitioner can identify the number of problems discovered by a sample and concurrently determine the effectiveness and efficiency of the evaluation process.

7.5.1 What Does It Mean to Monitor Problems?

We have already shown how practitioners can construct a table that tracks and presents a sample's behavior (Chapter 6, Table 6.1) by collecting data on a series of subjects' behaviors, with each instance able to be represented in a binary fashion—i.e. (1) 0 = Problem/error not found; (2) 1 = Problem/error found.

In order to understand how this kind of table can assist practitioners in their work, it could be useful to exemplify the complexity of an evaluation test as follows:

You might imagine that a practitioner invites a certain number of people for a particular kind of ramble in the woods. The practitioner assigns participants the following goal: Go in the woods and follow the pathway indicated by the map in order to identify and report to me where in the woods you see mushrooms without picking them up from the woods. You can note on the map the position of each mushroom you see. After each participant returns from the woods, the practitioner has a list of the mushrooms identified by each subject. It can so happen that some subjects will have identified the same mushrooms in the same positions; these mushrooms are probably the most visible. Other mushrooms, however—those in more hidden positions—are identified only by a small number of participants. When a mushroom is identified by a participant, the identification reported by the other participants adds nothing to the overall discovery behavior of the sample, while any new mushroom identified increases the overall effectiveness of the sample. The more participants to go into the woods the higher the probability that the sample will have identified a larger number of mushrooms, because a larger group has a greater scope for divergent behavior (i.e., more participants looking for mushrooms in hidden positions) as compared to a smaller group. Involving a large sample is quite expensive for the practitioner, however, and it is never the most efficient solution. It is in fact possible to identify the smallest group with the greatest quality of discovery behavior. In this context, the quality of the behavior is seen as the ability of a small sample to accurately represent the behavior of a larger sample. We can thus define the representativeness of a sample as the degree to which the mushrooms (i.e., the problems) accurately identified by the sample represent the mushrooms that can be identified by all possible participants in the woods ramble following the pathway indicated on the map (i.e., the task of the evaluation test).

Outside of this example, the organization of the problems identified by each user into a table can drive practitioners to observe two possible kinds of behaviors within the sample:

1. *Homogeneous behavior*: In this case, a practitioner can observe that the sample has a coherent rate of discovering problems. There are two cases of homogeneous behaviors:
   a. *Negative homogeneity*, in which all of the users have found all of the problems (Table 7.1)
      The *p*-value would be equal to 1, and the practitioner would have reliable information with which to argue that there are many evident and important problems with the product. The sample's homogeneously negative behavior could be cited in proposing a redesign of the product to solve these problems, with a subsequent new evaluation of the updated design.
   b. *Positive homogeneity*, in which none of the users identify any problems (Table 7.2)
      In this ideal condition, the *p*-value is equal to 0 and the evaluators can report to the client that the technology is ready for release or for a larger-scale evaluation. A *p*-value very close to 0 is usually the result of a test–retest process, in which the product has already been evaluated and redesigned, perhaps several times, thereby increasing the difficulties associated with, and reducing the likelihood of, problem identification.
2. *Heterogeneous behavior*: In this case, the practitioner observes that the sample has identified a certain number of problems with different weights (i.e., how many participants identified the same problems). This heterogeneous problem identification clearly shows practitioners that there are a certain number of problems in the product, but it cannot inform evaluators

TABLE 7.1

An Example of a Sample with Homogenous Negative Behavior

	Problems Perceived in *N* Tasks			
	Problem 1	Problem 2	Problem 3	*p*-Value
Participant 1	1	1	1	1
Participant 2	1	1	1	1
...	...	...	...	...
Weight of problems	2	2	2	
			Raw *p*-value	1

Note: The table has a "1" indicative of a problem identified, in each row and column, meaning that each problem has been identified by each participant, which in turn means that all problems were visible to all participants (i.e., a high weight of problems).

TABLE 7.2

An Example of a Sample with Homogenous Positive Behavior

	Problems Perceived in *N* Tasks	*p*-Value
Participant 1	0	0
Participant 2	0	0
...	...	...
Weight of problems	0	
	Raw *p*-value	0

Note: The table has a "0" in each row and column, meaning that no problems were identified in each task, and thus that there are no problems to be identified by participants in the interaction (i.e., a low weight of problems).

as to the representativeness of the sample and the reliability of the data; this can be analyzed only by testing the sample's *p*-value through the estimation models (see Section 7.5.2 for an example of a heterogeneous sample's behavior).

While homogeneous behavior by a sample can lead practitioners to obtain reliable information (prompting redesign or market release decisions), most evaluation studies will identify some degree of heterogeneity within the sample's behavior. When the sample exhibits heterogeneous behavior, practitioners lack sufficient information with which to make an informed redesign/release decision. Consequently, they must analyze the p-value and, in line with their aims and budget constraints, they must then consider adding more users to the sample in order to provide the quality of information needed to take an informed decision.

7.5.2 REFINING THE p-VALUE OF HETEROGENEOUS SAMPLES THROUGH ESTIMATION MODELS

In Chapter 6, we proposed an example (Table 6.1) of a heterogeneous sample's behavior with a raw p-value equal to 0.23. Practitioners may plugged this raw p-value (i.e., $p = 0.23$) into the error distribution formula (Chapter 6, Equation 6.1) obtained a result that affirmed the fact that the first eight users in the sample would be sufficient to identify more than the 85% of the interaction problems (Figure 7.5).

The return on investment (ROI) model is considered an optimistic method for estimating the p-value (Borsci et al., 2012a; Schmettow, 2008; Woolrych and Cockton, 2001), and several alternative estimation models have been proposed for obtaining more conservative estimations of the p-value. The first such alternative model, the Good–Turing (GT), was proposed in the HCI field by J. R. Lewis (2001), on the basis of the original formalization of Irving John Good in collaboration with Alan Mathison Turing during the Second World War at the United Kingdom's main decryption establishment of Bletchley Park (Good, 1953; for a review on statistical methods for speech recognition, refer to Jelinek, 1997). As Turner et al. (2006) well explain, GT model incorporates the adjustment proposed by Morten Hertzum and Niels Ebbe Jacobsen (2003)—respectively associate professor of Computer Science at Roskilde University of Denmark and

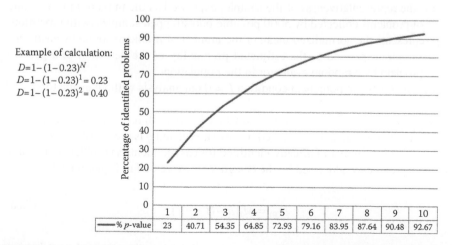

Example of calculation:

$D = 1 - (1 - 0.23)^N$
$D = 1 - (1 - 0.23)^1 = 0.23$
$D = 1 - (1 - 0.23)^2 = 0.40$

	1	2	3	4	5	6	7	8	9	10
% p-value	23	40.71	54.35	64.85	72.93	79.16	83.95	87.64	90.48	92.67

FIGURE 7.5 **(See color insert.)** Example of the error distribution formula application on the base of the return on investment model, in which the sample's discovery likelihood is estimated by the raw p-value of the cohort.

head of research at the Danish Consumer Council of Denmark—that seeks to normalize the p-value as follows:

$$padj = \frac{1}{2}\left[\left(\frac{P_{est}}{1+(E(M_1)/M)}\right) + \left[\left(P_{est}-\frac{1}{n}\right)\left(1-\frac{1}{n}\right)\right]\right] \tag{7.1}$$

where
   P_{est} is the initial estimate computed from the raw data of a usability study
   $E(M_1)$ is the number of usability problems discovered exactly once
   M is the total number of usability problems detected by all users
   n is the number of test participants

Second, the Monte Carlo resampling method is a statistical resampling technique that has been used to simulate the impact of the subjects taking part in the evaluation in different orders (for a complete review of the Monte Carlo application in HCI see Lewis, 2000).

   Third, the bootstrap discovery behavior (BDB) model proposed by Borsci et al. (2011), adopts a bootstrap approach (Efron, 1979; Fox, 2002) and modifies the classic error distribution formula (Chapter 6, Equation 6.1) as follows:

$$D_{(L)} = M_t[a-(1-p)^{L+q}] \tag{7.2}$$

where
   M_t represents the total number of problems present in the interface
   a is the representativeness of the sample, expressed as the maximum limit value
      of problems collected by 5000 possible bootstrapped samples (with repetition)
   p represents the normalized mean of the number of problems found by each sub-
      sample, expressed as the estimated probability of the detection of a generic
      problem by a random evaluator in the population
   q expresses the hypothetical condition $L = 0$ (an analysis without evaluators)

In other words, since D does not vanish when $L = 0$, $D(0)$ represents the number of evident problems that can be detected by any subject and q is the possibility that they detect a certain number of already identified (or easy to identify) problems that have not been previously addressed by the designer, as expressed in Equation 7.2a:

$$D_{(0)} = M_t[a-(1-p)^q] \tag{7.2a}$$

In Equation 7.2a, q represents the properties of the interface from the evaluation perspective, with its extreme value being the "zero condition," where no problems are found. A BDB model, such as that expressed in Equation 7.2, expands the scope of analysis by adding two new parameters not considered in the classic error distribution formula (see Chapter 6, Equation 6.1): (1) all of the possible discovery behaviors of participants (a) and (2) a rule that governs the selecting of the representative data (q). In this sense, a BDB model proposes a modification of the error distribution formula to include new factors within the sample discovery likelihood estimation.

Returning to our heterogeneous sample with a raw p-value equal to 0.23, when we apply the GT, the Monte Carlo analysis, or the BDB model, we arrive at more conservative p-value estimates (Table 7.3).

By using each model with an initial six subjects, practitioners can obtain a range of discovery likelihoods, from 0.11 (i.e., p_{GT}) to 0.23 (i.e., p_{Raw}) ($M = 0.128$). By using the lowest p-value (in this case, $p_{GT} = 0.11$) and the mean ($p_M = 0.18$), practitioners can argue that, in order to identify more than 85% of the problems, they require a sample composed of 8–10 subjects, with a discovery behavior that is in line with that of the current cohort.

In our case, the sample p-value is quite low—i.e., the first six participants have exhibited bad behavior. This usually happens when evaluators apply the wrong criteria in selecting subjects. We must also consider the fact that the results obtained from the estimation models should be considered true only when all new participants added to the cohort maintain the current sample's discovery behavior. In fact, if the evaluators can add new users with higher discovery behavior to the sample by checking and revising the selection criteria, the overall sample p-value will increase while the number of users needed to achieve the desired D will decrease.

Finally, when the sample behavior is heterogeneous, an evaluator should rely on a range of values rather than adopting a unique number estimated by one model (e.g., the ROI model). This range of p-values, as estimated by different models, can be used by the practitioner to revise the sample selection criteria when the starting cohort of users has a low p-value and for monitoring each new subject added to the sample after that, and whether the discovery behavior of the cohort increases or decreases.

TABLE 7.3

Estimation of the p-Values of a Heterogeneous Sample's Behavior as Calculated by Different Models

ROI		GT		MC Analysis		BDB Model	
p_{Raw}	>85% of the problems	p_{GT}	>85% of the problems	p_{MC}	> 85% of the problems	p_{BDB}	>85% of the problems
0.23	8 subjects	0.11	17 subjects	0.19	10 subjects	0.020	10 subjects

Note: Return on investment (ROI), Good–Turing (GT); Monte Carlo (MC); and bootstrap discovery behavior (BDB) model. The p-values estimated with the models (p_{Raw}, p_{GT}, p_{MC}, p_{BDB}) show that the discovery likelihood of this sample, composed of six subjects, is insufficient to identify more than the 85% of the problems in the product under evaluation.

7.5.3 MAKING A DECISION ON THE BASIS OF THE SAMPLE BEHAVIOR

As Borsci et al. (2013) have suggested, in the case of a sample that exhibits heterogeneous behavior, GP is a procedure that can be applied in the organizing of the data, in the calculation of the sample's behavior, and in conducting comparative analyses of different estimation models on the basis of the information collected from the sample. When the p-value is lower than the standard set as the evaluation goal (e.g., $p \leq 0.30$), the sample can be seen as offering the evaluators insufficient information to generate a valid report. In these cases, the evaluator, respecting the available budget, should enlarge the sample (i.e., add users), with the goal of discovering more problems until the aimed for percentage of identified problems has been achieved.

Without adhering to the GP model, for instance, an evaluator (whom we refer to here as $E1$), after the first five users' analysis, could estimate the cohort's p-value as being equal to 0.06. Since this result would mean that the sample has identified only 26% of the problems present within the product—which, according to $E1$'s budget, accounts for $2000—$E1$ should then be expected to recommend adding an additional 15 users into the sample without other estimations (i.e., at a cost of $100 for each test), assuming that the cohort will discover at least 71% of the problems.

On the other hand, another evaluator (whom we refer to here as $E2$) decides to apply the GP model in testing the same interface with the initial sample of five users ($p = 0.06$). In line with the procedure, the sample p-value is far from the standard (i.e., $p \geq 0.3$, for an aimed-for D of 80%–85%); $E2$ therefore revises the selection criteria and decides to analyze the changes to the p-value after each completed user test. After the analysis of three new users selected on the basis of the revised criteria, $E2$ discovers that the sample's p-value has increased to 0.20—meaning that, with a sample of eight users, $E2$ has discovered more problems (83%) than $E1$ while spending only $800 of a total budget of $2000.

This example shows how GP can be applied in a useful and pragmatic way to the estimation models and for determining the effectiveness and efficiency of the evaluation process.

In conclusion, the GP model allows practitioners to analyze the reliability of the data gathered and enables them to estimate the sample size needed to identify a given percentage of interaction problems. This procedure provides a new perspective on the discovery likelihood and gives the evaluator a tool for deciding when to enlarge the sample, or redesign or release the product. It also allows evaluators to control costs and objectively demonstrate the reliability of their evaluations.

7.6 CONCLUSION

In the present chapter, we have analyzed the rules and methods any evaluator should apply in order to test the usability and the UX of a system. By discussing the differences between the commonsense ideas of what an evaluation is and what a professional assessment entails, we have described the efforts any evaluator must undertake in order to control the evaluation variables. In particular, we have analyzed the importance of the evaluators controlling the users' processes of goal achievement for the assessment of the usability and the UX of a system. Furthermore, we have presented the UX as a dynamic process, during which users develop and engage in an intrasystemic dialogue with a product. We proposed that, in order to assess the UX, an evaluator must apply an IMIE composed by blending expert- and user-based analyses together with an analysis of the users' perceptions of the intrasystemic dialogue quality. The IMIE can be composed of different evaluation techniques (Figure 7.4), which can be applied by practitioners to assess the main aspects of the UX: the usability (quality traits), the emotional and affective aspects of the interaction (*Kansei*), and the meaningfulness of the product. In line with the presentation of the evaluation techniques that can compose an IMIE, we have discussed how practitioners can best manage and analyze the evaluation data in order to present and discuss both the effectiveness and the efficiency of their evaluation process, by showing to their clients and to the design team the representativeness of their data.

Finally, we have presented a systematic approach for the analysis and interpretation of qualitative data (GTA) and an innovative procedure for the management of said data and for sample-size estimation (GP). In particular, the steps included within the GP model have been discussed in depth, by remarking on the distance from the classic one-size-fits-all solution (Nielsen, 2000, 2012; Nielsen and Landauer, 1993; Virzi, 1990, 1992) and on the value of this procedure as a tool for analyzing the effectiveness and efficiency of an evaluation cohort test.

In the next chapter, the evaluation techniques for the UX and the usability assessment (summarily presented in this chapter, in Figure 7.4) and the role of experts and users in each technique are discussed and analyzed.

8 Evaluation Techniques, Applications, and Tools

8.1 INTRODUCTION

The use and application of evaluation techniques for measuring interaction is one of the key factors in successful (i.e., effective and efficient) evaluation processes. In our perspective, evaluation techniques are the tools that evaluators use for assessing a product and helping designers to transform it into an intrasystemic solution (i.e., a psychotechnology), facilitating and improving the dialogue between user and interface.

A corpus of gray literature on the Internet (Cygnis Media, 2012; Fredheim, 2011; Olyslager, 2012; Reichelt, 2008; ZURBlog, 2011) highlights the doubts of several designers and experts of interaction about the possibility of designing a user experience (UX) or a product for everyone. As Helge Fredheim (2011)—front-end developer at Bekk Consulting of Norway—claims, designers have no possibility of designing an experience, but they can only try to focus their attention on the design elements that can support and facilitate users during interactions:

> We can design the product or service, and we can have a certain kind of user experience in mind when we design it. However, there is no guarantee that our product will be appreciated the way we want it to be. (Fredheim, 2011)

The problems and the doubts expressed by the expert community are at the core of the psychotechnological approach. In fact, according to the psychotechnological perspective, a team of developers cannot directly design a UX nor directly design products for everyone, because, as explained in Chapters 5 and 6, users' mental model and their experience during an interaction cannot be completely captured and integrated in the interface by a simple simulation process. What developers can do, in order to achieve the Interface for All goal, is to design the product by considering all the aspects of the UX, and then, after evaluation of the interaction, redesign the product in collaboration with the evaluators, aiming to adapt the interface to the different kinds of user needs, attitudes, skills, and habits (i.e., design for all) by increasing its quality in use and the esthetic aspects of the product (i.e., UX).

In this chapter, we shall analyze the composition of the integrated evaluation process (i.e., IMIE) and discuss some of the possible techniques for assessing the different aspects of the interaction (see Chapter 7, Figure 7.4). As we clarified in Chapters 5 through 7, practitioners can assess all the different aspects of usability and UX (i.e., *Kansei*, quality traits, and meaningfulness) by creating their own IMIE for analyzing the dialogue between the user and the product. As we suggest in

Chapter 5 (Section 5.4.2.3), evaluators need to analyze three aspects of the intrasystemic dialogue through their IMIE:

1. *System evaluation*: The analysis of the objective aspects of the interface
2. *Subjective evaluation of the interaction*: The subjective evaluation and experience of the interaction, obtained by the analysis of the users' perception of the system functioning
3. *User evaluation of the interaction quality*: The overall quality perceived by the user in terms of satisfaction, workload, etc.

In Chapter 7, we have divided the evaluation techniques into three groups of methods: (1) the qualitative methods and subjective measurements required for the interaction analysis, (2) the usability testing and real interaction analysis, and (3) the inspection and analytic methods of expected interactions.

All the techniques belonging to these three groups provide reliable measures, and they are often used in human–computer interaction (HCI) assessment. Nevertheless, to compose an IMIE, practitioners cannot use a set of techniques that belongs to only one of these groups but must at least select one method per each group in order to compose a whole evaluation process.

For instance, a practitioner who wants to evaluate a website may decide to apply only evaluation techniques that belong to group (1), i.e., qualitative and subjective measurements. In particular, this evaluator intends to observe a sample of users during their interaction with the website through an eye-tracker device administering a satisfaction questionnaire to the users after their navigation. In this hypothetical case, the practitioner can only collect data about two of the three aspects of the intrasystemic dialogue according to the IMIE (Figure 8.1): (1) the subjective evaluation of the system functioning by means of the eye-tracking analysis and (2) the overall quality perceived by the users through the standardized questionnaire. Nevertheless, without an analysis of the system functioning, the evaluator cannot gather information about the objective problems that may affect the final user interaction. Moreover, although the evaluator can obtain reliable information about usability even without considering the system functioning—that is to say the *Kansei* aspects and the meaningfulness of the product (all aspects of the UX)—those data must to be considered as partial and somewhat questionable because a large part of the objective problems caused by the system functioning may remain hidden from the evaluation.

Figure 8.1 represents the relationship among the evaluation methods, the aspects of UX assessed by each method type, and the aspects of intrasystemic dialogue observed by a practitioner applying the methods.

In sum, when evaluators decide to evaluate the interaction without composing an IMIE, they may collect reliable data about the interaction, but these can only represent the intrasystemic dialogue in part. In fact, under a psychotechnological perspective (see Chapters 3 through 5), the only way of exhaustively assessing the interaction is to compose an IMIE with a set of techniques that can be used for obtaining data about all the elements of the intrasystemic dialogue (system functioning, perceived functioning of the product, and quality of the interaction) by taking into account as many UX aspects as possible (meaningfulness, quality traits, and *Kansei*).

Method class	Method type	UX — Meaning	Quality — Safety	Quality — Reliability, etc.	Usability — Effectiveness	Usability — Efficiency	Usability — Satisfaction	Kansei — Pleasure, joy, etc.	IMIE — Measured aspects of the intrasystemic dialogue
(1) Qualitative and subjective measurements for the interaction analysis	Interview	X	X	X			X	X	(i) The user evaluation of the interaction quality (i.e., the overall quality perceived)
	Observation	X	X		X		X	X	
	Diary	X	X	X			X	X	
	Satisfaction questionnaire	X	X	X			X	X	
	Psychometric questionnaire	X					X	X	
	Biofeedback analysis		X				X	X	
(2) Usability testing and analysis of real interaction	Eye-tracker		X		X	X	X	X	It can be used mostly for (i) but also for (ii)
	Concurrent think-aloud				X	X			(ii) The subjective evaluation of the interaction (i.e., perception of system functioning)
	Retrospective think-aloud				X		X		
	Remote testing				X	X			
(3) Inspection and simulation methods of expected interaction	Heuristic list				X	X			(iii) System evaluation
	Cognitive walkthrough				X	X			
	Task analysis				X	X			

FIGURE 8.1 Synoptic representation of the relationship among the evaluation methods and type, the UX, and the IMIE. The measures of the UX and usability are divided into three groups of methods: (1) qualitative and subjective measurements for the interaction analysis, (2) usability testing and real interaction analysis, and (3) inspection and simulation methods of expected interaction. By selecting only one technique from one of these three groups, the evaluator can cover only one aspect of a complete evaluation process (i.e., IMIE): (i) the user evaluation of the interaction quality, (ii) the subjective evaluation of the interaction, and (iii) system evaluation. In order to assess the interaction fully, an evaluator has to compose an IMIE by selecting, and mixing together, at least one evaluation technique per each group.

This chapter discusses some of the most frequently applied evaluation techniques for composing an IMIE and measuring the usability and the UX of a product. In order to achieve this goal, we organize the chapter in three macrosections as follows:

- In Section 8.2, we discuss the inspection and simulation methods of the expected interaction. By these methods, the evaluators can analyze the object functioning for defining a set of expected problems (Figure 8.1, IMIE—(iii) system evaluation). As we discussed in Chapter 5 (Sections 5.3 and 5.3.1), these expected problems are not to be considered as real ones because they have not been identified as such by users; in fact, only after a test with a sample of end users (the real interaction testing) can the evaluators observe how many expected problems are identified by real users (i.e., matched problems) and how many problems remain hidden to the users (false problems). The main advantages of the use of inspection and simulation methods is that these kinds of techniques allow evaluators to have an overview of the product functioning and to identify the most problematic tasks facing the users testing the interaction.

- In Section 8.3, we discuss the qualitative and subjective measures of the interaction. These methods are used for analyzing the overall perspective of the users (Figure 8.1, IMIE—(i) user evaluation of the interaction quality) about the interaction. Nevertheless, these methods are only based on users' overall perspective on the product and cannot be used by practitioners for collecting data about the interaction problems experienced by the users in a specific context of use.
- In Section 8.4, we discuss the real user interaction analysis (Figure 8.1, IMIE—(ii) subjective evaluation of the interaction). These methods are used by evaluators in order to compose the core phase of an evaluation process, that is, the recruitment of data about the problems experienced by users during an interaction: which and how many problems actually affect the interaction and where and when problems are experienced by users.

Each macrosection describes how the evaluation techniques work, their limits, and their strengths. In particular, for each technique, we consider which kind of participants (users or experts) an evaluator should include in a sample and, moreover, the involvement of users with disability in the UX and usability assessment. In fact, as we clarified in Chapter 6, the development and the diffusion of disabled user testing is an important strategy in terms of the future challenges of the pervasive presence of technology in everyday environments. In tune with this, we present and discuss the application of the evaluation techniques created for or adapted to test disabled users' interaction as a new resource for extending evaluation outcomes.

8.2   INSPECTION AND SIMULATION METHODS OF THE EXPECTED INTERACTION

In this macrosection, three evaluation techniques are discussed—the heuristic analysis, the cognitive walkthrough (CW), and the task analysis.

As we observed in Chapter 6 (Sections 6.1.1 and 6.2), an evaluator can predict the impact of the features and functioning of a psychotechnology in the real world by simulating the behavior, attitudes, habits, and reactions of the possible users (i.e., users' mental models) during the interaction. By using these methods and assuming the designer's perspective (the designers' mental model) on how the product has to be used, the evaluators can measure the product functioning.

As we suggested in Chapter 6, during the system evaluation, evaluators should reconstruct the model of users that the designer had in mind when developing the system functioning. In light of this, the inspection and simulation models should be used before the analysis of the users' interaction (i.e., subjective measurements and testing) in order to create a baseline for measuring the distance between the data of the expected (simulated) interaction with the system and the data deriving from the real experience with the product.

Through assessment of the system functioning, the evaluators obtain a measure that is the distance from the designer's mental model embedded in the image of the system—i.e., gathered by the inspection and simulation models—and the users' mental model of the product—that is, gathered by the real user testing (Section 8.4).

In the inspection and simulation analysis, the evaluators simulate the interaction by using a list of principles (empirical model of final users; see Chapter 6, Section 6.2) or simulating the users' behavior through specific predictive techniques based on a user model (such as GOMS; Chapter 1, Box 1.3 and Chapter 6, Section 6.2). Nevertheless, a user model is generally a limited representation of users' real behavior. For instance, a model cannot represent users' personalities, attitudes, habits, or impairments but only his or her expected interaction on the basis of a certain set of rules (Chapter 6, Section 6.2). Although some researchers have recently tried to create models for predicting the interaction behavior of users with disability (e.g., blind users; Schrepp, 2006; Tonn-Eichstädt, 2006), as we discussed in Chapter 6, it is clearly impossible to simulate the divergent perspective of final users and, moreover, of disabled ones.

In the next sections, we describe the evaluation techniques for inspecting the interaction (inspection methods) and decomposing the interaction tasks (task analysis methods) usually applied by evaluators to simulate the possible users' intrasystemic dialogue with a technology.

8.2.1 INSPECTION OF THE INTERACTION

The inspection methods (Nielsen and Mack, 1994) are a group of methods that usually do not need the participation of users and are conducted by usability experts who have at least 3–5 years of experience in usability testing. The assumption on the basis of the inspection methods is that evaluators skilled in measuring interactions have internalized a representation of the user to be able to make a predictive diagnosis of the dialogue among real users and the product under assessment, without recourse to the observation of a cohort of users during an interaction. Inspection methods are techniques for creating a representation of the system functioning that depicts how the system works when experts simulate the users' interaction.

The theoretical subjectivity and the impossibility of a complete simulation of users' behavior are the main disadvantages of this discounted interaction assessment process. For these reasons, the inspection of interaction is considered only as a starting point of the assessment and can be used by practitioners for finding possible problems during the interaction and preparing the scenario for usability testing with users.

The inspection methods family is quite large (for a complete review, refer to Nielsen and Mack, 1994) and includes heuristic evaluation and estimation, cognitive and pluralistic walkthrough, inspection of the product features, consistency and standards inspection, and formal usability inspection. In the next two sections, we explain the most frequently applied methods in usability and UX assessment—heuristics and CW analysis.

8.2.2 HEURISTIC EVALUATION

The basic idea behind the heuristic evaluation methods (HEMs) (Molich and Nielsen, 1990; Nielsen, 1994a; Nielsen and Molich, 1990) is that the experts inspect the functioning and usability of a product by using as an evaluation tool a list of principles (heuristics). These principles are used as a baseline (ideal model of perfect functioning) in order to compare the product under assessment with the ideal one. Accordingly, the evaluators can estimate the limitations and shortages of the product and provide designers with a list of suggestions to bridge the gap between the actual and the ideal system. Any heuristic list contains a set of features that a system has to respect and indirectly provides evaluators with a user model. For instance, among the principles proposed by Nielsen and Molich (1990) for website analysis, the heuristic "visibility of system status" suggests to evaluators that a good system should inform users about what is going on in the interface by means of appropriate feedbacks. Moreover, this heuristic assumes a user who needs to know his or her position in the interface during the navigation of a website, receiving information and feedbacks necessary for going ahead with the interaction.

During the evolution of the HCI, different kinds of heuristic lists have been produced. Examples include:

- The 10 heuristics for the web interface analysis created by J. Nielsen and Molich (1990). These heuristics are intended as rules of thumb for inspecting the product and concern different aspects of the interaction, such as the safety of the user, the flexibility and efficiency of use, the recoverability of the errors, etc. (Nielsen Norman Group, 2012).
- Principles of interaction design of Bruce Tognazzini—principal of the Nielsen Norman Group. These principles are presented as a list of 16 heuristics (http://www.asktog.com/basics/firstPrinciples.html), which can be used by evaluators for testing the effectiveness of interactions with software, website, or mobile devices interfaces, by considering different aspects of the interactions such as, for example, the chance for the users to reach easily any information in the interface (anticipation), the level of protection offered by the system in saving the users work (protect users' work), etc.
- Shneiderman's golden rules of interface design (Shneiderman, 1986). These eight rules can be used for assessing different kinds of interfaces by taking into account the consistency of the sequences of interactions (strive for consistency), the memory effort required of the users during the interaction (reduce short-term memory [STM] load), etc.

All these lists can be used for inspecting the product functioning by a team of experts. During the evaluation session, each expert is invited to analyze the product, separately or in a group. After the analysis, the experts separately write down the problems they have identified in the product, reporting, in line with each heuristic, the violations to each heuristic on a set of post-it (70 × 70 mm) notes or online forms. Then, all the experts of the evaluation group discuss together the identified violations to each heuristic, rating the severity of the identified problems. The final report can be used by designers for a first redesign of the interface, especially for solving serious problems, such as links or buttons that do not work, blank pages, functions that threaten the security of the final users, and so on.

Kurosu et al. (1997) showed that it is difficult for an evaluator to shift his or her focus of attention among the different heuristics during the assessment. In order to solve this problem, the authors proposed a structured procedure for applying the heuristic evaluation, called structured heuristic evaluation method (sHEM). During an sHEM, the evaluators are involved in different cycles of assessment by focusing on a set of coherent aspects of the product at each cycle. For instance, the evaluators' attention can focus on assessing the ergonomic aspects in the first cycle and on cognitive aspects in the second one. This means that in each cycle the evaluator can assess a reduced list of heuristics, by reducing both the attention shift and the effort that the evaluator has to perform during the assessment.

The heuristic analysis was developed to help evaluators with usability assessment; nevertheless, a group of researchers from the Tampere University of Finland (Väänänen-Vainio-Mattila et al., 2008; Väänänen-Vainio-Mattila and Wäljas, 2009) has recently claimed that it is possible to use the heuristic analysis for analyzing the UX of a service as well. For the assessment of a service in terms of both pragmatic and hedonic aspects, the researchers proposed the following six heuristics (Väänänen-Vainio-Mattila and Wäljas, 2009):

- *Usage and creation of composite services*: Users can add new service components offered to them through the service. In some cases, users can even create their own service components or applications.
- *Cross-platform service access*: Users can access the relevant service elements they need on their personal computers and mobile terminals.
- *Social interaction and navigation*: Users can interact with their relevant user communities and utilize other users' navigation histories in their interaction with the service.
- *Dynamic service features*: Users can perceive the changes in the service contents or user interface.
- *Context-aware services and contextually enriched content*: The service adapts to the user's context of use and offers meaningful contextual information associated with the media contents.
- *General UX-related issues*: The service user interface should be usable and esthetically pleasing, supporting users' trust and privacy, and other experiential aspects.

The model behind these principles and the outcomes of the application of this list of heuristics for the UX assessment are still under discussion, but the advantage of the application of this kind of heuristic analysis is that an evaluator can assess a service as positive or negative in terms of either pragmatic or hedonic features. For instance, by analyzing the heuristic number four (H4), the "dynamic service features," the evaluator can report suggestions in this way:

- H4—When users enter the service, although it is not possible to gain an overview of the recent changes in the service functioning and information structure (negative pragmatic), they can easily use the new functions of the interface (positive pragmatic).
- H4—The service is cumbersome, and it may be hard for a user to spend time navigating the service (negative hedonic). The service satisfies users' curiosity/seeking of knowledge by frequently offering interesting contents (positive hedonic).

Finally, the heuristic analysis has a large set of applications, and the challenge for evaluators is to apply this inspection method in UX assessment. Therefore, the main advantages of the heuristic analysis are the low cost and the quick assessment processes. Nevertheless, it only provides a limited and holistic analysis of the system functioning and, usually, the number of issues identified by evaluators with this technique is scant. Hence, there is a high possibility of false-positive identifications of interface problems especially in the analysis of complex interfaces. For this reason, as noted earlier, the heuristic analysis has to be considered as only the starting point of an interaction assessment.

8.2.3 COGNITIVE WALKTHROUGH METHOD

A CW is a technique for empirically simulating the user's interaction with a product (Lewis et al., 1990; Polson and Lewis, 1990).

In general, a CW starts with a task analysis (we discuss the task analysis in Section 8.2.4), in which the evaluators decompose an interaction task in a list of actions that a user has to perform to achieve the goal of the task. The task analysis is used for (1) specifying the sequence of the steps that a user should take to accomplish task and (2) observing the responses of the system to the user's actions. Once the task analysis is over, the experts simulate the actions of a hypothetical user by means of a question list, and for each item on the list on a scale from 0 to 100, rate the possibility of a user experiencing problems in performing each action of a task.

The original version of the CW was based on the exploratory learning (CE+) model of Polson and C. Lewis (1990). Thomas Mahatody and colleagues, of the University of Lille Nord (France), reviewing the evolution and the use of the CW in the interaction assessment, recently affirmed that:

CE+ model was the first cognitive learning theory to use HCI. Design guidelines, called "Design Principles for Successful Guessing", were derived from this theory to support the design of interactive systems requiring little or even no user training. The CE+ model has three main components: a learning component, a problem-solving component, and an execution component. The model operates as follows: A system user chooses an action among several alternatives based on the similarity between his or her goals and expected consequence of the action; after carrying out the action selected, the user evaluates the system response using the heuristics proposed by [C.] Lewis (1986, 1988). In this way, users evaluate their progress toward their goals. If the goal is achieved, the learning that occurs is registered by inscribing the steps taken by the system (i.e., the evaluated response) in the rule-based representation of procedural knowledge proposed by Kieras [and Polson] (1985). Otherwise, the problem-solving component is activated to discover appropriate action, and so forth. The execution component consists of triggering an applicable rule that matches the current context. (Mahatody et al., 2010, pp. 742–743)

During the evolution of the HCI, many modifications and extensions of the original CW have been proposed, which are intended to help experts to apply this technique or set the CW in different frameworks, such as the decision cycle model (DCM) (see Chapter 5, Section 5.4.1) by Hutchins et al. (1985). Mahatody et al. (2010) identified at least 11 variations of CW, such as the revision of the CW question list and its reorganization under the DCM proposed by Antonio Rizzo—professor at the Communication Science Department, University of Siena—and colleagues in the AVANTI project (1997, see also Chapter 1, Box 1.4).

In order to exemplify the use of this method, in this chapter, we describe only the application of the original CW question list in the framework of the DCM.

As Table 8.1 and Figure 8.2 show, evaluators may simulate all the possible users' actions for achieving a task by asking themselves nine questions (Lewis et al., 1990; Polson et al., 1992).

TABLE 8.1
Question List Originally Proposed by Lewis et al. (1990) for Conducting a Cognitive Walkthrough Evaluation Form for a Single User's Action

1. Description of user's immediate goal:
2. (First/next) atomic action user should take:
    2a. Obvious that action is available? Why/why not?
    2b. Obvious that action is appropriate to goal? Why/why not?
3. How will user access description of action?
    3a. Problem accessing? Why/why not?
4. How will user associate description with action?
    4a. Problem associating? Why/why not?
5. All other available actions less appropriate?
    5a. For each? Why/why not?
6. How will user execute the action?
    6a. Problems? Why/why not?
7. If timeouts, time for user to decide before timeout?
    7a. Why/why not?
8. Execute the action. Describe system response:
    8a. Obvious progress has been made toward goal? Why/why not?
    8b. User can access needed information in system response? Why/why not?
9. Describe appropriate modified goal, if any:
    9a. Obvious that goal should change? Why/why not?
    9b. If task completed, is it obvious? Why/why not?

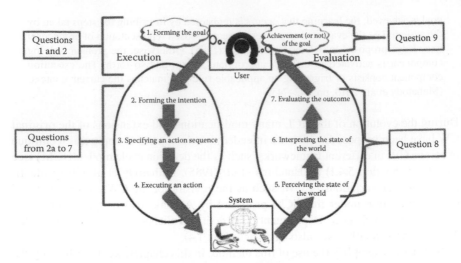

FIGURE 8.2 **(See color insert.)** Adapted representation of the decision cycle model of Hutchins et al. (1985), integrated with the nine questions of the original CW inspection. (From Polson, P.G. et al., *Int. J. Man-Mach. Stud.*, 36(5), 741, 1992.)

As Lewis and colleagues suggest, by using this list of questions a practitioner

> begins by giving a description of the user's current goals and the correct action ([…] Questions 1 and 2). The next series of questions (Questions 2a through 7) evaluate the ease with which the user will be able to correctly select that action and execute it. Next, the evaluator describes the system response and judges its adequacy (Question 8). The final question (Question 9) evaluates whether the user's ability to form an appropriate goal for the next action or detect that the task has been completed. If the task is not complete, the evaluator assumes that the goals have been correctly modified and proceeds to evaluate the next step. (Lewis et al., 1990, p. 238)

Finally, during the assessment, the practitioner can use the CW questions to analyze the decision cycle of the user interaction (i.e., the execution of the action and the evaluation of the action, Figure 8.2) (for a complete review, refer to Militello and Hutton, 1998; Norman, 1986).

In the middle of the 1990s, Cathleen Wharton and her colleagues (1994) at the University of Colorado produced a short list of questions to reduce the effort required of evaluators for a CW analysis (for a complete guide of the CW application and use, refer to Novick 1999). In the interaction analysis, this short version of CW is usually preferred because the evaluators involved in the users' actions simulation process have to consider only four questions:

1. Will the user try to achieve the right effect?
2. Will the user notice that the correct action is available?
3. Will the user associate the correct action with the effect that they are trying to achieve?
4. If the correct action is performed, will the user see that progress is being made toward their goal?

Although the CW can be considered as a powerful simulation tool, it requires practitioners (1) to possess substantial expertise for comprehending the application of the cognitive model behind the technique, such as the CE+ (Lewis et al., 1990; Polson and Lewis, 1990) and (2) to make an extraordinary effort to perform a task analysis followed by a deep analysis of each action of the users through a set of questions. Moreover, given that it is often considered too expensive compared with a heuristic analysis, and does not provide any information about the frequency or severity of the problems but only a long list of comments about the product and its interface functioning, many professionals prefer to apply the heuristic analysis instead of the CW.

8.2.4 TASK ANALYSIS

The task analysis is used by practitioners to decompose in a flow chart what a user is required to do to achieve a task in terms of actions. This kind of analysis is used by practitioners for obtaining data such as the duration of the task, the sequence, and the complexity of the actions that the users need to take. Moreover, there are some specific variations of this kind of analysis, such as the cognitive task analysis (for a complete review, refer to Militello and Hutton, 1998), which measure not only the total time and the number of user actions required during the interaction but also the cognitive processes for achieving a task by assessing, for instance, the time required by the users for thinking about each action, or for comprehending each interface feedback. These kinds of task analysis have been created for assessing the complexity of the task and also for comparing the user performance and consider, for instance, the differences in performance and decision-making processes between lay, novice, and expert users and the users' mental workload in complex actions, etc.

Although task analysis has a long history of application in different fields (Crystal and Ellington, 2004), in HCI studies the most commonly applied technique is the hierarchical one (Stanton, 2006). The hierarchical task analysis (HTA) (Annett and Duncan, 1967; Annett et al., 1971; Hodgkinson and Crawshaw, 1985; Stanton, 2006) breaks down the task into a hierarchy of goals, operations, and plans: goals are the objectives associated with operation of the device; operations are the observable behaviors or activities the user has to perform in order to accomplish the goals; and plans are unobservable decisions and planning on behalf of the operator. During the analysis, each task is described by a statement that reports the overall goal of the task and its associated subgoals (Stanton and Young, 1999).

Usually, experts apply the HTA to simulate the users' behavior before a testing session with real users; then, the end users are invited to analyze the interface by following the same set of tasks that have been previously analyzed by the evaluators (we discuss the real interaction of the users in Section 8.4). After the user test, the evaluators, by analyzing the recordings of the users' interaction, can compare the users' behavior with the results from the HTA such as the average time taken to achieve a certain goal, the difference between the number of clicks made by real users, and the number of clicks that the expert analysis estimated to be enough to perform the same action.

Task analysis is a central step for assessing the usability and the UX with different kinds of users, with and without disability. In fact, only this technique allows evaluators to define the tasks for users' evaluation and practitioners to assess the distance between the expected interaction and the real one.

8.2.5 Summary of Inspection and Simulation Methods of the Expected Interaction

In order to analyze the system functioning, the evaluators have to simulate the users' interaction behavior and need, by following the rules of the selected evaluation technique. This simulation allows practitioners to inspect the product without the involvement of the users by defining the functional shortages and errors of functioning. As Figure 8.3 shows, by applying the inspection and simulation techniques, the evaluators analyze the product functioning using an ideal model of system and user. Usually, this ideal model, embedded in standards and design principles, is the same model that the developers have used to design the system. Given this, the evaluators reconstruct the designers' perspective of the product (i.e., their mental model), by analyzing the image of the system with inspection and simulation techniques.

The inspection of the product functioning drives the evaluators to identify the actual errors in the functioning that may cause problems during the users' interaction, such as, for example, wrong links, functions, etc. Moreover, independent of the errors, this analysis may help evaluators in simulating the possible problems that a

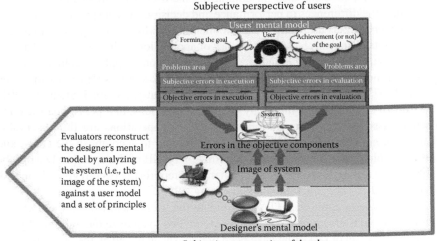

FIGURE 8.3 **(See color insert.)** Synoptic representation of the interaction observed through inspection and simulation methods. This figure represents the reconstruction of the designers' mental model done by evaluators and the assessment of the system functioning imagined by designers with a user model. When the evaluator analyzes the system by means of these methods, he or she can identify the actual errors of the product functioning (e.g., wrong links, functions that do not work, etc.), the possible problems that a user can experience in interacting the system, and also the distance between an ideal system and the product under assessment.

user (represented by an explicit model, personas, or indirectly by a set of principles or standards) can experience during the interaction.

The inspection and simulation techniques are usually the initial step of any IMIE. In fact, the evaluator can use the results of these analyses for a preliminary raw assessment of the product, and for identifying macroscopic issues that the designers should solve before usability testing. Because all these techniques are based on ideal models, it is quite clear that the reliability of the collected data depends on the model's representativeness of all the possible final users' behavior. Nevertheless, as discussed in Chapter 6, the different contexts of product use and the users with disability interaction behavior are often neglected in these models. Hence, for gathering useful information and data about the different interaction experiences and divergent behaviors of users, the evaluators should employ a mixed sample of users with and without disability.

In sum, the inspection and the simulation methods cannot be used as an ultimate solution for assessing the interaction, but have to be considered as the starting point of any evaluation process.

8.3 QUALITATIVE AND SUBJECTIVE MEASUREMENTS FOR INTERACTION ANALYSIS

This macrosection discusses all the qualitative and quantitative tools and techniques that can be used by a practitioner for collecting data about the users' perception of the quality of interaction and their subjective perspective on the system. Among these methods of UX and usability analysis, we include questionnaires, psychometric tools, interviews, observations, diaries, eye-tracking methodology, and biofeedback analysis.

These techniques require a sample of users that, in most cases, should include those with disability. Disabled users often interact with products by means of assistive technology. The assistive technology can be divided into software technologies, such as screen readers or magnifiers, and hardware devices, such as eye-trackers or BCIs, and they play a social function by contributing to the individual "body/self as it is experienced and presented to others" (Lupton and Seymour, 2000, p. 1861). Therefore, it is important to note that, when involving disabled users in the evaluation process and, in particular, in the analysis of the interaction by means of qualitative and subjective measurements, practitioners must pay attention to the impact of the product under assessment in the activities of the users' everyday life, where technologies often take part to users' personal meaning, interactional effects, needs, motivation, and occupational value (Krantz, 2012). Moreover, by including different kinds of users (with and without disability) in the assessment cohort and collecting information by qualitative and subjective measurements, evaluators can collect numerical data (or convert it into numerical data) and manipulate these data with statistical methods. These techniques are largely applied in the HCI, and the reliability of the gathered data depends on the consistency of the applied measures and the possibility normalizing the outcomes. Currently, although in HCI literature there is no empirical evidence that those methods cannot be used in a reliable way for testing usability and UX with disabled users, qualitative methods are seen in social science as particularly accessible for disabled users (Farmer and Macleod, 2011). Nevertheless, as Martin Farmer and Fraser Macleod—researchers at the Office for Disability Issues in the UK Government Department for Work and Pensions—observe, it is necessary to adapt or select the qualitative measure for a study on the basis of people's disabilities:

> [People with learning disabilities or more severe communication or neuro-diversity impairments] may prefer the flexibility associated with in-depth interviews or ethnography, where they are able to discuss issues in their own words rather than answering according to pre-defined response categories in a questionnaire. (Farmer and Macleod, 2011, p. 36)

As we discuss in Chapter 6, it may be quite difficult and expensive to recruit and test disabled users, and for these reasons professionals often prefer to exclude such users from the evaluation cohort. We believe that, apart from the logistical problems of recruiting disabled users, many professionals could have some concerns because they are not trained in adapting tools and instruments to users' individual functioning. This process of assessment tool adaptation, as Farmer and Macleod (2011) underline, is a necessary requirement to manage with "sensitivity" the relationship with disabled users. Therefore, it is important for usability and UX evaluators to acquire expertise in the interaction between disabled users and technology, or to collaborate with (or recruit to the evaluation teams) experts with these competences. In tune with this, Federici and Scherer recently proposed a new professional figure for the assistive technology evaluation process who can work in this multidisciplinary field: the psychotechnologist (Federici et al., 2011; Federici and Scherer, 2012b; Miesenberger et al., 2012).

Finally, we discuss in the next sections the qualitative and subjective measurements, bearing in mind that in most cases these techniques can be used for testing the interaction with a sample of users with and without disability. We show in each section how a technique presents specific barriers for disabled users, and how an evaluator can remove these limitations by using specific alternative instruments (e.g., head-mounted eye-trackers instead of remote eye-trackers for people with poor movement control, Section 8.3.5.2) or by changing the evaluation procedure, such as the administration of a usability questionnaire instead of an interview (Section 8.3.1).

8.3.1 QUESTIONNAIRE AND PSYCHOMETRIC TOOLS

Questionnaires allow evaluators to gain a great number of quantitative data about users' qualitative experience, such as satisfaction or pleasure.

As Bram Oppenheim—researcher at the London School of Economics—suggests

> A questionnaire is not just a list of questions or a form to be filled in. It is essentially a measurement tool, an instrument for the collection of particular kinds of data. Like all such instruments, the aims and the specifications of a questionnaire stem directly from the overall research design. (Oppenheim, 2000, p. 10)

Moreover, as Kirakowski explains, a questionnaire in the field of usability can generally be considered as "a method for the elicitation, and recording, and collecting of information" (Kirakowski, 2000).

During the HCI evolution, many standardized questionnaires have been created for measuring satisfaction and perceived usability. In what follows, we list some of the standardized questionnaires and scales applied by evaluators for interaction assessment.

- The *System Usability Scale* (SUS), developed in 1986 by the Digital Equipment Corporation Ltd, is a 10-item quick and dirty scale that provides a global assessment of the perceived usability that can be operatively defined as the subjective perception of interaction with a system (Brooke, 1996). The items in this questionnaire have been developed according to the three usability criteria of ISO 9241-11 (1998): (1) the ability of users to complete tasks using the system, and the quality of the output of those tasks (effectiveness), (2) the amount of resources consumed in performing tasks (efficiency), and (3) the users' subjective reactions using the system (satisfaction). One can use the SUS for assessing software and websites by simply replacing the word "system" in every item with the word "website." Each item allows users to answer on a five-point scale ranging from "strongly disagree" to "strongly agree." Even though John Brooke (1996)—the developer of the SUS at the Digital Equipment Corporation—has affirmed that this tool is based on a monodimensional scale, recent studies showed that this questionnaire is actually composed of two different factors that are correlated to each other—usability (eight items) and learnability (two items)—(Borsci et al., 2009; Lewis and Sauro, 2009).
- The *Questionnaire for User Interaction Satisfaction* (QUIS), created by the Human-Computer Interaction Lab at College Park of the University of Maryland, aims to gauge users' satisfaction with user–interface interaction. The QUIS was first implemented in a paper and pencil form using a nine-point Likert scale (Chin et al., 1988), and it is available in different languages (English, German, Italian, Brazilian Portuguese, and Spanish). Several computer-based versions have been created and have the same reliability as the paper and pencil version (Harper et al., 1997). The QUIS is composed of three main components: (1) a demographic questionnaire, (2) a measure of overall system satisfaction along six scales, and (3) nine measures of different interface factors such as screen factors, terminology and system feedback, learning factors, system capabilities, technical manuals, online tutorials, multimedia, teleconferencing, and software installation. Components (2) and (3) are measured on a nine-point Likert scale.
- The *Post Study System Usability Questionnaire* (PSSUQ) was designed by IBM to assess the satisfaction of users during interaction with computer software or web interfaces (Lewis, 2002). The PSSUQ is composed of an overall scale of 19 items and three subfactors measured on a seven-point Likert scale: system usefulness (items 1–8), information quality (items 9–15), and interface quality (items 16–18). As James R. Lewis (2002)—the developer

of the PSSUQ at IBM—reports on the basis of many years of experimental application, this questionnaire is very reliable (with a Cronbach's alpha ranging from 0.83 to 0.96).

- The *Software Usability Measurement Inventory* (SUMI) was created by the Human Factors Research Group, at the University College of Cork to assess the perceived quality of use of software. It consists of 50 statements (available in Dutch, English, French, German, Japanese, Greek, Italian, Japanese, Spanish, and Swedish) and three closed responses: "agree," "don't know," and "disagree." The SUMI has a specific data management software (SUMISCO, http://sumi.ucc.ie/), which can be used for estimating a global usability scale and five subscales: (1) efficiency, the degree to which users can achieve goals with the product; (2) affect, how much the product captures the users' emotional responses; (3) helpfulness, the extent to which the product seems to assist the users; (4) control, the degree to which the users feel that they own the interaction; and (5) learnability, the ease with which a user can get started and learn new features of the product. A specific and simplified version of the SUMI for website analysis is the Website Analysis and MeasureMent Inventory (WAMMI). WAMMI has the same psychometric structure and output as the SUMI, but it is composed of only 20 statements, with a very strong reliability index ranging from 0.90 to 0.93 (http://www.wammi.com/).

Practitioners can administrate these questionnaires to the user (usually at the end of the test) with a great level of confidence in the outcomes, because all these instruments are standardized and widely used in HCI studies. Nevertheless, a questionnaire is a set of limited items, and it can only measure a predetermined set of UX or usability aspects. As Kirakowski says

> a questionnaire tells you only the user's reaction as the user perceives the situation. Thus some kinds of questions, for instance, to do with time measurement or frequency of event occurrence, are not usually reliably answered in questionnaires. [...] A questionnaire is usually designed to fit a number of different situations (because of the costs involved). Thus a questionnaire cannot tell you in detail what is going right or wrong with the application you are testing. (Kirakowski, 2000)

Given this, the evaluators intending to use these instruments should adapt their assessment goals to the limits of the questionnaire. In fact, UX is a multidimensional concept, and it cannot be held to a "gold standard" valid for any kind of user, context, or purpose. Therefore, practitioners have to select the appropriate measure that best suits the purpose of the assessment.

Together with the questionnaires, evaluators can use a psychometric tool for measuring specific UX aspects. As Francis Galton claims, psychometrics is the "art of imposing measurement and number upon operations of the mind" (1879, p. 149). In light of this, we can define a psychometric tool as a standardized instrument (such as questionnaires or tests) that is designed, verified, and validated to test psychological variables (such as learning, decision making, etc.) by measuring the human responses and behavior (e.g., reaction time, workload, etc.).

Examples of psychometric tools are

- The *Subjective Workload Assessment Technique* (SWAT) is a commonly applied technique of workload analysis. It is composed of three main dimensions—time load, mental effort, and psychological stress load (Reid, 1985). The time load is associated with the time needed for a person to accomplish or fail to complete a task. The mental effort is an indicator of the amount of attention or mental demands required to accomplish a task and, generally, this is dependent on the complexity of the task. Finally, the psychological stress load refers to conditions that produce confusion, frustration, and/or anxiety during task performance and, therefore, make task accomplishment more difficult. In order to apply a SWAT analysis, evaluators should invite the users to analyze the product and rate each of the three dimensions (time load, mental effort, and psychological stress) by selecting one of three possible statements (positive or negative). For instance, the user can assess his or her perception of the time load during the task interaction by rating it by one of the following: (1) "Often have spare time"—interruptions or overlap among activities occur infrequently or not at all; (2) "Occasionally have spare time" —interruptions or overlap among activities occur frequently; (3) "Almost never have spare time" —interruptions or overlap among activities are frequent or occur all the time. At the end of the analysis, the evaluator has a list of positive or negative statements that can be used for reporting to the designers the level of workload experienced by users during the exploration and use of the product. The SWAT is a powerful technique, but "it has two main problems: it is not very sensitive for low mental workloads and it requires a time-consuming card sorting pre-task procedure" (Luximon and Goonetilleke, 2001, p. 229).
- The *Cooper–Harper Scale*, created by George Cooper and Robert Harper (1969)—respectively, scientists at the Ames Aeronautical Laboratory (today, Ames Research Center) and at Cornell Aeronautical Laboratory (today, Calspan Corporation)—for assessing aircraft-handling qualities. It can be used, with some modification to the original items, for assessing the users' workload during the interaction with computer systems and interfaces (Annett, 2002a). This scale is composed of a logical-graphic presentation of 10 items for measuring the overall perceived quality of the system and its deficiencies.
- The *NASA Task Load Index* (NASA-TLX) is a multidimensional measure of the workload, and it is considered a tool with a high level of reliability compared with SWAT analysis (Vidulich and Tsang, 1985, 1986). This instrument has six dimensions: (1) mental demand, (2) physical demand, (3) temporal demand, (4) performance, (5) effort, and (6) frustration level. All these dimensions are measured on a 20-point scale from low to high, except for performance, which ranges from good to poor (Human Performance Research Group, 2012). The mental demand scale aims to measure the mental and perceptual activity required of users and the easiness of the task, whereas the physical demand scale measures the

activity required. The time demand scale measures the time pressure felt by the user to rate or pace the tasks. The performance scale assesses how much the user is satisfied by his or her performance in achieving the goal (the success perceived). The effort dimension assesses how hard it is for the users to mentally and/or physically work to accomplish their level of performance. Finally, the frustration level scale assesses how users are insecure, discouraged, irritated, stressed, and annoyed versus secure, gratified, content, relaxed, and complacent during the task.

All the questionnaires and the instruments described earlier have been used mostly for assessing usability. Nevertheless, recently, Marc Hassenzahl and Andrew Monk (2010)—respectively professors at the Folkwang University of Germany and at the University of York in the United Kingdom—proposed a specific scale designed for surveying a large set of UX aspects, called *AttrakDiff* (see http://www.attrakdiff.de). *AttrakDiff* is composed of 23 seven-step items whose poles are opposite adjectives (e.g., confusing–clear, unusual–ordinary, good–bad), and its outcomes allow practitioners to obtain information about (1) the product pragmatic quality (PQ), (2) the product hedonic quality (HQ), and (3) the product attractiveness (ATT). The *AttrackDiff* can be used for testing a large group of participants online (only German and English users), with a very consistent scale (Cronbach's alpha equals 0.83 for PQ; 0.90 for HQ; and 0.93 for ATT; Hassenzahl, 2001). This kind of holistic survey, used together with a standardized tool, can be very useful for a practitioner who aims to obtain an overall qualitative measure of the UX.

We have to consider that all these tools are created for testing users without disabilities and that, in most cases, users with physical impairments can only fill out online surveys by means of specific technological supports (e.g., screen readers, track-ball, etc.). Hence, as we said in Section 8.3, when evaluators aim to involve cognitively impaired people in the assessments, they have to consider how to exemplify the administrations of these tools, for example by presenting the items in the form of a structured or semistructured interview (Section 8.3.2).

At the same time, in order to analyze a large set of UX aspects and minimize the barriers faced by the different kinds of users, practitioners could try to construct their own scale, but the results so obtained cannot be generalizable. Another strategy consists in adapting the standardized questionnaires by reducing or recalibrating/simplifying the items, for example by using a couple of scales of the QUIS as an interview for a sample of users with disability and the whole scale with nondisabled users.

Practitioners can also decide to use specific satisfaction questionnaires created for disabled users such as, for example, the *Quebec User Evaluation of Satisfaction with Assistive Technology* (QUEST2.0, see: Demers et al., 2002a). This questionnaire is usually applied for measuring assistive technology satisfaction, and it can also be easily adapted for a UX analysis. Moreover, the QUEST can be used as a self-administration questionnaire or as an interview, whose response categories range from 1 (not satisfied at all) to 5 (very satisfied). Three scales are provided to analyze the QUEST scores: device (from Q1 to Q8), services (from Q9 to Q12), and total score. All scores are calculated by summing and then averaging the valid responses to assigned items (Demers et al., 2002a,b).

Finally, in order to involve disabled users in the assessment, the evaluators should identify a way for comparing the outcomes of participants with and without disability, by selecting and adapting a specific set of measurements. Moreover, whereas collecting some descriptive data about participants without disability (e.g., expertise, skills, and attitudes) can be sufficient for discriminating the individual differences in their evaluation performances, when users with disabilities are added to the cohort, the evaluator also has to consider their individual functioning, along with their expertise, skills, and attitudes, in order to estimate the differences between all the evaluation participants. In other words, practitioners who want a reliable representation of the disabled users involved in the assessment could discriminate and compare the disabled users' performances by obtaining some measures or indexes about their individual functioning. As we discussed in Section 8.3, practitioners may collaborate with (or include in their assessment team) experts on disability in order to obtain those measures (e.g., psychologist, physiatrist, psychotechnologist, etc.) who are trained in collecting these kinds of measures by means of specific instruments such as the *World Health Organization Disability Assessment Schedule 2.0* (Federici and Meloni, 2010b; Üstün et al., 2010). Sometimes, participants with disability directly provide these kinds of measures to evaluators; in that case, the practitioners need only to collect and use these data for discriminating and comparing user performances.

8.3.2 INTERVIEW

We can identify three kinds of interviews that differ in terms of the organization and presentation of questions to participants (Patton, 1987): (1) structured interview, (2) semistructured interview, and (3) nonstructured interview. The structured interview is a set of research questions that is similar to a questionnaire and in which the interviewer presents one question at a time. In the semistructured interview, the interviewer uses a list of research questions in random order, varying them on the basis of the users' answers. In this kind of interview, evaluators can also add specific questions in tune with the users' comments. Otherwise, the nonstructured interview is similar to an informal conversation: The interviewer is focused on asking specific aspects about the product interaction by following the emerging dialogue with the users, in line with the aims of the product evaluation. The nonstructured interview may take a long time and it requires a high level of expertise, because the interviewer has to bear in mind the general questions about the issue and drive the participants during the discussion by adapting the questions to their answers. As we said before, the structured interview has the same limitations as the questionnaire, but it can be used easily by novice interviewers. As Tim May—researcher at the Centre for Sustainable Urban and Regional Futures at Salford University in the United Kingdom—underlines, the semistructured interview is particularly efficient when the "researcher has a specific focus for their interviews within a range of other methods employed in their study" (May, 2011, p. 135). In light of this, we suggest that, in most cases, a semistructured interview amply meets the practitioners' needs during usability and UX research that is usually carried out on a specific product tested by a multiple set of techniques. As Deborah Mayhew—usability consultant and co-founder and CEO of the Online User Experience Institute in the United States—reports (1999), in the usability and UX field practitioners may also discriminate an evaluation process carried out via interview on the basis of where and when the questions are administered to the participants. In fact, the participants can be interviewed for example in laboratories or at home, immediately after or sometime after the interaction, etc. Then, we can further discriminate them in two other different types of interview: off-site and on-site interview.

Off-site interviews can be conducted in artificial settings either before or after the users' interaction (e.g., for measuring their level of expectation). A typical example of this technique is the focus group, whereby a group of users are invited by a moderator to ask some questions about specific aspects of the product. A group interview is an efficient technique because evaluators can obtain many answers from only one question, and they can expect the mutually positive influence among users that can facilitate their answers. Since, however, the group interview is usually conducted in settings that are different from the real environment and not carried out during the users' interaction with the technology under evaluation, the evaluators have to assess the possible differences between what the participants answered in the session room and their perception of performances during interaction in the real context.

The on-site interview both depends on and is related to the environment where the users usually experience the interaction with a product. An example is the contextual inquiry (Beyer and Holtzblatt, 1998): an ethnographic method consisting of a combination of observation and interview. In this method, data are collected during the users' interactions in their contexts of use through the interviewer's observations. Although the interviewers should minimize the impact of their presence, they must interrupt the user interaction with the technology in order to administer to the participants a list of questions about the UX aspects under assessment (e.g., structured, semistructured interview). To avoid interrupting the flow of the user's behavior, evaluators should silently observe the interaction by video-recording it. Therefore, after the interaction session, the users should be invited to retrospectively analyze their previous actions by means of the interviewer's questions. The on-site interview is widely used in the assessment process since it allows practitioners to collect data during the interaction with the product.

All the different kinds of interview require a long time to prepare questions and test the users. For this reason, many researches in the HCI field (Consolvo et al., 2007; Hudson et al., 2002; Intille et al., 2003; Kubey and Csíkszentmihályi, 1990) have started to use a variation of the traditional interview method called the experience sampling method (ESM) (Larson and Csíkszentmihályi, 1983, 1992). This method consists in repeatedly requesting users to report their thoughts, feelings, and actions during their daily or weekly interactions, by using their phones, online tools, or mobile phone applications. Similarly to a structured interview, in the ESM, users are asked to answer questions and give a rating for their current feelings and experience regarding the product during a day or over a week.

Structured, semistructured, and nonstructured interviews can all be used with users with and without disability. Nevertheless, practitioners who want to interview disabled users should have at least a bachelor's degree or working experience in the field of disabilities (e.g., a psychotechnologist), and it might be useful to include two or more respondents (e.g., parents, siblings, direct-care staff) who have known the participant "for at least three months and have had recent opportunities to observe the person function in one or more environments for substantial periods of time" (Tassé et al., 2008, p. 2). In cases involving disabled persons with low intellectual functioning, the interviewer should administrate the questions to a proxy, i.e., parents or supporters, who will respond on behalf of the user. The involvement of a third person (proxy) can be useful in the evaluation of particular types of technologies for disability, such as assistive technology. In this case, when the evaluation aims to assess the match between the user and the assistive technology, the proxy plays an active role in the UX assessment since he or she is a fundamental part of the context of use (Borsci et al., 2012b). Although proxies' responses may reflect the disabled person's view, for the specific aim of the evaluation of interaction we recommend the use of other qualitative methods such as observation, because the data obtained by interviewing a third person on behalf of the participant are necessarily mediated by his or her own experience and mental model of the technology, and it can strongly affect the evaluation data.

8.3.3 OBSERVATION

Similarly to the interview, the observation allows evaluators to collect a great amount of information. The existing observation practices (Baber and Stanton, 1996) can be divided into two main groups—observation in controlled environments (experimental) and observation in uncontrolled environments.

Experimental observation is a practice that has to be conducted in controlled environments (e.g., laboratories) for direct observation of the user interaction. This type of observation is often applied along with other techniques such as the interview (contextual inquiry) or think-aloud tests (Hackos and Redish, 1998; Nielsen, 1993). When practitioners wish to analyze a large group of users in their everyday environments and have only a limited budget, they can arrange indirect (or remote) observation (Hartson et al., 1996; Ivory and Hearst, 2001) by means of an asynchronous analysis of the online data of the users' interaction performances. Of course, indirect observation does not guarantee complete control of the environmental variables. We discuss remote testing in greater detail in Section 8.4.4.

An example of observation that can be conducted in uncontrolled environments is naturalistic observation. This is an on-site assessment of users' interaction in their everyday environments. It is usually conducted by video-recording the user's everyday environment (e.g., user's office desk, kitchen, dining room, etc.). Since video-cameras are now able to record more than 20 consecutive hours and their size is less intrusive than before, the evaluators can register the users' interaction and leave them to perform their natural behavior with very little external influence. This observation can be used in public places, such as a ticket counter, a retail shop, or a restaurant.

Independent of the type of observation used (controlled or uncontrolled), practitioners can use the collected data to extrapolate information about the sequence, frequency, and duration of the users' interaction activities (Drury, 1990). To complete the overall picture of the UX analysis, all the gathered information can be analyzed by means of specific software for qualitative data analysis or a GTA approach (Chapter 7, Section 7.4.1.).

Observation is ubiquitous in the UX evaluation, because it serves as a basis for the usability testing (Section 8.4) and, moreover, it can also be used as an independent tool for gathering data about the users' everyday behavior. Of course, naturalistic observation could be very useful for evaluating the use of assistive or medical technology devices in the everyday environments of disabled users' interaction.

8.3.4 DIARY

The interview and the observation techniques often require the presence of an interviewer or observer, which could affect the users' interaction and their answers or reactions, thus affecting the reliability of the gathered information. In order to avoid the practitioner's direct intervention, the user interaction diary can help evaluators to capture the activities that occur during the interactions in real environments (Palen and Salzman, 2002; Rieman, 1993). Although the diary is considered a powerful ethological method for obtaining data about the time spent on each activity by users (Ericsson et al., 1990), guaranteeing evaluators "a relative high standard of objectivity" (Rieman, 1993, p. 321), the diary method is rarely used in interaction evaluation studies (Nørgaard and Hornbæk, 2006).

In traditional diary studies, users track their interaction activities for a certain period, usually 2 or 3 weeks, recording their actions by writing down a block note or by using tools such as audio-recorders, video-cameras, or digital cameras (photo-diary method). A variation of this method is the day reconstruction method (DRM) proposed by Kahneman—professor at the Woodrow Wilson School and Department of Psychology at Princeton University in the United States—and his colleagues (2004). In the DRM, users are asked to write a diary about their interaction experience the day before by completing a structured self-administered questionnaire. The questionnaire is structured to help users to construct a sequence of episodes focused on their emotions and feelings. The DRM has the advantage of being more focused than the traditional diary on the users' feelings and the emotional aspects of the interaction.

The main advantage of the diary, compared with other qualitative and subjective measurements, is that practitioners can ask users to register their impressions in textual, visual, or audio form for a long time, thus gathering a huge amount of information for each participant. Usually, the data diaries are a good basis for preparing for the interviews of the participants. Finally, the diary method can be considered an accessible evaluation technique for testing disabled users. In fact, it is a flexible procedure that allows a practitioner to easily adapt it to user needs, in line with Farmer and Macleod's suggestions (2011). For instance, practitioners can select the best and easiest way of recording (e.g., audio, video, etc.) information about users' experience by agreement with each participant.

8.3.5 EYE-TRACKING METHODOLOGY AND BIOFEEDBACK

Among qualitative and subjective measurements, eye-tracking systems and biofeedback devices are currently two of the most advanced and high-tech solutions.

These measurements can be used together with other evaluation techniques (e.g., observation and interview), and they offer practitioners the chance to collect objective data (e.g., user stress and frustration during the interaction, user gazing at the interface) from the users' physiological and sensory-motor reactions during the interaction. Evaluators can use such objective data for assessing the qualitative and the subjective point of view of users about their interaction with a product.

Both biofeedback and eye-tracking technologies have a long history in the HCI field (for a review, refer to Andreassi, 2006; Jacob, 1995; Poole and Ball, 2006), and they provide evaluators with a large set of analyses.

For instance, biofeedback analysis tracks different kinds of signals by means of electroencephalography, electrocardiography, and electromyography, which can be used for analyzing parameters such as cardiac frequency, brain activity, or event-related potential (Joyce et al., 2002; Maruta et al., 2010; Sereno and Rayner, 2003). In order to collect these kinds of data, evaluators have to apply to the users' bodies a set of sensors and electrodes for detecting signals. Similarly, the eye-tracking system can be used for analyzing eye movement components such as saccade movements, eye rotations, pupil diameter, convergence and divergence, etc. (Duchowski, 2007). For the evaluation process, two kinds of eye-tracking devices can be used—the remote eye-tracker, which is integrated in displays and monitors, or the head-mounted, which is usually integrated in helmets or glasses. The remote eye-trackers are composed of detection and recording devices that are usually hidden to users. They are particularly useful in indoor contexts with different kinds of screens. Otherwise, the head-mounted eye-tracking systems can be used in environmental contexts, as users can actually wear the device. Clearly, head-mounted eye-trackers are particularly intrusive but easily portable when user mobility is required (Mele and Federici, 2012a).

In the next sections, we discuss the biofeedback and the eye-tracking methodologies, with particular attention to the advantages and the limitations of their use for the evaluation process.

8.3.5.1 Biofeedback Usability and UX Testing

Biofeedback analysis requires a certain level of expertise in human factors and in cognitive sciences and great expertise in signal analysis for interpreting the meanings of data. A biofeedback device can be used to detect and record reliably the signal variations in users' physiology, measured as changes in skin conductivity, heart activity, blood pressure, respiration, voice quality, and electrical activities in muscle and brain (Andreassi, 2006; Sperry and Fernandez, 2008). These changes occur in response to thought processes and mental events and can be used as a reliable measure of users' emotional states, such as stress, frustration, or workload (Ward et al., 2001; Wastell and Newman, 1996; Wilson and Sasse, 2000).

Biofeedback usability and UX tests are conducted in laboratory environments, and the participants are invited to interact or observe the product interaction with different scenarios or in a free task condition while they are monitored by biofeedback devices using sensors and electrodes. After the biofeedback analysis, other techniques are usually employed, such as a questionnaire or an interview, in order to gather further details on user opinions about the product under evaluation (Mandryk et al., 2006; Yannakakis and Hallam, 2007).

The main advantage of the biofeedback analysis is the opportunity to collect reliable and objective data about user reactions during the interaction. Nevertheless, in order to interpret the users' physiological changes, practitioners have to carry out lengthy statistical analyses. In fact, although biofeedback detection devices are usually sold along with statistical analysis software, a large part of the interpretation has to be done manually. Moreover, biofeedback devices are often intrusive since the application of sensors to the user's body can affect the natural flow of the interaction, thus limiting the user's natural movements. Moreover, the reliability of the collected data could be affected by different factors such as the system setting or the right positioning of the sensors on the participants' bodies. In light of this, evaluators have to pay attention to the experimental setting, since a wrong procedure may decrease the quantity and the quality of the detected signals and, in consequence, of the collected data.

The use of biofeedback devices can be a very powerful resource for an evaluator; however, the complexity of these systems and the analysis of the collected data are often a barrier for professionals without the required level of expertise for conducting an assessment efficiently and effectively with these tools.

8.3.5.2 Eye-Tracking Usability and UX Testing

Nowadays, eye-tracking analysis is a widely applied methodology in the UX and usability field (Nielsen and Pernice, 2010; Poole and Ball, 2006). Eye-tracking devices are used in laboratories and in everyday environments for analyzing both the eye movements and the focus of the user during the interaction. As represented in Figure 8.1, eye-tracking methodology is mostly used for collecting data about the overall quality of the interaction, but it can be also adopted for usability testing. In fact, eye-trackers can collect data about effectiveness, efficiency, and (indirectly) user satisfaction. Use of the eye-tracker alone, however, cannot help evaluators to collect data regarding the kind of problems identified by the user. In light of this, eye-tracking systems have to be combined with other techniques for usability testing in order to be considered as a technique for analyzing user perception of the product functioning (see Section 8.4).

In the last 10 years, the use of eye-tracking methodology in evaluation assessment has increased, thanks to the diffusion of increasingly reliable, smart, and accurate detection and tracking technologies (Poole and Ball, 2006). Nowadays, eye-trackers are widely used for collecting data about visual search and visual information processing mechanisms, reading, behavior in natural tasks (e.g., driving, sports, etc.), or information processing in different domains (Mele and Federici, 2012a,b). Moreover, eye-tracking devices are also used in neuroscience research in combination with biofeedback devices such as positron emission tomography, magneto-encephalography, and functional magnetic resonance imaging, for testing subjects' brain functioning during specific activities such as word recognition (Joyce et al., 2002; Maruta et al., 2010; Sereno and Rayner, 2003).

As Seppo Nevalainen and Jorma Sajaniemi (2004)—researchers at the University of Joensuu in Finland—suggest, any evaluation with an eye-tracker is composed of at least four main phases:

1. The *setup* phase, in which the position of both the participant and the eye-tracker is adjusted. For instance, when using a remote eye-tracker, the user has to be positioned in front of the screen, with a certain distance from the device, according to the device features.
2. The *adjustment* phase, in which the practitioner analyzes the functionality of the device to detect the users' fixations and saccade.
3. The *calibration* phase, in which the user's eye calibration value is computed by analyzing the eye behavior when following a calibration target presented on the screen.
4. The *monitoring* phase, in which the experts analyze the functionality of the eye-tracker and the eventual deterioration of the calibration by readjustment during the experiment.

One of the main advantages for practitioners in using eye-tracking methodology is that it reliably collects objective data about the subjective overall perception of the interaction. These data can be used by evaluators to tell designers which parts of the product need to be adjusted to increase the users' interaction experience (Duchowski, 2007). Moreover, most eye-tracking devices come with specific software that provides visual data analysis (e.g., eye fixations, scan paths in eye movements, saliency) and statistical data analysis, to help evaluators to interpret the meaning of the data obtained on their products. Therefore, although eye-trackers are powerful and reliable tools for HCI assessment, the practitioners have to be aware of certain disadvantages and limitations in the application of these instruments. First, the thresholds used by the automatic software for the interpretation of the collected data (e.g., the minimum time of duration of a fixation) are not standardized and, as a consequence, the measures carried out by different devices on the same product can slightly vary (Poole and Ball, 2006). Moreover, the accuracy of the eye-trackers available on the market varies on the basis of their functioning and features; hence, the comparability of evaluation studies adopting eye-tracking methodology may depend on the features of the eye-tracker, such as the data collected in milliseconds, the saccade resolution of the device, etc. (for a list of some current eye-tracker features, refer to http://www.tobii.com, http://www.smivision.com, and http://www.sr-research.com/). Moreover, evaluators budgeting for the purchase of an eye-tracker must carefully consider the tool's physical characteristics, bearing in mind the different needs of users with and without disability and the features of the product they want to test. As noted earlier, practitioners can find many types of portable devices on the market (integrated in helmets and glasses) and devices that reduce and control head movements (i.e., head-mounted eye-trackers), which can be used to test products in different kinds of contexts (from an interface to a physical environment), and with different kinds of users, with and without disability. For instance, the evaluator testing a website interface with a sample of nondisabled users could use a remote eye-tracker, as it minimizes the influence of the camera on the natural behavior of the users. Conversely, when an evaluator aims to test the interaction with portable or physical products (tablets, mobile and smart phones, assistive technologies, etc.), in an everyday environment (house, workplace, shopping center, etc.), participants necessarily wear a portable eye-tracking device that may affect their natural interaction. These types of devices, by means of head movement compensation solutions, provide reliable binocular eye-tracking data in a highly mobile and flexible way, and they are easily integrated with other mobile technologies and sensors, such as EEG or GPS, regardless of the peculiarities of subjects involved in the experimentation (e.g., eye color, age, glasses, contact lenses) or environmental conditions (e.g., light in the room, position of the screen) (Mele and Federici, 2012a). Consequently, when a sample of users with a low level of either motor control or attentional focus is involved in an evaluation test conducted by eye-tracking methodology, the evaluators may use portable devices to facilitate the participant analysis. Nevertheless, as Jacob and Kean—respectively, professor of computer science at Tufts University and researcher on usability strategies at the Xerox corporation of Rochester—suggest, portable eye-trackers "still have the discomfort of the head-mounted systems and add the burden of the backpack" (Jacob and Karn, 2003, p. 578), thus affecting the natural interaction of the users. In conclusion, the use of the eye-tracker requires less expertise than a biofeedback device, since it can automatically analyze the collected data. Evaluators should, however, be able to use both types of device, paying attention to the limitations of the software analysis in order to avoid misinterpretation of the results.

8.3.6 SUMMARY OF THE QUALITATIVE AND SUBJECTIVE MEASUREMENTS FOR INTERACTION ANALYSIS

In order to collect data about the subjective evaluation of an interaction, evaluators have to select one or more qualitative and subjective measurements (Figure 8.1, IMIE—user evaluation of the interaction quality). As Figure 8.4 shows, qualitative and subjective measurements allow evaluators to observe the users' reaction to the problems that they experience while interacting with a technology and evaluate the product output.

Therefore, qualitative and subjective techniques are not able to collect data about the type of problems experienced by users (Section 8.4), but only the user reaction to those problems.

Although qualitative and subjective measurements are techniques for observing the user point of view on the product through a holistic assessment of the interaction, usability testing and analysis of the user interaction (Section 8.4) offer a deep analysis of the quality of the interaction. Consequently, there is a link between qualitative measurements and usability testing, because both are methods that extrapolate data about an interaction by involving the users.

Finally, whereas qualitative measurements investigate quality in use by considering the overall satisfaction or other subjective aspects that are useful for assessing UX, usability testing is focused on the effectiveness and efficiency of quality in use, as we explain in the next section.

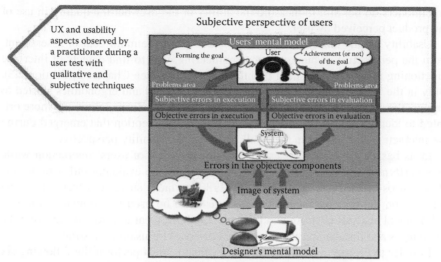

FIGURE 8.4 (**See color insert.**) Synoptic representation of the interaction observed by qualitative and subjective methods. It represents the users' perspective on their interaction with a product (subjective perspective of users, at the top) and the designer's perspective on the product functioning (subjective perspective of developer, at the bottom). When the evaluator involves a sample of users in the assessment, by using a qualitative and subjective technique, he or she can only measure the reaction of the users and their qualitative point of view.

8.4 USABILITY TESTING AND ANALYSIS OF REAL INTERACTION

In this macrosection, we discuss two main evaluation techniques for testing UX and usability: the think-aloud protocol and the remote testing. By means of these techniques, practitioners can collect data about the number, kind, and location of problems experienced by users during the interaction with a product. The participants involved can be either nonexperts (novice) in the use of the product or experts in the use of similar products. For instance, in usability testing, participants are usually all novices, whereas in the UX evaluation process, the assessment of quality in use occurs initially when the participants are novices (first use of the product) and then when they have become experts. In these UX analyses, the participants' previous expertise with similar products is an important variable for discriminating differences among users. Usability testing is mostly conducted in laboratories, although it is also possible to conduct it in the everyday environment, whereas remote testing is a less controllable type of test mostly conducted in natural environments, as discussed in Section 8.3.3.

8.4.1 USABILITY TESTING

We use the term "usability testing," instead of "user testing," because the target is not the user but the product perceived by the user. In fact, in usability testing, practitioners do not aim to measure the ability of the user but the quality in use of the product perceived by user.

Usability testing has been used since 1960s when the main goal of assessment, from the perspective of human factor engineering, was to find defects of interface functioning in line with a small usability perspective (see Chapter 2, Section 2.3). Only in the 1980s, however, when cognitive psychology and ergonomics started to support the design and manufacturing field, did testing become more and more oriented to identifying the cognitive aspects and user perception that emerged during the interaction, shifting from the small to the bigger usability perspective.

In its basic form, usability testing is an observation of users' interaction while they perform a series of tasks that are mandated by the evaluator either by means of scenarios or in free condition. In the 1980s, a more structured form of testing centered on the user interaction process started to be used by evaluators: the verbal protocol analysis (Ericsson and Simon, 1980). In what follows, we describe the advantages and disadvantages of the verbal protocol for usability testing.

In order to prepare a usability test, an evaluator must perform the following six steps: (1) set up the test environment and recruit participants, (2) decide on the testing procedure, (3) prepare the instructions for the users, (4) draw up the task list, (5) schedule the test, and (6) prepare useful material such as the consent form and remuneration schedule. Usually, the total time needed for a test should be 1 or 2 h.

After the data analysis, the evaluator should create a report for the design team. In order to report their data, the evaluator can use a standardized template called the Common Industry Format for Usability, which follows ISO/IEC 25062 (2006). This template allows practitioners to describe the analysis carried out on the product and the context of use tested during the assessment. In the UX evaluation process, the information obtained from the usability testing is used as a baseline for the user testing that should be carried out after a certain time of product use to improve the next version of the product. Moreover, in the usability design process, the information is immediately discussed with the design team to revise the product before another test (formative testing) or to revise the final version of the product (summative testing).

Usability testing is usually performed in well-structured laboratories; nevertheless, today, thanks to the portability of devices for testing and recording user interaction, the evaluator can also test users in their everyday environments. In traditional testing, the participants analyze a functional mock-up or a prototype of the product. Nevertheless, the mock-up or trial device often become available in the later stage of the development, so sometimes the testing is carried out on a paper prototype, especially for the web or software interfaces.

When the prototype (or its paper version) is tested in a laboratory, the analysis is carried out in a large room (Figure 8.5) divided by a half-mirror (Figure 8.5). On the right side of the room, as in Figure 8.5, the experimental setting is set up for participant interaction. In order to create a tension-releasing environment, practitioners usually decorate the space with a painting on the wall, a potted plant, a carpet, and a desk and chair of good quality. The participant receives instructions from an audio-speaker or from a facilitator who sits behind her or him. The participant's behavior is then video-recorded by means of a small video-camera positioned on the ceiling and observed by the design stakeholders behind the half-mirror. On the left side of

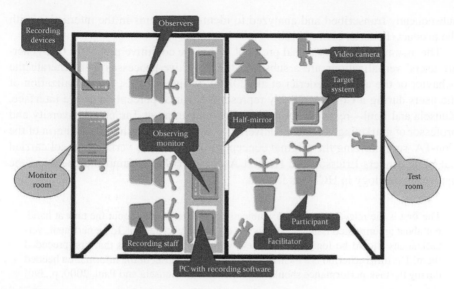

FIGURE 8.5 The Usability Testing Laboratory setting is located in two rooms separated by a half-mirror (in the middle of the figure). On the right side, there is a room for the participant testing, in which the user interacts with the system and the facilitator observes the interaction. The user's verbalizations and behavior are video-recorded. On the left side, behind the half-mirror, a group of developers and marketing experts observe the user's interaction, and the screen actions of the user are recorded by a recording system.

the room, as in Figure 8.5, hidden by the half-mirror, marketing people, designers, sales personnel, other stakeholders, and the testing staff assisting in the trials discuss reasons for and possible solutions to the difficulties verbalized or shown by the participants during the trial.

In conclusion, usability testing is a complex and detailed analysis of real user interaction. The value of the collected data strictly depends on the way in which the test is organized and managed by the evaluator. In fact, the evaluator should support participants in identifying interaction problems.

After the 1980s, verbal protocols became the main method of testing usability, and even today this technique is the one most frequently applied to collect users' descriptions of problems experienced during interaction. Two main types of verbal protocol are commonly used in HCI, concurrent thinking aloud (Con-TA) and retrospective thinking aloud (Retro-TA). In the next section, we describe the advantages and the limitations of these two types of verbal protocols.

8.4.2 Concurrent Thinking Aloud in Usability Testing

The Con-TA is a structured form of the traditional usability testing that can be performed in a laboratory or in less structured environments (e.g., users' workplace, house, classroom, etc.). By means of the Con-TA, participants are asked to verbalize every action and any problem they perceive during their interaction. The participants' behavior and verbalizations that occur during the test should be video-recorded and subsequently transcribed and analyzed to identify problems in the interaction with the product (Federici et al., 2010b).

The assumption of any verbal protocol is that the cognitive processes that generate users' verbalizations are a subset of the cognitive processes that generate the behavior or the action (Federici et al., 2010b). In light of this, the verbalization of the users during a Con-TA reliably represents the user perception of the interface. Kuusela and Paul—respectively professor of marketing at Tampere University and professor of marketing at Denver University—amply explain the three criteria of the Con-TA, summarizing the original conceptualization of the verbal protocol carried out by K. Anders Ericsson and Herbert A. Simon (1993)—famous pioneers of the applied psychology in HCI—as follows

> The first is the relevance criterion: Subjects should be talking about the task at hand, not about an unrelated issue. Second is the consistency criterion: To be pertinent, verbalizations should be logically consistent with the verbalizations that just preceded them. The third criterion is a memory requirement: A subset of the information heeded during the task performance should be remembered. (Kuusela and Paul, 2000, p. 390)

The Con-TA helps practitioners to understand the behavior of and the reasons for user actions. During the analysis, however, the participants quite often forget to verbalize their thoughts and actions, and they perform some operations silently. In this case, the facilitators should help the users by reminding them of the task instructions. During a Con-TA session, the evaluator acts as a facilitator by supporting the users' verbalization or answering their requests. Moreover, the facilitator should be prepared to help users by minimizing their influence to the natural interaction flow. It can be useful for facilitators to prepare a list of stereotyped indications for answering participants' questions during the Con-TA. For instance, if a user asks about the correctness of his or her action, the facilitator could answer: "Do you think it is in line with the goal of the task?" or "There are no right answers; It depends on what you are experiencing. Do you think it is in line with the goal are your trying to achieve?"

In the Con-TA, the user's working memory (WM) and STM (Johnstone et al., 2006) play an important role. The WM is a cognitive system for processing transitory information to manage and execute verbal and nonverbal tasks during actions (Baddeley and Hitch, 1974). The WM can be considered as a function of the STM that is specialized to process information before it is stored in the long-term memory (LTM) or discharged for functional reasons (Becker and Morris, 1999). Of course, the functioning of the WM, STM, and LTM and their relationships involves a sophisticated and complex process that we do not discuss here. For better understanding of the Con-TA and its limitations, however, we describe the process behind user verbalizations.

As Figure 8.6 shows, in the Con-TA, user attention is focused on interaction (action in Figure 8.6). The participant spends just a few seconds (usually fewer than five) during the interaction from thinking about the action to performing it to the verbalization of problems encountered, strategies adopted, and impressions gained. In light of this, the users' verbalizations during a Con-TA are pertinent to the

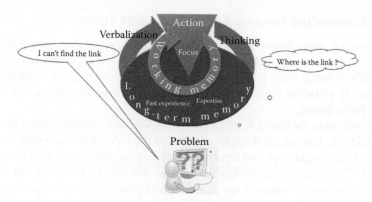

FIGURE 8.6 (See color insert.) The users pay attention to the action while they are forced to verbalize their thoughts. By maintaining a short time between the perception of the action, the thoughts, and the verbalization actions, practitioners can prevent participants using their experiences and expertise (in the long-term memory) to solve a problem before they verbalize it. In concurrent thinking aloud, the working memory is the primary process that helps users to produce pertinent verbalizations.

technology under analysis because the attention focus of users is on the actions and problems they are experiencing in the interaction. For that reason, whether the users forget to verbalize or spend a long time between action and elicitation, the facilitator should remind the users "to think aloud" in order to avoid their being affected by previous experience stored in their LTM, and by maintaining a short time between the actions and the verbalizations.

The Con-TA is a reliable evaluation technique, although the effort required of users is considerable since they are forced to make verbalizations while they are thinking and performing actions. Therefore, the Con-TA may affect the natural flow of the interaction and can strongly stress the users. Moreover, the Con-TA cannot be used with participants with visual impairment who use a screen reader for interacting with the system. In fact, as Federici and colleagues underline, during an interaction assessment with screen reader users, the closeness

> between action and verbalization is lost: the use of the screen reader, in fact, increases the time for verbalization (i.e., in order to verbalize, blind users must first stop the screen reader and then restart it). (Federici et al., 2010b, p. 266)

Moreover, during a Con-TA, a screen reader user should concurrently (1) interact with the product, (2) listen to the screen reader, and (3) verbalize the problems. This switching process between different actions and cognitive processes is stressful for the user, and it produces a reduced number of verbalizations by blind users compared with sighted and poor reliability of the collected data (Guan et al., 2006). At the same time, given the effort required of the sighted user to switch between the instructions, the verbalization process, and the interaction with the product, the Con-TA cannot be applied with people with cognitive disabilities or with attention and memory disorders (Guan et al., 2006; van den Haak et al., 2003), and evaluators often use an alternative technique for the interaction analysis: the Retro-TA.

8.4.3 RETROSPECTIVE THINKING ALOUD IN USABILITY TESTING

In the Retro-TA, users first silently complete the tasks and only afterward verbalize the process, analyzing the video of their interaction (Guan et al., 2006; van den Haak et al., 2003). When it is not possible to use video-recording support, evaluators can invite users to verbalize the problems that occurred during the interaction of their previous performance.

Differently from the Con-TA, in the Retro-TA, the users' verbalizations are based on their LTM. In fact, the participants, looking at the video, make a cognitive reconstruction of their experience and report their actions, strategies, and problems to the evaluators. This cognitive reconstruction can be affected by proactive interference (Still, 1969) caused by events or learning that occurred prior to the experience with the system under evaluation. A proactive interference occurs when past memories inhibit an individual's full potential to retain new memories in any given context (Wikipedia contributors, 2012b).

As shown in Figure 8.7, in the Retro-TA, the interaction experience is stored by users in their LTM (target experience) and mixed with their judgments, previous experiences, and expertise.

In the Retro-TA, the user is largely relieved of the effort of interacting and verbalizing concurrently. This strong advantage allows practitioners to use this technique with people with visual (Strain et al., 2007) and cognitive disabilities

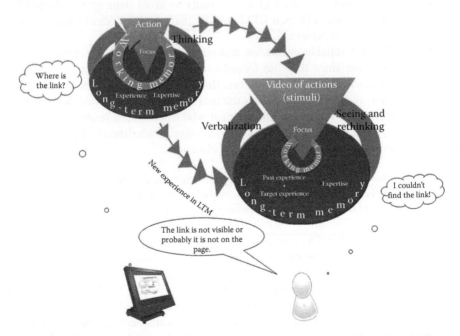

FIGURE 8.7   (See color insert.) Memory processes in the Retro-TA. The users, by observing the video, can remember and recover the details of their experience from their long-term memory (LTM). The users rethink the target experience and verbalize the problems through the lens of previous experiences and expertise.

(Johnstone et al., 2006). Nevertheless, with the Retro-TA, user verbalizations are influenced by user opinions and judgments about the entire navigation of the product. For instance, if a user considers the overall interaction with the product unsatisfactory, his or her verbalizations during the analysis of the video could reflect this judgment. Therefore, there is a strong proactive influence of the LTM in the Retro-TA: the user's previous experiences with similar technologies can influence the reconstruction of the interaction experienced with the product under assessment.

Maaike van den Haak and Menno de Jong (2003)—researchers at the Faculty of Behavioral Sciences of the University of Twente in the Netherlands—show that the participants in Retro-TA identify fewer problems than those in the Con-TA, and that the Retro-TA provides less accurate data than the concurrent procedure. Moreover, in the retrospective condition, the users' verbalizations are more focused on explanations and less on the interaction procedures, therefore resulting in less pertinent verbalizations than those produced by the concurrent condition (Bowers and Snyder, 1990; Kuusela and Paul, 2000).

In sum, although the Retro-TA overcomes some of the limitations of the Con-TA by relieving users of the effort of interacting and verbalizing concurrently, it does not maintain the same level of reliability as the latter. In fact, the verbalizations collected in the retrospective protocol are less pertinent to the technology under assessment than those of the concurrent one. In light of this, data collected by evaluators from a Retro-TA are not comparable with those obtained in a Con-TA session.

Finally, when evaluators want to test user interaction with a verbal protocol, they should select either a Con-TA or a Retro-TA depending on their evaluation aims. In particular, when evaluators aim to test the interface with a group of people with visual disabilities, a Retro-TA seems the only reliable solution for obtaining a comparable set of data. Some alternative techniques for testing disabled users with a verbal protocol have been developed, as we discuss in the next section.

8.4.4 Alternative Verbal Protocols for Disabled Users and Partial Concurrent Thinking Aloud

Philip Strain, Dawn Shaikh—researchers at Google—and Richard Boardman (2007)—UX consultant at Upstart User Experience—suggest that, in order to overcome the problems caused by screen reader use evaluators can apply two variants of the Retro-TA:

1. Modified stimulated Retro-TA, in which the participants interact with the product without interruptions; after each task, the facilitator may stop the screen reader and ask participants to walk through the interface to describe their actions and problems.
2. Synchronized concurrent think aloud, in which the facilitator explains to participants that every time they want to verbalize a problem they can pause the screen reader audio in the middle of an interaction and discuss what they have experienced.

These two variants of the Retro-TA have been tested and are considered to be reliable measures (Strain et al., 2007). Nevertheless, as Federici et al. (2010b) underline, these are only functional solutions. In fact, these two modified protocols allow evaluators to test a sample of disabled users conveniently, but they cannot collect data about the user performance during the interaction. Therefore, the user verbalizations also remain less pertinent to actual interaction in Strain and colleagues' variants of the Retro-TA than those obtained by a Con-TA test.

In order to provide a technique for testing blind and cognitive disabled users and collect data comparable to those obtained by means of the Con-TA, Federici and colleagues developed and tested (Borsci et al., 2011; Federici et al., 2010a,b) a specific protocol called partial concurrent thinking aloud (PCTA).

The PCTA comprises two main steps (Figure 8.8). In the first step, the participant analyzes the interface silently. When the participant identifies a problem, he or she has to ring a desk-bell near the mouse, thus creating a memory sign. This step is a variation of the Con-TA, in which memory signs and screen actions (or screen reader actions) are audio–video recorded. The second step is a variation of the Retro-TA, in which the participant, by observing the audio–video recorded actions and listening to the memory signs, verbalizes the problems that he or she experienced during the interaction.

The main advantage of the PCTA is that the users are driven by the memory signs to retrieve from the LTM only the information that is pertinent to the assessment. In fact, in the second step of the PCTA (Figure 8.9), when a participant

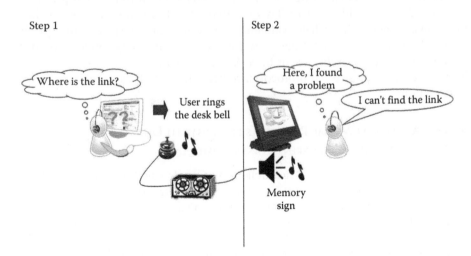

FIGURE 8.8   (See color insert.) Evaluation process of partial concurrent thinking aloud. In the first step (step 1, on the left side of the figure), the user creates a memory sign during the interaction (ringing a desk bell) each time he or she finds a problem. In this step, memory signs and screen actions (or screen reader actions) are audio–video recorded. In the second step (step 2, on the right side of the figure), the memory signs and the recorded stimuli help the user to recall the problems they previously identified. In this second step, the user is involved in a retrospective analysis whereby he or she is invited to verbalize the problems found. (Adapted from Federici, S. et al., *Cogn. Process.*, 11(3), 263, 2010b.)

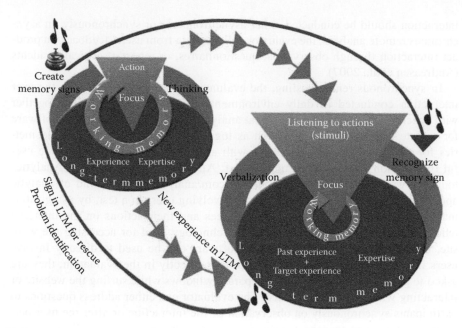

FIGURE 8.9   (See color insert.) The memory processes in the PCTA. Participants can recognize the audio-recorded memory signs, while listening to the screen reader interaction or observation of the screen actions. The memory signs and the audio–video recording can help users to retrieve relevant information from their long-term memory (LTM).

listens to a memory sign, he or she is alerted that, at a certain point during the interaction, there was a problem. Hence, participants can use the memory sign as a rescue tool, extrapolating from their LTM only the information pertaining to the interaction experience (Sign Experience in Figure 8.9) by minimizing the interference of previous experiences. As in the Con-TA, in the PCTA, the users can immediately indicate when and where they found a problem during the interaction with the product, and the audio–video recording encourages pertinent evaluation of the interaction.

In conclusion, the main advantage of the PCTA is that it allows practitioners to test users with visual and cognitive disabilities (Borsci et al., 2011; Federici et al., 2010a,b) by obtaining evaluation performances comparable to those of a Con-TA. Nevertheless, like the Retro-TA, the PCTA is a process of usability testing that requires more investment, in terms of time, than the Con-TA.

8.4.5   Remote Testing

Remote testing of the interaction is considered cheaper than traditional usability testing, and it is nowadays a protocol that is widely applied to test large sample of users in interaction studies (Andreasen et al., 2007; Waterson et al., 2002). As discussed in Section 8.3.3, in remote testing, evaluators and users should be separated from each other in both time and space (Castillo et al., 1998), or at least in one of these two (only in time or only in space), and the observation of the interaction should be conducted either asynchronously or synchronously. In asynchronous remote analysis, the evaluator collects data from users' feedback on product interaction through observation, questionnaires, or report of critical incidents (Andreasen et al., 2007).

In synchronous remote testing, the evaluator collects information on the user interaction conducted in daily environments by using questionnaires together with specific software applications that analyze the users' behavior. The software for remote testing collects data such as logs and other more sophisticated metrics for analyzing users' performance with an interface, in order to provide useful information for improving the product. An example is the Google Analytics tools for websites (see http://www.google.com/analytics/). This kind of analytic application extracts data without directly involving users in a test, by using information about users' interaction performances and their actions on the interface (clicks, time of web navigation, type of technology used for accessing the website, etc.). Nevertheless, other types of software can be used to directly involve users in remote testing. When users take part directly in the evaluation, they are asked to perform tasks presented in separate windows while surfing the website or interacting with a product interface. The evaluator can either address questions to participants synchronously on observation of the interaction or after the user performance, i.e., in an asynchronous way. Concurrently, the software collects analytics about participant behavior, time of performance, task completion, failure rates, etc. In the last few years, a wide variety of software has been developed to help practitioners arrange remote evaluation tests. These applications, however, have the primary disadvantage of reducing the level of controllability of the test environment. In fact, although remote testing tools reduce the costs of the evaluation and provide good data reliability, the detail of data collected, especially compared with the results collected by traditional usability testing, is poor. To the identification of fewer usability problems is added another limitation—the process is time-consuming for the users (Andreasen et al., 2007). These limitations are also confirmed by a comparative study carried out by Hellen Petrie—professor of HCI at the University of York—and colleagues (Petrie et al., 2006), in which a sample of blind users assessed two interfaces in both local and remote conditions. The results of this study showed that the number of problems identified by the users "in the local evaluations is over four times as many as in the remote evaluations" (Petrie et al., 2006, p. 1139).

In conclusion, although remote testing can be considered as a valuable evaluation resource and a cheap way of recruiting a large set of data about real user interaction, it cannot be used as an ultimate solution, but only as a technique that has to be combined with other methods to achieve good reliability of the collected data. In fact, in remote testing, it is difficult to supervise and help users to report problems concerning the interaction, as happens in the Con-TA or in the Retro-TA. Furthermore, in remote testing, the practitioners may find many limitations in the comprehension of users' experience, personal differences, styles, and attitudes. For instance, in remote testing involving disabled users, it may be quite difficult to assess the role of assistive technology in user interaction (Petrie et al., 2006).

8.4.6 SUMMARY OF USABILITY TESTING AND THE ANALYSIS OF REAL USER INTERACTION

The analysis of real user interaction is essential in any interaction evaluation to assess the functioning of the product perceived by the user (Figure 8.1). In particular, through these techniques, practitioners can collect data about both user performance and perceived problems by observing users' attitudes, skills, and reactions during the interaction (see Figure 8.10). These data should be used by practitioners to analyze which problems are perceived by the user during the interaction, the user reactions that occur during the execution of the input, and their problems in comprehending the product output/feedbacks. In this way, the evaluators can identify the position of each interaction problem and the possible errors related to the product (objective error) that can cause problems during the interaction (objective errors in execution or in evaluation).

Whereas qualitative and subjective measurements are techniques for observing the user point of view on the product through a holistic assessment of the interaction, usability and remote testing of the user interaction offer a deeper analysis of product functioning as perceived by end users. Therefore, there is a relationship between qualitative measurements and usability testing, because both of them are methods

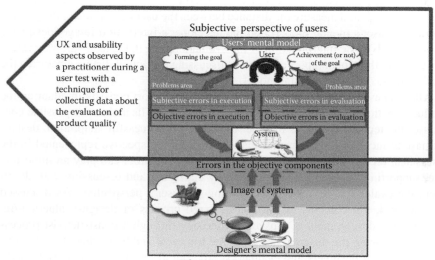

FIGURE 8.10 **(See color insert.)** Synoptic representation of the interaction observed through methods of evaluating the product quality (user evaluation of quality). It represents the user's perspective on the interaction with a product (subjective perspective of users, at the top) and the designer's perspective about the product functioning (subjective perspective of developers, at the bottom). When the evaluator involves a sample of users in the assessment by using either usability or real interaction testing, he or she can measure user reaction, time of performance, success, and failure rate. Furthermore, the evaluator also identifies where the problems are discovered by the participant during the interaction (i.e., which parts of the product are experienced as problematic) and the probable errors of the object causing them.

involving users to extrapolate data about the interaction. Moreover, the testing methods allow practitioners to identify the problems perceived by the users in the context of use and where and when the problems occur during the interaction, necessary data for report to designers. To analyze the reliability findings of the evaluation process, the evaluator may resort to the grounded procedure (Chapter 7).

In sum, the analysis of the real user interaction is the core phase of any evaluation process, because it allows practitioners to observe the user interaction and identify the real problems of use in an empirical way.

8.5 CONCLUSION

In the present chapter, we have presented the methods that can be used by practitioners to compose an IMIE and assess three main dimensions of the intrasystemic dialogue: (1) the system functioning as it is designed (the system evaluation), (2) the system functioning as it is perceived by the users (subjective evaluation), and (3) the overall perception of the interaction quality. In order to fully assess the usability and the UX of a product, an evaluator should measure all three dimensions—selecting specific methods in line with the design phase (formative or summative), the aim of the evaluation, and the available budget (Chapter 6, Figure 6.1).

As discussed in Chapter 5 (Section 5.2.2.3 and Figure 5.8), the aim of the evaluators is to observe and measure the distance between the user perception of the product interaction (user's mental model) and the developer's interaction image (designer's mental models). The interpretation of the evaluation data (Chapter 7) allows evaluators to create the global report needed for discussing the actual distance between the user's and the designer's mental model.

After the evaluation process, the designer's main effort consists in adapting the product functioning to the users' needs, attitude, and skills and to the possible contexts of the technology's use. In order to produce a successful adaptation, designers have to include in their mental model the users' perspective represented in the assessment report. In this adaptation process, the evaluators can play an important role, supporting designers in this context by clarifying and discussing with developers the evaluation results and advocating the user's perspective. As discussed in Chapter 4, the outcome of the user-centered process of design-evaluation-(re) design is the development of a psychotechnology through a constructivist process in which—during the different phases of the life cycle and by means of an iterative dialogue among designers and evaluators—the initial product is recursively modified and tested until the evaluation data confirm that the product guarantees a high level of usability and UX to the final users.

The goal of the User Interface for All can be reached only when there is strong collaboration and exchange of information between designer and evaluator, since the only way for a developer to design a usable and accessible interaction experience is to have a clear comprehension of the user's perspective by means of the evaluation. Therefore, the design of a product on the basis of a model or an empirical list of users' needs, attitudes, and skills is only the starting point of a life cycle, as the product can be improved only after several cycles of assessment and redesign in which it is iteratively adapted to the different nuances of human functioning and contexts of use, becoming an intrasystemic system.

Ideally, the adaptations of the initial product to real users' needs, attitudes, habits, and skills should transform the system to a psychotechnology that can be used in any context of use and by any user. In the real world, however, the final level of usability and UX of the product and the user perception of the product as a psychotechnology will depend on the investment in terms of assessment and design. The released product will be perceived and used as a psychotechnology only by those users and contexts of use that the evaluators have taken into account during the assessment process on the basis of the available budget. In fact, the designer may redesign and adapt the product only for those users and contexts of use that have been previously represented and analyzed by the collected evaluation data. Evaluators and designers have an equal role in determining and increasing the level of the usability and UX of a product and in contributing to attempts to achieve the ideal goal of the Design for All. Therefore, to transform a technology into a psychotechnological one, investments in terms of designing and evaluating the product functioning should be considered as equally important for reaching the shared goal—the intrasystemic solution.

References

Abrams, D. and Hogg, M. A. (1990). *Social Identity Theory: Constructive and Critical Advances*. Hemel Hempstead, U.K.: Harvester Wheatsheaf.

Abramson, L. Y., Seligman, M. E., and Teasdale, J. D. (1978). Learned helplessness in humans: Critique and reformulation. *Journal of Abnormal Psychology, 87*(1), 49–74. doi:10.1037//0021-843X.87.1.49.

Alben, L. (1996). Quality of experience: Defining the criteria for effective interaction design. *Interactions, 3*(3), 11–15. doi:10.1145/235008.235010.

Altman, B. M. and Gulley, S. P. (2009). Convergence and divergence: Differences in disability prevalence estimates in the United States and Canada based on four health survey instruments. *Social Science and Medicine, 69*(4), 543–552. doi:10.1016/j.socscimed.2009.06.017.

American Psychiatric Association. (2000). *Diagnostic and Statistical Manual of Mental Disorders: DSM-IV-TR®* (4th edn.). Arlington, VA: American Psychiatric Association.

Amiel, T. and Sargent, S. L. (2004). Individual differences in Internet usage motives. *Computers in Human Behavior, 20*(6), 711–726. doi:10.1016/j.chb.2004.09.002.

Andersen, P. B. (2001). What semiotics can and cannot do for HCI. *Knowledge-Based Systems, 14*(8), 419–424.

Anderson, J. R. (1996). *The Architecture of Cognition*. Cambridge, MA: Lawrence Erlbaum Associates.

Andreasen, M. S., Nielsen, H. V., Schrøder, S. O., and Stage, J. (2007, April 30–May 3). What happened to remote usability testing? An empirical study of three methods. Paper presented at the *SIGCHI Conference on Human Factors in Computing Systems: CHI '07*, San Jose, CA. doi:10.1145/1240624.1240838.

Andreassi, J. L. (2006). *Psychophysiology: Human Behavior and Physiological Response* (5th edn.). Mahwah, NJ: Lawrence Erlbaum Associates.

Annett, J. (2002a). Subjective rating scales in ergonomics: A reply. *Ergonomics, 45*(14), 1042–1046. doi:10.1080/00140130210166762.

Annett, J. (2002b). Subjective rating scales: Science or art? *Ergonomics, 45*(14), 966–987. doi:10.1080/0014013021016695.

Annett, J. and Duncan, K. D. (1967). Task analysis and training design. *Occupational Psychology, 41*(4), 211–221.

Annett, J., Duncan, K. D., Stammers, R., and Gray, M. J. (1971). *Task Analysis*. London, U.K.: HMSO.

Ark, W. S. and Selker, T. (1999). A look at human interaction with pervasive computers. *IBM Systems Journal, 38*(4), 504–507. doi:10.1147/sj.384.0504.

Armano, D. (2012). The future isn't about mobile; it's about mobility. Retrieved September 15, 2012, from http://blogs.hbr.org/cs/2012/07/the_future_isnt_about_mobile_its.html

Ashforth, B. E. and Mael, F. (1989). Social identity theory and the organization. *Academy of Management Review, 14*(1), 20–39. doi:10.5465/AMR.1989.4278999

Aspinwall, L. G. and Staudinger, U. M. (Eds.). (2003). *A Psychology of Human Strengths: Fundamental Questions and Future Directions for a Positive Psychology*. Washington, DC: American Psychological Association.

Audouze, F. (1999). Technology and human evolution. In R. A. Wilson and F. C. Keil (Eds.), *The MIT Encyclopedia of the Cognitive Sciences* (pp. 828–829). Cambridge, MA: MIT Press.

Baber, C. (2002). Subjective evaluation of usability. *Ergonomics, 45*(14), 1021–1025. doi:10.1080/00140130210166807.

Baber, C. (2004). Critical path analysis for multimodal activity. In N. Stanton, A. Hedge, K. Brookhuis, E. Salas, and H. Hendrick (Eds.), *Handbook of Human Factors and Ergonomics Methods* (pp. 41.41–41.48). Boca Raton, FL:CRC Press. doi:10.1201/9780203489925.ch41.

Baber, C. and Stanton, N. A. (1996). Observation as a technique for usability evaluations. In P. W. Jordan (Ed.), *Usability in Industry* (pp. 85–94). London, U.K.: Taylor & Francis Group.

Baddeley, A. D., Eysenck, M. W., and Anderson, M. C. (2009). *Memory*. New York: Psychology Press.

Baddeley, A. D. and Hitch, G. (1974). Working memory. In G. H. Bower (Ed.), *The Psychology of Learning and Motivation: Advances in Research and Theory* (Vol. 8, pp. 47–89). New York: Academic Press. doi:10.1016/S0079-7421(08)60452-1.

Ball, L. J., Evans, J. S. B. T., and Dennis, I. (1994). Cognitive processes in engineering design: A longitudinal study. *Ergonomics, 37*(11), 1753–1786. doi:10.1080/00140139408964950.

Bandura, A. (1986). *Social Foundations of Thought and Action: A Social Cognitive Theory.* Upper Saddle River, NJ: Prentice-Hall.

Bandura, A. (1997). *Self-Efficacy: The Exercise of Control.* New York: W.H. Freeman.

Bandura, A. (1999). A social cognitive theory of personality. In L. A. Pervin and O. P. John (Eds.), *Handbook of Personality: Theory and Research* (2nd edn., pp. 154–196). New York: Guilford Press.

Batra, D. and Davis, J. G. (1992). Conceptual data modelling in database design: Similarities and differences between expert and novice designers. *International Journal of Man-Machine Studies, 37*(1), 83–101. doi:10.1016/0020-7373(92)90092-y.

Becker, J. T. and Morris, R. G. (1999). Working memory(s). *Brain and Cognition, 41*(1), 1–8. doi:10.1006/brcg.1998.1092.

Berger, C. R. and Calabrese, R. J. (1975). Some explorations in initial interaction and beyond: Toward a developmental theory of interpersonal communication. *Human Communication Research, 1*(2), 99–112. doi:10.1111/j.1468-2958.1975.tb00258.x.

Berners-Lee, T. (1989). Information Management: A Proposal. Retrieved September 15, 2012, from http://www.w3.org/History/1989/proposal.html

Berners-Lee, T. (1990a). Pre-W3C web and internet background. Retrieved September 15, 2012, from http://w3.org/2004/Talks/w3c10-HowItAllStarted/?n = 15

Berners-Lee, T. (1990b). World Wide Web. Retrieved September 15, 2012, from http://www.w3.org/History/19921103-hypertext/hypertext/WWW/TheProject.html

Berners-Lee, T. and Cailliau, R. (1990). World Wide Web: Proposal for a hypertexts project. Retrieved September 15, 2012, from http://w3.org/Proposal.html

Berners-Lee, T. and Fischetti, M. (1999). *Weaving the Web: The Original Design and Ultimate Destiny of the World Wide Web by Its Inventor.* London, U.K.: Orion Business.

von Bertalanffy, L. (1950). An outline of general system theory. *The British Journal for the Philosophy of Science, 1*(2), 134–165. doi:10.1093/bjps/I.2.134.

Bevan, N. (2001). Quality in use for all. In C. Stephanidis (Ed.), *User Interfaces for All: Concepts, Methods, and Tools* (pp. 353–317). Mahwah, NJ: Lawrence Erlbaum Associates.

Beyer, H. and Holtzblatt, K. (1998). *Contextual Design: Defining Customer-Centered Systems.* San Francisco, CA: Morgan Kaufmann.

Bias, R. G. (1991). Walkthroughs: Efficient collaborative testing. *IEEE Software, 8*(5), 94–95. doi:10.1109/52.84220.

Bias, R. G. and Mayhew, D. J. (2005). *Cost-Justifying Usability: An Update for an Internet Age* (2nd edn.). San Francisco, CA: Morgan Kaufmann.

Bickenbach, J. E., Chatterji, S., Badley, E. M., and Üstün, T. B. (1999). Models of disablement, universalism and the international classification of impairments, disabilities and handicaps. *Social Science and Medicine, 48*(9), 1173–1187. doi:10.1016/S0277-9536(98)00441-9.

Bindé, J. (2005). Towards knowledge societies: UNESCO world report. SHS.2005/WS/44. Retrieved September 15, 2012, from UNESDOC website. http://unesdoc.unesco.org/images/0014/001418/141843e.pdf

Biswas, P. and Langdon, P. (March 29–April 2, 2011). Towards an inclusive world—A simulation tool to design interactive electronic systems for elderly and disabled users. Paper presented at the *2011 Annual SRII Global Conference*. San Jose, CA. doi:10.1109/SRII.2011.18.

Boguta, K. (2011). Computational history. Retrieved September 15, 2012, from http://www.kovasboguta.com

Bohman, P. R. and Anderson, S. (May 10–14, 2005). A conceptual framework for accessibility tools to benefit users with cognitive disabilities. Paper presented at the *International Cross-Disciplinary Workshop on Web Accessibility: W4A '05*. Chiba, Japan. doi:10.1145/1061811.1061828.

Borsci, S., Federici, S., and Lauriola, M. (2009). On the dimensionality of the System Usability Scale (SUS): A test of alternative measurement models. *Cognitive Processing, 10*(3), 193–197. doi:10.1007/s10339-009-0268-9.

Borsci, S., Federici, S., Mele, M. L., Polimeno, D., and Londei, A. (2012a). The bootstrap discovery behaviour model: Why five users are not enough to test user experience. In E. M. Alkhalifa and K. Gaid (Eds.), *Cognitively Informed Intelligent Interfaces: Systems Design and Development* (pp. 258–279). Hershey, PA: IGI Global. doi:10.4018/978-1-4666-1628-8.ch015.

Borsci, S., Kurosu, M., Federici, S., and Mele, M. L. (2012b). Systemic user experience. In S. Federici and M. J. Scherer (Eds.), *Assistive Technology Assessment Handbook* (pp. 337–359). Boca Raton, FL: CRC Press. doi:10.1201/b11821-19.

Borsci, S., Londei, A., and Federici, S. (2011). The bootstrap discovery behaviour (BDB): A new outlook on usability evaluation. *Cognitive Processing, 12*(1), 23–31. doi:10.1007/s10339-010-0376-6.

Borsci, S., Macredie, R. D., Barnett, J., Martin, J., Kuljis, J., and Young, T. (Accepted on July 22, 2013). *Reviewing and Extending the Five–User Assumption: A Grounded Procedure for Interaction Evaluation. ACM Transactions on Computer-Human Interaction (TOCHI)*.

Botella, C., Riva, G., Gaggioli, A., Wiederhold, B. K., Alcaniz, M., and Baños, R. M. (2012). The present and future of positive technologies. *Cyberpsychology, Behavior, and Social Networking, 15*(2), 78–84. doi:10.1089/cyber.2011.0140.

Bovair, S., Kieras, D. E., and Polson, P. G. (1990). The acquisition and performance of text-editing skill: A cognitive complexity analysis. *Human–Computer Interaction, 5*(1), 1–48. doi:http://dx.doi.org/10.1207/s15327051hci0501_1

Bowers, V. A. and Snyder, H. L. (1990). Concurrent versus retrospective verbal protocol for comparing window usability. *Proceedings of the Human Factors and Ergonomics Society Annual Meeting, 34*(17), 1270–1274. doi:10.1177/154193129003401720.

Bradford, J. S. (1994). Evaluating high-level design: Synergistic use of inspection and usability methods for evaluating early software designs. In J. Nielsen and R. L. Mack (Eds.), *Usability Inspection Methods* (pp. 235–253). New York: John Wiley & Sons.

Brandon, D. P. and Hollingshead, A. B. (2004). Transactive memory systems in organizations: Matching tasks, expertise, and people. *Organization Science, 15*(6), 633–644. doi:10.1287/orsc.1040.0069.

Brewer, J. (2004, May 17–22). Web accessibility highlights and trends. Paper presented at the *International Cross-Disciplinary Workshop on Web Accessibility: W4A '04*. New York. doi:10.1145/990657.990667.

Brooke, J. (1996). SUS: A "quick and dirty" usability scale. In P. W. Jordan, B. Thomas, B. A. Weerdmeester, and I. L. McClelland (Eds.), *Usability Evaluation in Industry* (pp. 189–194). London, U.K.: Taylor & Francis.

Bruner, J. S. (1977). *The Process of Education: A Landmark in Educational Theory*. Cambridge, MA: Harvard University Press.

Buccino, G., Binkofski, F., Fink, G. R., Fadiga, L., Fogassi, L., Gallese, V. et al. (2001). Action observation activates premotor and parietal areas in a somato-topic manner: An fMRI study. *European Journal of Neuroscience, 13*(2), 400–404. doi:10.1046/j.1460-9568.2001.01385.x.

Build for All project. (2006). *The Build For All Reference Manual.* Retrieved September 15, 2012, from Build-for-all.net website: www.build-for-all.net

Buller, D. B., Woodall, W. G., Zimmerman, D. E., Heimendinger, J., Rogers, E. M., Slater, M. D. et al. (2001). Formative research activities to provide web-based nutrition education to adults in the Upper Rio Grande Valley. *Family and Community Health, 24*(3), 1–12.

Bunge, M. (1977). Emergence and the mind. *Neuroscience, 2*(4), 501–509. doi:10.1016/0306-4522(77)90047-1.

Caldwell, B., Cooper, M., Guarino Reid, L., and Vanderheiden, G. (2008). Web content accessibility guidelines (WCAG) 2.0—W3C recommendation. Retrieved September 15, 2012, from http://www.w3.org/TR/WCAG20

Card, S. K., Moran, T. P., and Newell, A. (1980). The keystroke-level model for user performance time with interactive systems. *Communications of the ACM, 23*(7), 396–410. doi:10.1145/358886.358895.

Card, S. K., Moran, T. P., and Newell, A. (1983). *The Psychology of Human-Computer Interaction.* Hillsdale, NJ: Lawrence Erlbaum Associates.

Card, S. K., Moran, T. P., and Newell, A. (1986). The model human processor: An engineering model of human performance. In K. R. Boff, L. Kaufman, and J. P. Thomas (Eds.), *Handbook of Perception and Human Performance: Cognitive Processes and Performance* (Vol. 2, pp. 1–35). New York: John Wiley & Sons.

Casasanto, D. (2011). Different bodies, different minds: The body specificity of language and thought. *Current Directions in Psychological Science, 20*(6), 378–383. doi:10.1177/0963721411422058.

Castillo, J. C., Hartson, H. R., and Hix, D. (April 18–23, 1998). Remote usability evaluation: Can users report their own critical incidents? Paper presented at the *Conference on Human Factors in Computing Systems: CHI '98.* Los Angeles, CA. doi:10.1145/286498.286736.

Caulton, D. (2001). Relaxing the homogeneity assumption in usability testing. *Behaviour & Information Technology, 20*(1), 1–7. doi:10.1080/01449290010020648.

Central Statistics Office. (2008). *National Disability Survey 2006: First Results.* Retrieved September 15, 2012, from http://www.cso.ie/en/media/csoie/releasespublications/documents/otherreleases/nationaldisability/National%20Disability%20Survey%202006%20First%20Results%20full%20report.pdf

Charlton, J. I. (1998). *Nothing About Us Without Us: Disability Oppression and Empowerment.* Berkeley, CA: University of California Press.

Charmaz, K. (2000). Grounded theory: Objectivist and constructivist methods. In N. K. Denzin and Y. S. Lincoln (Eds.), *Handbook of Qualitative Research* (2nd edn., pp. 509–535). Thousand Oaks, CA: Sage.

Charmaz, K. (2006). *Constructing Grounded Theory: A Practical Guide through Qualitative Analysis.* London, U.K.: Sage.

Cheatham, L. P. (2012). Effects of Internet use on well-being among adults with physical disabilities: A review. *Disability and Rehabilitation: Assistive Technology, 7*(3), 181–188. doi:10.3109/17483107.2011.625071.

Chi, M. T. H., Feltovich, P. J., and Glaser, R. (1981). Categorization and representation of physics problems by experts and novices. *Cognitive Science, 5*(2), 121–152. doi:10.1207/s15516709cog0502_2.

Chin, J. P., Diehl, V. A., and Norman, K. L. (May 15–19, 1988). Development of an instrument measuring user satisfaction of the human-computer interface. Paper presented at the *Conference on Human Factors in Computing Systems: SIGCHI '88.* Washington, DC. doi:10.1145/57167.57203.

Chisholm, W., Vanderheiden, G., and Jacobs, I. (1999). Web content accessibility guidelines 1.0—W3C Recommendation. Retrieved September 15, 2012, from http://www.w3.org/TR/WCAG10/

Chou, J.-R. and Hsiao, S.-W. (2007). A usability study on human-computer interface for middle-aged learners. *Computers in Human Behavior, 23*(4), 2040–2063. doi:10.1016/j.chb.2006.02.011.

Clark, J. (2006). To hell with WCAG 2. *A List Apart,* (217). Retrieved from http://www.alistapart.com/articles/tohellwithwcag2

Clark, A. (2010). *Memento*'s revenge: The extended mind, extended. In R. Menary (Ed.), *The Extended Mind* (pp. 43–66). Cambridge, MA: MIT Press.

Clark, A. and Chalmers, D. (1998). The extended mind. *Analysis, 58*(1), 7–19. doi:10.1093/analys/58.1.7.

Coffman, K. G. and Odlyzko, A. M. (2002). Growth of the internet. In I. P. Kaminow and T. Li (Eds.), *Optical Fiber Telecommunications IV-B: Systems and Impairments* (pp. 17–56). Waltham, MA: Academic Press.

Collins, M. A. and Quillian, M. R. (1972). How to make a language user. In E. Tulving and W. Donaldson (Eds.), *Organization of Memory* (pp. 309–351). New York: Academic Press.

Consolvo, S., Harrison, B., Smith, I., Chen, M. Y., Everitt, K., Froehlich, J. et al. (2007). Conducting in situ evaluations for and with ubiquitous computing technologies. *International Journal of Human–Computer Interaction, 22*(1–2), 103–118. doi:10.1080/10447310709336957.

Constantine, L. L. (2004). Beyond user-centered design and user experience: Designing for user performance. *Cutter It, 17*(2), 16–25.

Cooper, G. E. and Harper, R. P. (1969). The use of pilot rating in the evaluation of aircraft handling qualities. (AD 689722 Report 567). Retrieved September 15, 2012, from North Atlantic Treaty Organization website. http://www.dtic.mil/cgi-bin/GetTRDoc?AD = AD0689722

Cooper, A., Reimann, R., and Cronin, D. (2007). *About Face 3: The Essentials of Interaction Design* (3rd edn.). Indianapolis, IN: Wiley.

CORDIS. (1994). TIDE ACCESS project: Development platform for unified access to enabling environments. Retrieved September 15, 2012, from http://cordis.europa.eu/search/index.cfm?fuseaction = proj.document&PJ_LANG = EN&PJ_RCN = 1237003

CORDIS. (1995). AVANTI: Adaptive and adaptable interactions for multimedia telecommunications applications. Retrieved September 22, 2011, from http://cordis.europa.eu/infowin/acts/rus/trials/ac042.htm

Correa, T., Hinsley, A. W., and de Zúñiga, H. G. (2010). Who interacts on the Web?: The intersection of users' personality and social media use. *Computers in Human Behavior, 26*(2), 247–253. doi:10.1016/j.chb.2009.09.003.

Costa, P. T., Jr. and McCrae, R. R. (1992). *Revised NEO Personality Inventory (NEO-PI-R) and NEO Five-Factor Inventory (NEO-FFI) Manual.* Odessa, FL: Psychological Assessment Resources.

Craik, J. W. K. (1943). *The Nature of Exploration.* Cambridge, U.K.: Cambridge University Press.

Crystal, A. and Ellington, B. (August 6–8, 2004). Task analysis and human-computer interaction: Approaches, techniques, and levels of analysis. Paper presented at the *10th Américas Conference on Information Systems: AMCIS '04.* New York.

Csikszentmihalyi, M. (1990). *Flow: The Psychology of Optimal Experience.* New York: HarperCollins.

Cygnis Media. (2012). User experience cannot be designed. Retrieved December 1, 2012, from http://www.cygnismedia.com/blog/ux-cannot-be-designed/

Davis, I. (2012). Talis, Web 2.0 and all that—Internet alchemy. Retrieved September 15, 2012, from http://internetalchemy.org/2005/07/talis-web-20-and-all-that

De Kerckhove, D. (1991). Communication arts for a new spatial sensibility. *Leonardo, 24*(2), 131–135. doi:10.2307/1575281.

De Kerckhove, D. (1995). *The Skin of Culture: Investigating the New Electronic Reality.* Toronto, Ontario, Canada: Somerville.

De Kerckhove, D. (2010). *The Augmented Mind (The Stupid Ones Are Those Who Do Not Use Google).* Milan, Italy: 40k books.

Decety, J. and Jackson, P. L. (2004). The functional architecture of human empathy. *Behavioral and Cognitive Neuroscience Reviews, 3*(2), 71–100. doi:10.1177/1534582304267187.

Demers, L., Monette, M., Lapierre, Y., Arnold, D. L., and Wolfson, C. (2002a). Reliability, validity, and applicability of the Quebec User Evaluation of Satisfaction with assistive Technology (QUEST 2.0) for adults with multiple sclerosis. *Disability and Rehabilitation, 24*(1–3), 21–30. doi:10.1080/09638280110066352.

Demers, L., Weiss-Lambrou, R., and Ska, B. (2002b). The Quebec User Evaluation of Satisfaction with Assistive Technology (QUEST 2.0): An overview and recent progress. *Technology and Disability, 14*(3), 101–105.

Di Battista, G., Eades, P., Tamassia, R., and Tollis, I. G. (1999). *Graph Drawing: Algorithms for the Visualization of Graphs.* Upper Saddle River, NJ: Prentice-Hall.

Di Blas, N., Paolini, P., and Speroni, M. (June 28–29, 2004). "Usable Accessibility" to the web for blind users. Paper presented at the *8th ERCIM Workshop on User Interfaces for All.* Vienna, Austria. Retrieved September 15, 2012, from http://www.ui4all.gr/workshop2004/files/ui4all_proceedings/adjunct/accessibility/109.pdf

Didimo, W. and Liotta, G. (2012). The crossing angle resolution in graph drawing. In J. Pach (Ed.), *Thirty Essays on Geometric Graph Theory.* Berlin, Germany: Springer.

Dillon, A. (2001). Beyond usability: Process, outcome, and affect in human computer interactions [Au delà de la convivialité: processus, résultats, et affect, dans les interactions personne-machine]. *Canadian Journal of Information and Library Science, 26*(4), 57–69.

Diodati, M. (2007). *Accessibilità. Guida Completa* [Accessibility. Complete Guide]. Milano, IT: Apogeo.

Dion, B., Balcazar de laCruz, A., Rapson, D., Svensson, E., Peters, M., and Dion, P. (2006). *International Best Practices in Universal Design: A Global Review.* Ottawa, Ontario, Canada: Canadian Human Rights Commission.

Dix, A., Finlay, J., Abowd, G. D., and Beale, R. (2004). *Human-Computer Interaction.* Harlow, U.K.: Pearson Education.

Drury, C. G. (1990). Methods for direct observation of performance. In J. R. Wilson and E. N. Coriett (Eds.), *Evaluation of Human Work: A Practical Ergonomics Methodology* (pp. 35–57). London, U.K.: Taylor & Francis.

Drury, C. G. (2002). Measurement and the practising ergonomist. *Ergonomics, 45*(14), 988–990. doi:10.1080/00140130210166915.

Duchowski, A. T. (2007). *Eye Tracking Methodology: Theory and Practice* (2nd edn.). London, U.K.: Springer.

Durkheim, É. (1982). *The Rules of Sociological Method.* New York: Free Press.

Efron, B. (1979). Bootstrap methods: Another look at the jackknife. *Annals of Statistics, 7*(1), 1–26. doi:10.1214/aos/1176344552.

EIDD Design for All Europe. (2004). Stockholm declaration. Adopted on May 9, 2004, at the *Annual General Meeting of the European Institute for Design and Disability in Stockholm.* Retrieved September 15, 2012, from Design for All Europe.org website: http://www.designforalleurope.org/Design-for-All/EIDD-Documents/Stockholm-Declaration/

Ellison, N. B., Steinfield, C., and Lampe, C. (2007). The benefits of Facebook "Friends:" Social capital and college students' use of online social network sites. *Journal of Computer-Mediated Communication, 12*(4), 1143–1168. doi:10.1111/j.1083-6101.2007.00367.x.

Engel, G. L. (1977). The need for a new medical model: A challenge for biomedicine. *Science, 196*(4286), 129–136. doi:10.1126/science.847460.

Ericsson, K. A. and Simon, H. A. (1980). Verbal reports as data. *Psychological Review, 87*(3), 215–251. doi:10.1037/0033-295X.87.3.215.

Ericsson, K. A. and Simon, H. A. (1984). *Protocol Analysis: Verbal Reports as Data.* Cambridge, MA: MIT Press.

Ericsson, K. A. and Simon, H. A. (1987). Verbal reports on thinking. In C. Faerch and G. Kasper (Eds.), *Introspection in Second Language Research* (pp. 24–53). Clevedon, New Zealand: Multilingual Matters.

Ericsson, K. A. and Simon, H. A. (1993). *Protocol Analysis, Revised Edition: Verbal Reports as Data.* Cambridge, MA: MIT Press.

Ericsson, K. A., Tesch-Römer, C., and Krampe, R. T. (1990). The role of practice and motivation in the acquisition of expert-level performance in real life: An empirical evaluation of a theoretical framework. In M. J. A. Howe (Ed.), *Encouraging the Development of Exceptional Skills and Talents* (pp. 109–130). Leicester, U.K.: British Psychological Society.

Erikson, E. H. (1959). *Identity and the Life Cycle: Selected Papers.* New York: International Universities Press.

European Commission. (2003). *i2010—A European Information Society for Growth and Employment.* Retrieved from EU website. http://eur-lex.europa.eu/LexUriServ/ LexUriServ.do?uri = COM:2005:0229:FIN:EN:PDF

European Commission. (2008). i2010—Strategy for an innovative and inclusive European Information Society. Retrieved September 15, 2012, from http://ec.europa.eu/ information_society/doc/factsheets/035-i2010-en.pdf

European Commission. (2012a). eAccessibility—Opening up the information society. Retrieved September 15, 2012, from http://ec.europa.eu/information_society/activities/ einclusion/policy/accessibility/index_en.htm

European Commission. (2012b). Web accessibility. Retrieved September 15, 2012, from http://ec.europa.eu/information_society/activities/einclusion/policy/accessibility/ web_access/index_en.htm

European Union. (2001). Council resolution of 13 July 2001 on e-learning. *Official Journal of the European Communities, C*(204), 3–5. Retrieved from ec.europa.eu website: http://ec.europa.eu/education/archive/elearning/reso_en.pdf

European Union. (2003a). Council Resolution 6 February 2003: 'eAccessibility'— Improving the access of people with disabilities to the knowledge based society. *Official Journal of the European Union, C*(39), 5–7. Retrieved from ec.europa.eu website: http://eur-lex.europa.eu/LexUriServ/LexUriServ.do?uri = OJ:C:2003:039:0005:0007:EN:PDF

European Union. (2003b). Council resolution of 5 May 2003 on equal opportunities for pupils and students with disabilities in education and training. *Official Journal of the European Union, C*(134), 4–7. Retrieved from http://eur-lex.europa.eu/LexUriServ/LexUriServ. do?uri = OJ:C:2003:134:0006:0007:EN:PDF

Fairweather, P. and Trewin, S. (2010). Cognitive impairments and Web 2.0. *Universal Access in the Information Society, 9*(2), 137–146. doi:10.1007/s10209-009-0163-2.

Farmer, M. and Macleod, F. (2011). Involving disabled people in social research: Guidance by the office for disability issues. Retrieved September 15, 2012, from http://odi.dwp.gov. uk/docs/res/research/involving-disabled-people-in-social-research.pdf

Faulkner, L. (2003). Beyond the five-user assumption: Benefits of increased sample sizes in usability testing. *Behavior Research Methods, 35*(3), 379–383. doi:10.3758/ BF03195514.

Federici, S. (2002). *Sessualità alterabili. Indagine sulle influenze socioambientali nello sviluppo della sessualità di persone con disabilità in Italia* [*Alter*-able sexuality: Survey of socio-environmental influences in the development of the sexuality of people with disabilities in Italy]. Roma, Italy: Kappa.

Federici, S. and Borsci, S. (2010). Usability evaluation: Models, methods, and applications. In J. Stone and M. Blouin (Eds.), *International Encyclopedia of Rehabilitation* (pp. 1–17). Buffalo, NY: Center for International Rehabilitation Research Information and Exchange (CIRRIE). Retrieved September 15, 2012, from http://cirrie.buffalo.edu/encyclopedia/article.php?id = 277&language = en

Federici, S., Borsci, S., and Mele, M. L. (2010a). Usability evaluation with screen reader users: A video presentation of the PCTA's experimental setting and rules. *Cognitive Processing, 11*(3), 285–288. doi:10.1007/s10339-010-0365-9.

Federici, S., Borsci, S., and Stamerra, G. (2010b). Web usability evaluation with screen reader users: Implementation of the partial concurrent thinking aloud technique. *Cognitive Processing, 11*(3), 263–272. doi:10.1007/s10339-009-0347-y.

Federici, S., Corradi, F., Mele, M. L., and Miesenberger, K. (2011). From cognitive ergonomist to psychotechnologist: A new professional profile in a multidisciplinary team in a centre for technical aids. In G. J. Gelderblom, M. Soede, L. Adriaens, and K. Miesenberger (Eds.), *Everyday Technology for Independence and Care: AAATE 2011* (Vol. 29, pp. 1178–1184). Amsterdam, the Netherlands: IOS Press. doi:10.3233/978-1-60750-814-4-1178.

Federici, S. and Meloni, F. (2010a). A note on the theoretical framework of World Health Organization disability assessment schedule II. *Disability and Rehabilitation, 32*(8), 687–691. doi:10.3109/09638280903290012.

Federici, S. and Meloni, F. (2010b). WHODAS II: Disability self-evaluation in the ICF conceptual frame. In J. Stone and M. Blouin (Eds.), *International Encyclopedia of Rehabilitation* (pp. 1–22). Buffalo, NY: Center for International Rehabilitation Research Information and Exchange (CIRRIE). Retrieved from http://cirrie.buffalo.edu/encyclopedia/en/article/299/

Federici, S., Meloni, F., and Corradi, F. (2012a). Measuring individual functioning. In S. Federici and M. J. Scherer (Eds.), *Assistive Technology Assessment Handbook* (pp. 25–48). Boca Raton, FL: CRC Press. doi:10.1201/b11821-4.

Federici, S., Micangeli, A., Ruspantini, I., Borgianni, S., Corradi, F., Pasqualotto, E. et al. (2005). Checking an integrated model of web accessibility and usability evaluation for disabled people. *Disability and Rehabilitation, 27*(13), 781–790. doi:10.1080/09638280400014766.

Federici, S. and Olivetti Belardinelli, M. (2006). Un difficile accordo tra prevenzione e promozione [A difficult agreement between prevention and promotion]. *Psicologia clinica dello sviluppo, 10*(2), 330–334. doi:10.1449/22608.

Federici, S. and Scherer, M. J. (2012a). The assistive technology assessment model and basic definitions. In S. Federici and M. J. Scherer (Eds.), *Assistive Technology Assessment Handbook* (pp. 1–10). Boca Raton, FL: CRC Press. doi:10.1201/b11821-2.

Federici, S. and Scherer, M. J. (Eds.). (2012b). *Assistive Technology Assessment Handbook.* Boca Raton, FL: CRC Press. doi:10.1201/b11821.

Federici, S., Scherer, M. J., Meloni, F., Corradi, F., Adya, M., Samant, D. et al. (2012b). Assessing individual functioning and disability. In S. Federici and M. J. Scherer (Eds.), *Assistive Technology Assessment Handbook* (pp. 11–24). Boca Raton, FL: CRC Press. doi:10.1201/b11821-3.

Feng, J., Lazar, J., Kumin, L., and Ozok, A. (October 12–15, 2008). Computer usage by young individuals with down syndrome: An exploratory study. Paper presented at the *10th International ACM SIGACCESS Conference on Computers and Accessibility: ASSETS '08.* Halifax, Nova Scotia, Canada. doi:10.1145/1414471.1414480.

Feng, J., Lazar, J., Kumin, L., and Ozok, A. (2010). Computer usage by children with down syndrome: Challenges and future research. *Transactions on Accessible Computing, 2*(3), 1–44. doi:10.1145/1714458.1714460.

Fink, J., Kobsa, A., and Nill, A. (1996, October 30). User-oriented adaptivity and adaptability in the AVANTI project. Paper presented at the *Designing for the Web: Empirical Studies*. Redmond, WA. Retrieved September 15, 2012, from http://www.ics.uci.edu/hci/projects/avanti/publications/ms96.html

Fitts, P. M. (1954). The information capacity of the human motor system in controlling the amplitude of movement. *Journal of Experimental Psychology, 47*(6), 381–391. doi:10.1037/h0055392

Fox, J. (2002). *An R and S-Plus Companion to Applied Regression.* Thousand Oaks, CA: SAGE.

Fredheim, H. (2011). Why user experience cannot be designed. Retrieved December 1, 2012, from http://uxdesign.smashingmagazine.com/2011/03/15/why-user-experience-cannot-be-designed/

Fredrickson, B. L. (2001). The role of positive emotions in positive psychology. The broaden-and-build theory of positive emotions. *American Psychologist, 56*(3), 218–226. doi:10.1037/0003-066X.56.3.218.

Fredrickson, B. L. (2004). The broaden-and-build theory of positive emotions. *Philosophical Transactions of the Royal Society of London. Series B, Biological Sciences, 359*(1449), 1367–1378. doi:10.1098/rstb.2004.1512.

del Galdo, E. M., Williges, R. C., Williges, B. H., and Wixon, D. R. (1986). An evaluation of critical incidents for software documentation design. *Human Factors and Ergonomics Society Annual Meeting Proceedings, 30*(1), 19–23. doi:10.1177/154193128603000105.

Galimberti, U. (2002). *Psiche e techne: l'uomo nell'età della tecnica* [Psiche and techne: The man in the age of the technique]. Milano, Italy: Feltrinelli.

Galton, F. (1879). Psychometric experiments. *Brain, 2*(2), 149–162. doi:10.1093/brain/2.2.149.

Gangadharbatla, H. (2008). Facebook me: Collective self-esteem, need to belong, and internet self-efficacy as predictors of the iGeneration's attitudes toward social networking sites. *Journal of Interactive Advertising, 8*(5), 5–15. Retrieved September 15, 2012, from Jiad. org website: http://jiad.org/article100

Gazzaniga, M. S. (2008). *Human: The Science behind What Makes Your Brain Unique.* New York: Harper Collins.

Gentner, D. and Nielsen, J. (1996). The anti-Mac interface. *Communications of the ACM, 39*(8), 70–82. doi:10.1145/232014.232032.

Gerhardt-Powals, J. (1996). Cognitive engineering principles for enhancing human-computer performance. *International Journal of Human–Computer Interaction, 8*(2), 189. doi:10.1080/10447319609526147.

Gibson, J. J. (1977). The theory of affordances. In R. Shaw and J. Bransford (Eds.), *Perceiving, Acting, and Knowing: Toward an Ecological Psychology* (pp. 67–82). Hillsdale, NJ: Lawrence Erlbaum Associates.

Gibson, J. J. (1979). *The Ecological Approach to Visual Perception.* Boston, MA: Houghton Mifflin.

Gillies, J. and Cailliau, R. (2000). *How the Web Was Born: The Story of the World Wide Web.* New York: Oxford University Press.

Glaser, B. G. and Strauss, A. L. (1967). *The Discovery of Grounded Theory: Strategies for Qualitative Research.* Chicago, IL: Aldine Publishing Company.

Godwin-Jones, B. (2001). Emerging technologies: Accessibility and web design, why does it matter? *Language Learning & Technology, 5*(1), 11–19. Retrieved September 15, 2012, from Llt.msu.edu website: http://llt.msu.edu/vol5num1/emerging/default.pdf

Goffman, E. (1963). *Stigma: Notes on the Management of Spoiled Identity.* Englewood Cliffs, NJ: Spectrum Book.

Gonzales, A. L. and Hancock, J. T. (2011). Mirror, mirror on my Facebook wall: Effects of exposure to Facebook on self-esteem. *Cyberpsychology, Behavior, and Social Networking, 14*(1–2), 79–83. doi:10.1089/cyber.2009.0411.

Good, I. J. (1953). The population frequencies of species and the estimation of population parameters. *Biometrika, 40*(3–4), 237–264. doi:10.1093/biomet/40.3-4.237.

Gray, W., Duhl, F. J., and Rizzo, N. D. (1969). *General Systems Theory and Psychiatry.* Boston, MA: Little Brown.

Gray, W. D. and Salzman, M. C. (1998). Damaged merchandise? A review of experiments that compare usability evaluation methods. *Human–Computer Interaction, 13*(3), 203–261. doi:10.1207/s15327051hci1303_2.

Greenbaum, J. and Kyng, M. (1994). *Design at Work: Cooperative Design of Computer Systems.* Hillsdale, NJ: Lawrence Erlbaum Associates.

Guan, Z., Lee, S., Cuddihy, E., and Ramey, J. (2006, April 22–27). The validity of the stimulated retrospective think-aloud method as measured by eye tracking. Paper presented at the *Conference on Human Factors in Computing Systems: SIGCHI '06.* Montreal, Quebec, Canada. doi:10.1145/1124772.1124961.

Gugerty, L. and Olson, G. (1986). Debugging by skilled and novice programmers. *ACM SIGCHI Bulletin, 17*(4), 171–174. doi:10.1145/22339.22367.

Gunn, C. (1995, May 7–11). An example of formal usability inspections in practice at Hewlett-Packard company. Paper presented at the *Conference Companion on Human Factors in Computing Systems: CHI '95.* Denver, CO. doi:10.1145/223355.223451.

Gurven, M., von Rueden, C., Massenkoff, M., Kaplan, H., and Lero Vie, M. (2013). How universal is the big five? Testing the five-factor model of personality variation among forager-farmers in the Bolivian Amazon. *Journal of Personality and Social Psychology, 104*(2), 354–370. doi:10.1037/a0030841.

Gutmair, U. and Flor, C. (1998). Hysteria and cyberspace: Interview with Slavoj Žižek. *Telepolis.* Retrieved September 15, 2012, from Heise.de website: http://www.heise.de/tp/artikel/2/2492/1.html

Hackos, J. T. and Redish, J. C. (1998). *User and Task Analysis for Interface Design.* New York: John Wiley & Sons.

Hamburger, Y. A. and Ben-Artzi, E. (2000). The relationship between extraversion and neuroticism and the different uses of the Internet. *Computers in Human Behavior, 16*(4), 441–449. doi:10.1016/S0747-5632(00)00017-0.

Hancock, P. A., Weaver, J. L., and Parasuraman, R. (2002). Sans subjectivity—Ergonomics is engineering. *Ergonomics, 45*(14), 991–994. doi:10.1080/00140130210166898.

Harper, S. and Bechhofer, S. (2007). SADIe: Structural semantics for accessibility and device independence. *ACM Transactions on Computer–Human Interaction, 14*(2), 1–27. doi:10.1145/1275511.1275516.

Harper, S., Bechhofer, S., and Lunn, D. (2006, October 18–20). Taming the inaccessible web. Paper presented at the *24th Annual ACM International Conference on Design of Communication: SIGDOC '06.* Myrtle Beach, SC. doi:10.1145/1166324.1166340.

Harper, B., Slaughter, L., and Norman, K. (1997, November 1–5). Questionnaire administration via the WWW: A validation and reliability study for a user satisfaction questionnaire. Paper presented at the *World Conference on the WWW, Internet & Intranet: WebNet '97.* Toronto, Ontario, Canada. Retrieved September 15, 2012, http://www.lap.umd.edu/webnet/paper.html

Hart, S. G. and Staveland, L. E. (1988). Development of NASA-TLX (Task Load Index): Results of empirical and theoretical research. In P. A. Hancock and N. Meshkati (Eds.), *Human Mental Workload* (pp. 139–184). Amsterdam, the Netherlands: North-Holland.

Hartson, H. R., Andre, T. S., and Williges, R. C. (2003). Criteria for evaluating usability evaluation methods. *International Journal of Human–Computer Interaction, 15*(1), 145–181. doi:10.1207/S15327590IJHC1304_03.

Hartson, H. R., Castillo, J. C., Kelso, J., and Neale, W. C. (1996, April 13–18). Remote evaluation: The network as an extension of the usability laboratory. Paper presented at the *SIGCHI Conference on Human Factors in Computing Systems: CHI '90.* Vancouver, CA. doi:10.1145/238386.238511.

Hartson, H. R. and Hix, D. (1989). Toward empirically derived methodologies and tools for human-computer interface development. *International Journal of Man-Machine Studies, 31*(4), 477–494. doi:10.1016/0020-7373(89)90005-9.

Hassenzahl, M. (2001). The effect of perceived hedonic quality on product appealingness. *International Journal of Human–Computer Interaction, 13*(4), 481–499. doi:10.1207/s15327590ijhc1304_07.

Hassenzahl, M. (2005). The thing and I: Understanding the relationship between user and product. In M. Blythe, K. Overbeeke, A. Monk, and P. Wright (Eds.), *Funology: From Usability to Enjoyment* (Vol. 3, pp. 31–42). Berlin, Germany: Springer. doi:10.1007/1-4020-2967-5_4.

Hassenzahl, M. and Monk, A. (2010). The inference of perceived usability from beauty. *Human–Computer Interaction, 25*(3), 235–260. doi:10.1080/07370024.2010.500139.

Hassenzahl, M. and Tractinsky, N. (2006). User experience—A research agenda. *Behaviour & Information Technology, 25*(2), 91–97. doi:10.1080/01449290500330331.

Heider, F. (1958). *The Psychology of Interpersonal Relations.* Hillsdale, NJ: Lawrence Erlbaum Associates.

Henry, S. L. (2007). *Just Ask: Integrating Accessibility Throughout Design.* Raleigh, NC: Lulu.com.

Hertzum, M. and Jacobsen, N. E. (2003). The evaluator effect: A chilling fact about usability evaluation methods. *International Journal of Human–Computer Interaction, 15*(4), 183–204. doi:10.1207/S15327590IJHC1501_14.

Higgins, E. T. (1987). Self-discrepancy: A theory relating self and affect. *Psychological Review, 94*(3), 319–340. doi:10.1037/0033-295X.94.3.319.

Higgins, E. T. (1991). Development of self-regulatory and self-evaluative processes: Costs, benefits, and tradeoffs. In M. R. Gunnar and L. A. Sroufe (Eds.), *Self Processes and Development* (pp. 125–166). Hillsdale, NJ: Erlbaum.

Hix, D. and Hartson, H. R. (1993). *Developing User Interfaces: Ensuring Usability through Product and Process.* New York: Wiley & Sons.

Hodgkinson, G. P. and Crawshaw, C. M. (1985). Hierarchical task analysis for ergonomics research: An application of the method to the design and evaluation of sound mixing consoles. *Applied Ergonomics, 16*(4), 289–299. doi:10.1016/0003-6870(85)90094-8.

Hollan, J., Hutchins, E., and Kirsh, D. (2000). Distributed cognition: Toward a new foundation for human-computer interaction research. *ACM Transactions on Computer–Human Interaction, 7*(2), 174–196. doi:10.1145/353485.353487.

Horton, S. (2005). *Access by Design: A Guide to Universal Usability for Web Designers.* New York: New Riders Press.

Howard, P. E. N., Rainie, L., and Jones, S. (2001). Days and nights on the internet: The impact of a diffusing technology. *American Behavioral Scientist, 45*(3), 383–404. doi:10.1177/0002764201045003003.

Huang, W. (February 5–7, 2007). Using eye tracking to investigate graph layout effects. Paper presented at the *6th International Asia-Pacific Symposium on Visualization: APVIS '07.* Sydney, New South Wales, Australia. doi:10.1109/apvis.2007.329282.

Huang, W., Hong, S.-H., and Eades, P. (2008, March 5–7). Effects of crossing angles. Paper presented at the *IEEE Pacific Visualization Symposium: PacificVIS '08.* Kyoto, Japan. doi:10.1109/pacificvis.2008.4475457.

Hudson, J. M., Christensen, J., Kellogg, W. A., and Erickson, T. (2002, April 20–25). "I'd be overwhelmed, but it's just one more thing to do": Availability and interruption in research management. Paper presented at the *SIGCHI Conference on Human Factors in Computing Systems: CHI '02.* Minneapolis, MN. doi:10.1145/503376.503394.

Human Performance Research Group. (2012). *NASA TLX Paper and Pencil Version Instruction Manual.* Retrieved December 8, 2012, from http://humansystems.arc.nasa.gov/groups/TLX/paperpencil.html

Hutchins, E. L. (1980). *Culture and Inference: A Trobriand Case Study*. Cambridge, MA: Harvard University Press.

Hutchins, E. L. (1995). *Cognition in the Wild*. Cambridge, MA: MIT Press.

Hutchins, E. L. (2001). Distributed cognition. In J. S. Neil and B. B. Paul (Eds.), *International Encyclopedia of the Social & Behavioral Sciences* (pp. 2068–2072). Oxford, U.K.: Pergamon. doi:10.1016/b0-08-043076-7/01636-3.

Hutchins, E. L., Hollan, J. D., and Norman, D. A. (1985). Direct manipulation interfaces. *Human–Computer Interaction, 1*(4), 311–338. doi:10.1207/s15327051hci0104_2.

Hvannberg, E. T., Law, E. L.-C., and Lárusdóttir, M. K. (2007). Heuristic evaluation: Comparing ways of finding and reporting usability problems. *Interacting with Computers, 19*(2), 225–240. doi:10.1016/j.intcom.2006.10.001.

International Telecommunication Union. (September 15, 2011). The world telecommunication/ICT indicators database. From http://www.itu.int/ITU-D/ict/publications/world/world.html

International Telecommunications Union. (2010). The world in 2010: ICT facts and figures. Retrieved September 15, 2012, from http://www.itu.int/ITU-D/ict/material/FactsFigures2010.pdf

International Telecommunications Union. (2011). *Measuring the Information Society*. Geneva, Switzerland: ITU.

Internet World Stats. (2011). World internet users and population stats. Retrieved September 15, 2012, from http://www.internetworldstats.com/stats.htm

Intille, S. S., Rondoni, J., Kukla, C., Ancona, I., and Bao, L. (2003, April 5–10). A context-aware experience sampling tool. Paper presented at the *Human Factors in Computing Systems: CHI '03*. Ft. Lauderdale, FL. doi:10.1145/765891.766101.

ISO 13407. (1999) Human-centred design processes for interactive systems. International Organization for Standardization (ISO), Geneva, Switzerland.

ISO 20282-1. (2006) Ease of operation of everyday products—Part 1: Design requirements for context of use and user characteristics. International Organization for Standardization (ISO), Geneva, Switzerland.

ISO 9241-11. (1998) Ergonomic requirements for office work with visual display terminals—Part 11: Guidance on usability. International Organization for Standardization (ISO), Geneva, Switzerland.

ISO 9241-171. (2008) Ergonomics of human-system interaction—Part 171: Guidance on software accessibility. International Organization for Standardization (ISO), Geneva, Switzerland.

ISO 9241-20. (2009) Ergonomics of human-system interaction—Part 20: Accessibility guidelines for information/communication technology (ICT) equipment and services. International Organization for Standardization (ISO), Geneva, Switzerland.

ISO 9241-210. (2010) Ergonomics of human-system interaction—Part 210: Human-centered design for interactive systems. International Organization for Standardization (ISO), Geneva, Switzerland.

ISO/IEC 25010. (2011) Systems and software engineering—Systems and software quality requirements and evaluation (SQuaRE)—System and software quality models. International Organization for Standardization (ISO), Geneva, Switzerland.

ISO/IEC 25062. (2006) Software engineering—Software product quality requirements and evaluation (SQuaRE)—Common industry format (CIF) for usability test reports. International Organization for Standardization (ISO), Geneva, Switzerland.

ISO/IEC 62366. (2007) Medical devices—Application of usability engineering to medical devices. International Organization for Standardization (ISO), Geneva, Switzerland.

ISO/IEC 9126-1. (2001) Information technology—Software product evaluation: Quality characteristics and guidelines for their use. International Organization for Standardization (ISO), Geneva, Switzerland.

ISO/TR 16982. (2002) Ergonomics of human-system interaction—Usability methods supporting human-centred design. International Organization for Standardization (ISO), Geneva, Switzerland.

ISO/TR 18529. (2000) Ergonomics—Ergonomics of human-system interaction—Human-centred lifecycle process descriptions. International Organization for Standardization (ISO), Geneva, Switzerland.

Istituto Nazionale di Statistica (ISTAT). (2007). *Condizioni di salute, fattori di rischio e ricorso ai servizi sanitari: Anno 2005* [Health conditions, risk factors and use of health services: Year 2005]. Retrieved September 15, 2012, from http://www.salute.gov.it/imgs/C_17_pubblicazioni_650_allegato.pdf

Ivory, M. Y. and Hearst, M. A. (2001). The state of the art in automating usability evaluation of user interfaces. *ACM Computing Surveys, 33*(4), 470–516. doi:10.1145/503112.503114.

Jacob, R. J. K. (1995). Eye tracking in advanced interface design. In W. Barfield and T. A. Furness (Eds.), *Virtual Environments and Advanced Interface Design* (pp. 258–288). New York: Oxford University Press.

Jacob, R. J. K. and Karn, K. S. (2003). Eye tracking in human-computer interaction and usability research: Ready to deliver the promises. In J. Hyönä, R. Radach, and H. Deubel (Eds.), *The Mind's Eye: Cognitive and Applied Aspects of Eye Movement Research* (pp. 573–603). Oxford, U.K.: Elsevier Science.

Jarke, M., Bui, X. T., and Carroll, J. M. (1998). Scenario management: An interdisciplinary approach. *Requirements Engineering, 3*(3), 155–173. doi:10.1007/s007660050002.

Jasmin, K. and Casasanto, D. (2012). The QWERTY effect: How typing shapes the meanings of words. *Psychonomic Bulletin and Review, 19*, 499–504. doi:10.3758/s13423-012-0229-7.

Jay, C., Stevens, R., Glencross, M., Chalmers, A., and Yang, C. (2007). How people use presentation to search for a link: Expanding the understanding of accessibility on the Web. *Universal Access in the Information Society, 6*(3), 307–320. doi:10.1007/s10209-007-0089-5.

Jelinek, F. (1997). *Statistical Methods for Speech Recognition*. Cambridge, MA: MIT Press.

Jenkins, H. (2006). *Convergence Culture: Where Old and New Media Collide*. New York: University Press.

John, B. E. (April 1–5, 1990). Extensions of GOMS analyses to expert performance requiring perception of dynamic visual and auditory information. Paper presented at the *SIGCHI Conference on Human Factors in Computing Systems—Empowering People: CHI '90*. Seattle, WA. doi:10.1145/97243.97262.

John, B. E. and Kieras, D. E. (1996a). The GOMS family of user interface analysis techniques: Comparison and contrast. *ACM Transactions on Computer–Human Interaction, 3*(4), 320–351. doi:10.1145/235833.236054.

John, B. E. and Kieras, D. E. (1996b). Using GOMS for user interface design and evaluation: Which technique? *ACM Transactions on Computer–Human Interaction, 3*(4), 287–319. doi:10.1145/235833.236050.

John, O. P., Naumann, L. P., and Soto, C. J. (2008). Paradigm shift to the integrative big five trait taxonomy: History, measurement, and conceptual issues. In O. P. John, R. W. Robins, and L. A. Pervin (Eds.), *Handbook of Personality: Theory and Research* (3rd edn., pp. 114–158). New York: Guilford Press.

Johnson-Laird, P. N. (1989). Mental models. In M. I. Posner (Ed.), *Foundations of Cognitive Science* (pp. 469–499). Cambridge, MA: MIT Press.

Johnstone, C., Bottsford-Miller, N. A., and Thompson, S. J. (2006). *Using the Think Aloud Method (Cognitive Labs) to Evaluate Test Design for Students with Disabilities and English Language Learners*. (Technical Report 44). Retrieved September 15, 2012, from University of Minnesota, Minneapolis, MN, National Center on Educational Outcomes website. http://www.cehd.umn.edu/nceo/OnlinePubs/Tech44/

Jordan, P. W. (1994). What is usability? In S. A. Robertson (Ed.), *Contemporary Ergonomics* (pp. 454–458). London, U.K.: Taylor & Francis.

Joyce, C. A., Gorodnitsky, I. F., King, J. W., and Kutas, M. (2002). Tracking eye fixations with electroocular and electroencephalographic recordings. *Psychophysiology, 39*(5), 607–618. doi:10.1111/1469-8986.3950607.

Jünger, M. and Mutzel, P. (Eds.). (2004). *Graph Drawing Software*. Berlin, Germany: Springer.

Kahn, M. J. and Prail, A. (1994). Formal usability inspections. In J. Nielsen and R. L. Mack (Eds.), *Usability Inspection Methods* (pp. 141–172). Hoboken, NJ: John Wiley & Sons.

Kahneman, D., Krueger, A. B., Schkade, D. A., Schwarz, N., and Stone, A. A. (2004). A survey method for characterizing daily life experience: The day reconstruction method. *Science, 306*(5702), 1776–1780. doi:10.1126/science.1103572.

Karwowski, W. (2000). Symvatology: The science of an artifact-human compatibility. *Theoretical Issues in Ergonomics Science, 1*(1), 76–91. doi:10.1080/146392200308480.

Kelly, B., Sloan, D., Brown, S., Seale, J., Petrie, H., Lauke, P. et al. (2007, May 7–8). Accessibility 2.0: People, policies and processes. Paper presented at the *International Cross-Disciplinary Conference on Web Accessibility: W4A '07*. Banff, Alberta, Canada. doi:10.1145/1243441.1243471.

Kelly, B., Sloan, D., Phipps, L., Petrie, H., and Hamilton, F. (2005, May 10–14). Forcing standardization or accommodating diversity? A framework for applying the WCAG in the real world. Paper presented at the *International Cross-Disciplinary Workshop on Web Accessibility: W4A '05*. Chiba, Japan. doi:10.1145/1061811.1061820.

Kieras, D. (1988). Towards a practical GOMS model methodology for user interface design. In M. Helander (Ed.), *Handbook of Human-Computer Interaction* (1st edn., pp. 135–158). Amsterdam, the Netherlands: Elsevier.

Kieras, D. and Polson, P. G. (1985). An approach to the formal analysis of user complexity. *International Journal of Man-Machine Studies, 22*(4), 365–394. doi:10.1016/S0020-7373(85)80045-6.

Kirakowski, J. (2000). *Questionnaires in Usability Engineering: A List of Frequently Asked Questions* (3rd edn.). Retrieved September 15, 2012, from Human Factors Research Group website. http://www.ucc.ie/hfrg/resources/qfaq1.html

Kirakowski, J. (2002). Is ergonomics empirical? *Ergonomics, 45*(14–15), 995–997. doi:10.1080/00140130210166889.

Knecht, B. (2004). Accessibility regulations and a universal design philosophy inspire the design process. *Architectural Record, 192*, 145–150. Retrieved September 15, 2012, from Archrecord.construction.com website: http://archrecord.construction.com/resources/conteduc/archives/0401edit-1.asp

Koffka, K. (1935). *Principles of Gestalt Psychology*. New York: Harcourt Brace.

Krantz, O. (2012). Assistive devices utilisation in activities of everyday life—A proposed framework of understanding a user perspective. *Disability and Rehabilitation: Assistive Technology, 7*(3), 189–198. doi:10.3109/17483107.2011.618212.

Krug, S. (2000). *Don't Make Me Think! A Common Sense Approach to Web Usability*. Indianapolis, IN: New Riders.

Kubey, R. W. and Csíkszentmihályi, M. (1990). *Television and the Quality of Life: How Viewing Shapes Everyday Experience*. Hillsdale, NJ: Lawrence Erlbaum Associates.

Kurosu, M. (2007). Concept of usability revisited. In J. Jacko (Ed.), *12th International Conference on Human–Computer Interaction: Interaction Design and Usability* (Vol. 4550, pp. 579–586). Berlin, Germany: Springer. doi:10.1007/978-3-540-73105-4_64.

Kurosu, M. (2010, August 3–5). Concept structure of UX (user experience) and its measurement. Paper presented at the *Joint International Conference of Asia Pacific Computer Human Interaction and Ergofuture: APCHI & Ergofuture '10*. Bali, Indonesia. http://iea.cc/upload/Ergofuture%202010%20Brochure.pdf

Kurosu, M. (2012a, May 5–10). Psychological considerations on behavior and UX. Paper presented at the *Conference on Human Factors in Computing Systems: CHI '12*. Austin, TX. Retrieved June 15, 2012, from http://di.ncl.ac.uk/uxtheory/files/2011/11/6_Kurosu.pdf

Kurosu, M. (2012b, September 4–7). Three dimensions of artefact design—Meaning, quality and Kansei. Paper presented at the *Human Interface Symposium 2012*. Fukuoka City, Japan.

Kurosu, M. and Ando, M. (2008, September 20–22). The psychology of non-selection and waste: A tentative approach for constructing the user behavior theory based on the Artifact Development Analysis. Paper presented at the *74th Annual Convention of Japanese Psychological Association*. Osaka University, Osaka, Japan. Retrieved September 15, 2012, http://www.wdc-jp.biz/jpa/conf2010/

Kurosu, M. and Hashizume, A. (2012, May 22–25). Describing experiences in different mode of behavior—GOB, POB and SOB. Paper presented at the *Kansei Engineering and Emotion Research: KEER '12*. Penghu, Taiwan.

Kurosu, M., Matsuura, S., and Sugizaki, M. (October 12–15, 1997). Categorical inspection method—Structured heuristic evaluation (sHEM). Paper presented at the *International Conference on Systems, Man, and Cybernetics and Computational Cybernetics and Simulation: IEEE '97*. Orlando, FL. doi:10.1109/icsmc.1997.635329.

Kuusela, H. and Paul, P. (2000). A comparison of concurrent and retrospective verbal protocol analysis. *American Journal of Psychology, 113*(3), 387–404.

Lambie, T. (2006). Cognitive engineering. In W. Karwowski (Ed.), *International Encyclopedia of Ergonomics and Human Factors* (2nd edn., Vol. 1, pp. 15–18). Boca Raton, FL: CRC Press.

Larkin, J. H. (1983). The role of problem representation in physics. In D. Gentner and A. L. Stevens (Eds.), *Mental Models* (pp. 75–98). Hillsdale, NJ: Lawrence Erlbaum Associates.

Larson, R. and Csíkszentmihályi, M. (1983). The experience sampling method. In H. T. Reis (Ed.), *Naturalistic Approaches to Studying Social Interaction: New Directions for Methodology of Social and Behavioral Science* (Vol. 15, pp. 41–56). San Francisco, CA: Jossey-Bass.

Larson, R. and Csíkszentmihályi, M. (1992). Validity and reliability of the experience sampling method the experience of psychopathology. In R. Larson and M. Csíkszentmihályi (Eds.), *Validity and Reliability of the Experience Sampling Method: Investigating Mental Disorders in Their Natural Settings* (pp. 43–57). New York: Cambridge University Press. doi:10.1017/CBO9780511663246.006.

Lassila, O. and Hendler, J. (2007). Embracing "Web 3.0". *IEEE Internet Computing, 11*(3), 90–93. doi:10.1109/MIC.2007.52.

Law, E., Schaik, P., and Roto, V. (October 14, 2012). To measure or not to measure UX: An interview study. Paper presented at the *I-UxSED 2012*. Copenhagen, Denmark.

Law, E. L.-C., Vermeeren, A. P. O. S., Hassenzahl, M., and Blythe, M. (2007, September 3–7). Towards a UX manifesto. Paper presented at the *Proceedings of the 21st British HCI Group Annual Conference on People and Computers: HCI '07*. University of Lancaster, Lancaster, U.K.

Lazar, J. (Ed.). (2007). *Universal Usability: Designing Computer Interfaces for Diverse User Populations*. West Sussex, U.K.: Wiley & Sons.

Legrenzi, P. and Girotto, V. (1996). Mental models in reasoning and decision making. In J. Oakhill and A. Garnham (Eds.), *Mental Models in Cognitive Science* (pp. 95–118). Hove, U.K.: Psychology Press.

Lemay, R. (1994). A review of the standard rules on the equalization of opportunities for persons with disabilities, 1994, United Nations Department for Policy Coordination and Sustainable Development. *International Social Role Valorization Journal, 1*(2), 47–52.

Leroi-Gourhan, A. (1993). *Gesture and Speech*. Cambridge, MA: MIT Press.

Lewis, C. (1986). A model of mental model construction. *ACM SIGCHI Bulletin, 17*(4), 306–313. doi:10.1145/22339.22388.

Lewis, C. (1988). Why and how to learn why: Analysis-based generalization of procedures. *Cognitive Science, 12*(2), 211–256. doi:10.1207/s15516709cog1202_3.

Lewis, J. R. (1994). Sample sizes for usability studies: Additional considerations. *Human Factors, 36*(2), 368–378.

Lewis, D. (1999). Psychophysical and theoretical identifications. In D. Lewis (Ed.), *Papers in Metaphysics and Epistemology* (Vol. 2, pp. 248–261). New York: Cambridge University Press. doi:10.1017/CBO9780511625343.

Lewis, J. R. (2000). Validation of Monte Carlo estimation of problem discovery likelihood. (Tech. Rep. No. 29.3357). Retrieved from IBM website. http://drjim.0catch.com/pcarlo1-ral.pdf

Lewis, J. R. (2001). Evaluation of procedures for adjusting problem-discovery rates estimated from small samples. *International Journal of Human–Computer Interaction, 13*(4), 445–479. doi:10.1207/S15327590IJHC1304_06.

Lewis, J. R. (2002). Psychometric evaluation of the PSSUQ using data from five years of usability studies. *International Journal of Human–Computer Interaction, 14*(3–4), 463–488. doi:10.1080/10447318.2002.9669130.

Lewis, J. R. (2006). Sample sizes for usability tests: Mostly math, not magic. *Interactions, 13*(6), 29–33. doi:10.1145/1167948.1167973.

Lewis, C., Polson, P. G., Wharton, C., and Rieman, J. (April 1–5, 1990). Testing a walkthrough methodology for theory-based design of walk-up-and-use interfaces. Paper presented at the *SIGCHI Conference on Human Factors in Computing Systems: CHI '90*. Seattle, WA. doi:10.1145/97243.97279.

Lewis, C. and Rieman, J. (1993). *Task-Centered User Interface Design: A Practical Introduction.* Retrieved September 15, 2012, from http://users.cs.dal.ca/~jamie/TCUID/tcuid.pdf

Lewis, J. R. and Sauro, J. (2009, July 19–24). The factor structure of the system usability scale. Paper presented at the *1st International Conference on Human Centered Design '09*. San Diego, CA. doi:10.1007/978-3-642-02806-9_12.

Long, F. (2009, July 14–15). Real or imaginary: The effectiveness of using personas in product design. Paper presented at the *Irish Ergonomics Society Annual Conference 2009*. Dublin, Ireland. Retrieved September 15, 2012, from http://www.ergonomics.ie/Documents/Irish%20Ergonomics%20Review/Irish%20Ergonomics%20Review%202009.pdf

Lumsden, C. J. (1988). Gene-culture coevolution: Culture and biology in Darwinian perspective. In D. De Kerckhove and C. J. Lumsden (Eds.), *The Alphabet and the Brain: The Lateralization of Writing* (pp. 17–42). Berlin, Germany: Springer-Verlag.

Lumsden, C. J. (1999). Gene-culture coevolution. *Telepolis*. Retrieved September 15, 2012, from Heise.de website: http://www.heise.de/tp/druck/mb/artikel/2/2768/1.html

Lumsden, C. J. and Wilson, E. O. (1981). *Genes, Mind, and Culture: The Coevolutionary Process.* Cambridge, MA: Harvard University Press.

Lupton, D. and Seymour, W. (2000). Technology, selfhood and physical disability. *Social Science and Medicine, 50*(12), 1851–1862. doi:10.1016/S0277-9536(99)00422-0.

Luximon, A. and Goonetilleke, R. S. (2001). Simplified subjective workload assessment technique. *Ergonomics, 44*(3), 229–243. doi:10.1080/00140130010000901.

Mace, R. L. (1985). *Universal Design, Barrier-Free Environments for Everyone.* Los Angeles, CA: Designers West.

MacKenzie, I. S. (1992). Fitts' law as a research and design tool in human-computer interaction. *Hum.-Comput. Interact., 7*(1), 91–139. doi:http://dx.doi.org/10.1207/s15327051hci0701_3

Madans, J. H. and Altman, B. M. (2006, December 13–15). Purposes of disability statistics. Paper presented at the *Training Workshop on Disability Statistics for SPECA Countries: UN Special Programme for the Economies of Central Asia*. Bishkek, Kyrgyzstan. Retrieved September 15, 2012, from http://www.unece.org/stats/documents/2006.12.health.htm

Mahatody, T., Sagar, M., and Kolski, C. (2010). State of the art on the cognitive walkthrough method, its variants and evolutions. *International Journal of Human–Computer Interaction, 26*(8), 741–785. doi:10.1080/10447311003781409.

Malle, B. F. and Knobe, J. (1997). The folk concept of intentionality. *Journal of Experimental Social Psychology, 33*(2), 101–121. doi:10.1006/jesp.1996.1314.

Manago, A. M., Graham, M. B., Greenfield, P. M., and Salimkhan, G. (2008). Self-presentation and gender on MySpace. *Journal of Applied Developmental Psychology, 29*(6), 446–458. doi:10.1016/j.appdev.2008.07.001.

Mandryk, R. L., Atkins, M. S., and Inkpen, K. M. (2006, April 22–27). A continuous and objective evaluation of emotional experience with interactive play environments. Paper presented at the *SIGCHI Conference on Human Factors in Computing Systems: CHI '06*. Montreal, Quebec, Canada. doi:10.1145/1124772.1124926.

Marchetti, R. (1994, October 17–19). Using usability inspections to find usability problems early in the lifecycle. Paper presented at the *Pacific Northwest Software Quality Conference*. Portland, OR. Retrieved September 15, 2012, from http://www.uploads.pnsqc.org/1994/pnsqc1994.pdf

Mark, W. (1991). The computer for the 21st century. *Scientific American, 265*(30), 94–104.

Marsh, T. (2003). Staying there: An activity-based approach to narrative design and evaluation as an antidote to virtual corpsing. In G. Riva, F. Davide, and W. A. IJsselsteijn (Eds.), *Being There: Concepts, Effects and Measurements of User Presence in Synthetic Environments* (pp. 85–96). Amsterdam, the Netherlands: IOS Press.

Maruta, J., Lee, S. W., Jacobs, E. F., and Ghajar, J. (2010). A unified science of concussion. *Annals of the New York Academy of Sciences, 1208*(1), 58–66. doi:10.1111/j.1749-6632.2010.05695.x.

Marzouki, Y., Skandrani-Marzouki, I., Béjaoui, M., Hammoudi, H., and Bellaj, T. (2012). The contribution of Facebook to the 2011 Tunisian revolution: A cyberpsychological Insight. *Cyberpsychology, Behavior, and Social Networking, 15*(5), 237–244. doi:10.1089/cyber.2011.0177.

Mauri, M., Cipresso, P., Balgera, A., Villamira, M., and Riva, G. (2011). Why is Facebook so successful? Psychophysiological measures describe a core flow state while using Facebook. *Cyberpsychology, Behavior and Social Networks, 14*(12), 723–731. doi:10.1089/cyber.2010.0377.

May, T. (2011). *Social Research: Issues, Methods and Research.* New York: McGraw-Hill.

Mayhew, D. J. (1999). *The Usability Engineering Lifecycle: A Practitioner's Handbook for User Interface Design.* San Francisco, CA: Morgan Kaufmann.

McKenna, F. P. (2002). Subjective measures: Not perfect but what is? *Ergonomics, 45*(14), 998–1000. doi:10.1080/00140130210166870.

McLuhan, M. (1964). *Understanding Media: The Extensions of Man.* London, U.K.: Routledge & Kegan Paul.

Mele, M. L. and Federici, S. (2012a). Gaze and eye-tracking solutions for psychological research. *Cognitive Processing, 13*(Suppl. 1), S261–S265. doi:10.1007/s10339-012-0499-z.

Mele, M. L. and Federici, S. (2012b). A psychotechnological review on eye-tracking systems: Towards user experience. *Disability and Rehabilitation: Assistive Technology, 7*(4), 261–281. doi:10.3109/17483107.2011.635326.

Meltzoff, A. N. and Decety, J. (2003). What imitation tells us about social cognition: A rapprochement between developmental psychology and cognitive neuroscience. *Philosophical Transactions of the Royal Society of London. Series B, Biological Sciences, 358*(1431), 491–500. doi:10.1098/rstb.2002.1261.

Menary, R. (Ed.). (2010). *The Extended Mind.* Cambridge, MA: MIT Press.

Mendelson, A. and Papacharissi, Z. (2004, May 24). Users and manipulators: A typology of Internet usage styles. Paper presented at the *Annual Meeting of the International Communication Association.* New Orleans, LA.

Michell, J. (2002). Do ratings measure latent attributes? *Ergonomics, 45*(14), 1008–1010. doi:10.1080/00140130210166843.

Microsoft Corporation. (2012). Microsoft research. Retrieved September 15, 2012, from http://research.microsoft.com/en-us/

Miesenberger, K., Corradi, F., and Mele, M. L. (2012). The psychotechnologist: A new profession in the assistive technology assessment. In S. Federici and M. J. Scherer (Eds.), *Assistive Technology Assessment Handbook* (pp. 179–200). Boca Raton, FL: CRC Press. doi:10.1201/b11821-12.

Militello, L. G. and Hutton, R. J. B. (1998). Applied cognitive task analysis (ACTA): A practitioner's toolkit for understanding cognitive task demands. *Ergonomics, 41*(11), 1618–1641. doi:10.1080/001401398186108.

Mirza, M., Gossett Zakrajsek, A., and Borsci, S. (2012). The assessment of the environments of use: Accessibility, sustainability, and universal design. In S. Federici and M. J. Scherer (Eds.), *Assistive Technology Assessment Handbook* (pp. 67–81). Boca Raton, FL: CRC Press. doi:10.1201/b11821-6.

Molich, R. and Nielsen, J. (1990). Improving a human-computer dialogue. *Communications of the ACM, 33*(3), 338–348. doi:10.1145/77481.77486.

Mont, D. (2007). *Measuring Disability Prevalence. Special Protection Discussion Paper No. 0706.* Retrieved September 15, 2012, from The World Bank website. http://siteresources.worldbank.org/DISABILITY/Resources/Data/MontPrevalence.pdf

Moore, K. and McElroy, J. C. (2012). The influence of personality on Facebook usage, wall postings, and regret. *Computers in Human Behavior, 28*(1), 267–274. doi:10.1016/j.chb.2011.09.009.

Muller, M. J. and Kogan, S. (2010). Grounded theory method in HCI and CSCW. (10-09). Retrieved September 15, 2012, from IBM Watson Research Center website. http://domino.watson.ibm.com/cambridge/research.nsf/58bac2a2a6b05a1285256b30005b3953/818eb1454a54b9348525777d0071c35c!OpenDocument

Nadkarni, A. and Hofmann, S. G. (2012). Why do people use Facebook? *Personality and Individual Differences, 52*(3), 243–249. doi:10.1016/j.paid.2011.11.007.

Nagamachi, M. (1995). Kansei engineering: A new ergonomic consumer-oriented technology for product development. *International Journal of Industrial Ergonomics, 15*(1), 3–11. doi:10.1016/0169-8141(94)00052-5.

National Telecommunication and Information Administration (NTIA). (1999). Falling through the net: Defining the digital divide. Retrieved Setember 15, 2012, from U.S. Department of Commerce website. http://www.ntia.doc.gov/ntiahome/fttn99/contents.html

Nevalainen, S. and Sajaniemi, J. (2004, April 5–7). Comparison of three eye tracking devices in psychology of programming research. Paper presented at the *16th Annual Psychology of Programming Interest Group Workshop: PPIG'04.* Carlow. Ireland.

Newell, A. and Simon, H. A. (1972). *Human Problem Solving.* Englewood Cliffs, NJ: Prentice-Hall.

Nielsen, J. (1993). *Usability Engineering.* San Diego, CA: Morgan Kaufmann.

Nielsen, J. (1994a, April 24–28). Enhancing the explanatory power of usability heuristics. Paper presented at the *SIGCHI Conference on Human Factors in Computing Systems: CHI '94.* Boston, MA. Retrieved September 15, 2012, http://doi.acm.org/10.1145/191666.191729, doi:10.1145/191666.191729.

Nielsen, J. (1994b). Guerrilla HCI: Using discount usability engineering to penetrate the intimidation barrier. Retrieved September 15, 2012, from http://www.useit.com/papers/guerrilla_hci.html

Nielsen, J. (1995a). Card sorting to discover the users' model of the information space. Retrieved September 15, 2012, from http://www.useit.com/papers/sun/cardsort.html

Nielsen, J. (1995b). Severity ratings for usability problems. Retrieved September 15, 2012, from http://www.useit.com/papers/heuristic/severityrating.html

Nielsen, J. (1995c). Ten usability heuristics. Retrieved September 15, 2012, from http://www.useit.com/papers/heuristic/heuristic_list.html

Nielsen, J. (2000). Why you only need to test with 5 users. Retrieved September 15, 2012, from www.useit.com/alertbox/20000319.html

Nielsen, J. (2012). How many test users in a usability study? Retrieved September 15, 2012, from http://www.useit.com/alertbox/number-of-test-users.html

Nielsen, J. and Landauer, T. K. (1993, April 24–29). A mathematical model of the finding of usability problems. Paper presented at the *Conference on Human Factors in Computing Systems: INTERACT and CHI '93*. Amsterdam, the Netherlands. doi:10.1145/169059.169166.

Nielsen, J. and Mack, R. L. (Eds.). (1994). *Usability Inspection Methods*. New York: John Wiley & Sons.

Nielsen, J. and Molich, R. (1990, April 1–5). Heuristic evaluation of user interfaces. Paper presented at the *SIGCHI Conference on Human Factors in Computing Systems: CHI '90*. Seattle, WA. doi:10.1145/97243.97281.

Nielsen, J. and Pernice, K. (2010). *Eyetracking Web Usability*. Berkeley, CA: New Riders.

Nielsen Norman Group. (2012). Ten usability heuristics. Retrieved December 1, 2012, from http://www.nngroup.com/articles/ten-usability-heuristics/

Nishizeki, T. and Rahman, M. S. (2004). *Planar Graph Drawing*. Singapore: World Scientific.

Nørgaard, M. and Hornbæk, K. (2006, June 26–28). What do usability evaluators do in practice? An explorative study of think-aloud testing. Paper presented at the *6th Conference on Designing Interactive Systems: DIS '06*. University Park, PA. doi:10.1145/1142405.1142439.

Norman, D. A. (1983). Some observations on mental models. In D. Gentner and A. L. Steven (Eds.), *Mental Models* (pp. 7–14). Hillsdale, NJ: Lawrence Erlbaum Associates.

Norman, D. A. (1986). Cognitive engineering. In D. A. Norman and S. W. Draper (Eds.), *User Centered System Design: New Perspectives on Human-Computer Interaction* (pp. 31–61). London, U.K.: Lawrence Erlbaum Associates.

Norman, D. A. (1988). *The Psychology of Everyday Things*. New York: Basic Books.

Norman, D. A. (1990). *The Design of Everyday Things*. New York: Doubleday.

Norman, D. A. (1991). Cognitive artifacts. In J. M. Carroll (Ed.), *Designing Interaction: Psychology at the Human-Computer Interface* (pp. 17–38). New York: Cambridge University Press.

Norman, D. A. (1998). *The Invisible Computer: Why Good Products Can Fail, the Personal Computer Is So Complex, and Information Appliances are the Solution*. Cambridge, MA: MIT Press.

Norman, D. A. and Draper, S. W. (Eds.). (1986). *User Centered System Design: New Perspectives on Human-Computer Interaction*. London, U.K.: Lawrence Erlbaum Associates.

Norman, D. A., Miller, J., and Henderson, A. (1995, May 7–11). What you see, some of what's in the future, and how we go about doing it: HI at Apple computer. Paper presented at the *Conference companion on Human Factors in Computing Systems: CHI '95*. Denver, CO. doi:10.1145/223355.223477.

Novick, D. G. (1999). Using the cognitive walkthrough for operating procedures. *Interactions, 6*(3), 31–37. doi:10.1145/301153.301166.

Odlyzko, A. M. (2003, September 8–11). Internet traffic growth: Sources and implications. Paper presented at the *Optical Transmission Systems and Equipment for WDM Networking II*. Orlando, FL.

Olivetti Belardinelli, M. (1973). *La costruzione della realtà* [The construction of reality]. Torino, Italy: Boringhieri.

Olson, G. M. and Moran, T. P. (1998). Commentary on "Damaged merchandise?". *Human–Computer Interaction, 13*(3), 263–323. doi:10.1207/s15327051hci1303_3.

Olyslager, P. (2012). Why the user experience can or cannot be designed. Retrieved December 1, 2012, from http://blog.usabilla.com/how-to-design-for-the-user-experience/

Oppenheim, A. N. (2000). *Questionnaire Design, Interviewing and Attitude Measurement.* New York: Continuum.

Oppenheimer, D. M. (2008). The secret life of fluency. *Trends in Cognitive Sciences, 12*(6), 237–241. doi:10.1016/j.tics.2008.02.014.

O'Reilly, T. (2007). What is web 2.0: Design patterns and business models for the next generation of software. *Communications & Strategies, 65*(1st Quarter), 17–37.

Ovaska, S. and Räihä, K.-J. (1995, May 7–11). Parallel design in the classroom. Paper presented at the *Conference Companion on Human Factors in Computing Systems: CHI '95.* Denver, CO. doi:10.1145/223355.223666.

Oxford Dictionaries. (2010). meme. Retrieved September 15, 2012, from http://oxforddictionaries.com/definition/meme

Palen, L. and Salzman, M. (2002, November 16–20). Voice-mail diary studies for naturalistic data capture under mobile conditions. Paper presented at the *Conference on Computer Supported Cooperative Work: CSCW '02,* New Orleans, LA. doi:10.1145/587078.587092.

Patton, M. Q. (1987). *How to Use Qualitative Methods in Evaluation.* Newbury Park, CA: Sage.

di Pellegrino, G., Fadiga, L., Fogassi, L., Gallese, V., and Rizzolatti, G. (1992). Understanding motor events: A neurophysiological study. *Experimental Brain Research, 91*(1), 176–180.

Petrie, H. and Bevan, N. (2009). The evaluation of accessibility, usability, and user experience. In C. Stephanidis (Ed.), *The Universal Access Handbook* (pp. 299–314). Boca Raton, FL: CRC Press.

Petrie, H., Hamilton, F., King, N., and Pavan, P. (2006, April 22–27). Remote usability evaluations with disabled people. Paper presented at the *SIGCHI Conference on Human Factors in Computing Systems: CHI '06.* Montreal, Quebec, Canada. doi:10.1145/1124772.1124942.

Petrie, H. and Kheir, O. (2007, April 30–May 3). The relationship between accessibility and usability of websites. Paper presented at the *Conference on Human Factors in Computing Systems: 'CHI 07.* San Jose, CA. doi:10.1145/1240624.1240688.

Ping, R. M., Dhillon, S., and Beilock, S. L. (2009). Reach for what you like: The body's role in shaping preferences. *Emotion Review, 1*(2), 140–150. doi:10.1177/1754073908100439.

Plotkin, H. (1997). *Evolution in Mind: An Introduction to Evolutionary Psychology.* London, U.K.: Allen Lane & Penguin.

Polson, P. G. and Lewis, C. (1990). Theory-based design for easily learned interfaces. *Human–Computer Interaction, 5*(2), 191–220. doi:10.1207/s15327051hci0502&3_3.

Polson, P. G., Lewis, C., Rieman, J., and Wharton, C. (1992). Cognitive walkthroughs: A method for theory-based evaluation of user interfaces. *International Journal of Man-Machine Studies, 36*(5), 741–773. doi:10.1016/0020-7373(92)90039-N.

Poole, A. and Ball, L. (2006). Eye tracking in human-computer interaction and usability research: Current status and future prospects. In C. Ghaoui (Ed.), *Encyclopedia of Human Computer Interaction* (pp. 211–219). London, U.K.: Idea Group Reference.

Purchase, H. C. (2000). Effective information visualisation: A study of graph drawing aesthetics and algorithms. *Interacting with Computers, 13*(2), 147–162. doi:10.1016/s0953-5438(00)00032-1.

Purchase, H. C., Carrington, D., and Allder, J.-A. (2002). Empirical evaluation of aesthetics-based graph layout. *Empirical Software Engineering, 7*(3), 233–255. doi:10.1023/a:1016344215610.

Ramaprasad, A. (1987). Cognitive process as a basis for MIS and DSS design. *Management Science, 33*(2), 139–148. doi:10.1287/mnsc.33.2.139.

Regan, B. (2004, May 17–22). Accessibility and design: A failure of the imagination. Paper presented at the *International Cross-Disciplinary Workshop on Web Accessibility: W4A '04*. New York. doi:10.1145/990657.990663.

Reichelt, L. (2008). The general public myth (or, the whole world is not your user). Retrieved December 1, 2012, from http://www.disambiguity.com/the-general-public-myth/

Reid, G. B. (1985). Current status of the development of the subjective workload assessment technique. *Proceedings of the Human Factors and Ergonomics Society Annual Meeting, 29*(3), 220–223. doi:10.1177/154193128502900303.

Reid, L. G. and Snow-Weaver, A. (April 21–22, 2008). WCAG 2.0: A web accessibility standard for the evolving web. Paper presented at the *International Cross-Disciplinary Conference on Web Accessibility: W4A '08*. Beijing, China. doi:10.1145/1368044.1368069.

Reitman, J. S. (1971). Mechanisms of forgetting in short-term memory. *Cognitive Psychology, 2*(2), 185–195. doi:10.1016/0010-0285(71)90008-9.

Renfrow, D. G. (2004). A cartography of passing in everyday life. *Symbolic Interaction, 27*(4), 485–506. doi:10.1525/si.2004.27.4.485.

Ribera, M., Porras, M., Boldu, M., Termens, M., Sule, A., and Paris, P. (2009). Web content accessibility guidelines 2.0: A further step towards accessible digital information. *Program: Electronic Library and Information Systems, 43*(4), 392–406. doi:10.1108/00330330910998048.

Rieman, J. (1993, April 24–29). The diary study: A workplace-oriented research tool to guide laboratory efforts. Paper presented at the *Conference on Human Factors in Computing Systems: INTERACT '93 and CHI '93*. Amsterdam, the Netherlands. doi:10.1145/169059.169255.

Riva, G. (2009). Presence as cognitive process. In D. Benyon, M. Smyth, and I. Helgason (Eds.), *Presence for Everyone: A Short Guide to Presence Research* (pp. 29–31). Edinburgh, U.K.: Napier University.

Riva, G., Baños, R. M., Botella, C., Wiederhold, B. K., and Gaggioli, A. (2012). Positive technology: Using interactive technologies to promote positive functioning. *Cyberpsychology, Behavior, and Social Networking, 15*(2), 69–77. doi:10.1089/cyber.2011.0139.

Riva, G. and Mantovani, F. (2012). From the body to the tools and back: A general framework for presence in mediated interactions. *Interacting with Computers, 24*(4), 203–210. doi:10.1016/j.intcom.2012.04.007.

Riva, G., Waterworth, J. A., Waterworth, E. L., and Mantovani, F. (2011). From intention to action: The role of presence. *New Ideas in Psychology, 29*(1), 24–37. doi:10.1016/j.newideapsych.2009.11.002.

Rizzo, A., Marchigiani, E., and Andreadis, A. (1997, August 18–20). The AVANTI project: Prototyping and evaluation with a cognitive walkthrough based on the Norman's model of action. Paper presented at the *2nd Conference on Designing Interactive Systems: Processes, Practices, Methods, and Techniques: DIS '97*. Amsterdam, the Netherlands. doi:10.1145/263552.263629.

Rizzolatti, G. and Arbib, M. A. (1998). Language within our grasp. *Trends in Neuroscience, 21*(5), 188–194. doi:10.1016/S0166-2236(98)01260-0.

Robinson, D. and Fitter, M. (1992). Supportive evaluation methodology: A method to facilitate system development. *Behaviour & Information Technology, 11*(3), 151–159. doi:10.1080/01449299208924332.

Rogers, Y., Sharp, H., and Preece, J. (2011). *Interaction Design: Beyond Human-Computer Interaction* (3rd edn.). New York: John Wiley & Sons.

Ross, C., Orr, E. S., Sisic, M., Arseneault, J. M., Simmering, M. G., and Orr, R. R. (2009). Personality and motivations associated with Facebook use. *Computers in Human Behavior, 25*(2), 578–586. doi:10.1016/j.chb.2008.12.024.

Roto, V., Law, E., Vermeeren, A., and Hoonhout, J. (2011). *User Experience White Paper. Result from Dagstuhl Seminar on Demarcating User Experience*, September 15–18, 2010. Retrieved September 15, 2012, from http://www.allaboutux.org/files/UX-WhitePaper.pdf

Rotter, J. B. (1954). *Social Learning and Clinical Psychology*. Upper Saddle River, NJ: Prentice-Hall.

Rotter, J. B. (1966). Generalized expectancies for internal versus external control of reinforcement. *Psychological Monographs, 80*(1), 1–28. doi:10.1037/h0092976.

Roulstone, A. (2010). Access and accessibility. In J. Stone and M. Blouin (Eds.), *International Encyclopedia of Rehabilitation* (pp. 1–12). Buffalo, NY: Center for International Rehabilitation Research Information and Exchange (CIRRIE). Retrieved September 15, 2012, from http://cirrie.buffalo.edu/encyclopedia/article.php?id = 153&language = en

Rubin, J. and Chisnell, D. (2008). *Handbook of Usability Testing: How to Plan, Design, and Conduct Effective Tests* (2nd edn.). New York: John Wiley & Sons.

Rumhelhart, D. E., Lindsay, P. H., and Norman, D. A. (1972). A process model for long-term memory. In E. Tulving and W. Donaldson (Eds.), *Organization of Memory* (pp. 197–246). New York: Academic Press.

Russell, J. A. (2003). Core affect and the psychological construction of emotion. *Psychological Review, 110*(1), 145–172. doi:10.1037//0033-295X.110.1.145.

Ryan, T. and Xenos, S. (2011). Who uses Facebook? An investigation into the relationship between the Big Five, shyness, narcissism, loneliness, and Facebook usage. *Computers in Human Behavior, 27*(5), 1658–1664. doi:10.1016/j.chb.2011.02.004.

Rydin, Y., Bleahu, A., Davies, M., Dávila, J. D., Friel, S., De Grandis, G. et al. (2012). Shaping cities for health: Complexity and the planning of urban environments in the 21st century. *Lancet, 379*(9831), 2079–2108. doi:10.1016/S0140-6736(12)60435-8.

Saha, D. and Mukherjee, A. (2003). Pervasive computing: A paradigm for the 21st century. *Computer, 36*(3), 25–31. doi:10.1109/MC.2003.1185214.

Salimkhan, G., Manago, A. M., and Greenfield, P. M. (2010). The construction of the virtual self on MySpace. *Cyberpsychology, 4*(1), Art. 1. Retrieved September 15, 2012, from http://cyberpsychology.eu/view.php?cisloclanku = 2010050203&article = 1

Salvendy, G. (2002). Use of subjective rating scores in *ergonomics* research and practice. *Ergonomics, 45*(14), 1005–1007. doi:10.1080/00140130210166852.

Sánchez, M. C. and Schlossberg, L. (2001). *Passing: Identity and Interpretation in Sexuality, Race, and Religion*. New York: New York University Press.

Sauro, J. and Lewis, J. R. (2012). *Quantifying the User Experience*. Waltham, MA: Morgan Kaufmann.

Schacter, D. L. (1989). Memory. In M. I. Posner (Ed.), *Foundation of Cognitive Science* (pp. 683–725). Cambridge, MA: Bradford Books.

Schmettow, M. (2008, September 1–5). Heterogeneity in the usability evaluation process. Paper presented at the *22nd British HCI Group Annual Conference on People and Computers: Culture, Creativity, Interaction: BCS-HCI '08*. Liverpool, U.K. Retrieved September 15, 2012, from http://portal.acm.org/citation.cfm?id = 1531514.1531527&coll = Portal&dl = GUIDE&CFID = 102664816&CFTOKEN = 12988936

Schmettow, M. (2012). Sample size in usability studies. *Communications of the ACM, 55*(4), 64–70. doi:10.1145/2133806.2133824.

Schrepp, M. (2006). On the efficiency of keyboard navigation in Web sites. *Universal Access in the Information Society, 5*(2), 180–188. doi:10.1007/s10209-006-0036-x.

Schuler, D. and Namioka, A. (1993). *Participatory Design: Principles and Practices*. Hillsdale, NJ: Lawrence Erlbaum Associates.

Sears, A. (1997). Heuristic walkthroughs: Finding the problems without the noise. *International Journal of Human–Computer Interaction, 9*(3), 213–234. doi:10.1207/s15327590ijhc0903_2.

Seligman, M. E. P. and Csikszentmihalyi, M. (2000). Positive psychology. *American Psychologist, 55*(1), 5–14. doi:10.1037//0003-066X.56.1.89.

Sen, A. (1998). Mortality as an indicator of economic success and failure. *The Economic Journal, 108*(446), 1–25. doi:10.1111/1468-0297.00270.

Sen, A. (2002). Health: Perception versus observation. *British Medical Journal (Clinical Research Edition), 324*(7342), 860–861. doi:10.1136/bmj.324.7342.860.

Sereno, S. C. and Rayner, K. (2003). Measuring word recognition in reading: Eye movements and event-related potentials. *Trends in Cognitive Sciences, 7*(11), 489–493. doi:10.1016/j.tics.2003.09.010.

Shaw, L. H. and Gant, L. M. (2002). In defense of the Internet: The relationship between Internet communication and depression, loneliness, self-esteem, and perceived social support. *Cyberpsychology and Behavior, 5*(2), 157–171. doi:10.1089/109493102753770552.

Sheldon, P. (2009). "I'll poke you. You'll poke me!" Self-disclosure, social attraction, predictability and trust as important predictors of Facebook relationships. *Cyberpsychology, 3*(2), Art. 1. Retrieved September 15, 2012, from http://www.cyberpsychology.eu/view.php?cisloclanku = 2009111101article = 1

Shneiderman, B. (1983). Direct manipulation: A step beyond programming languages. *Computer, 16*(8), 57–69. doi:10.1109/MC.1983.1654471.

Shneiderman, B. (1986). *Designing the User Interface: Strategies for Effective Human-Computer Interaction.* Boston, MA: Addison-Wesley.

Shneiderman, B. (1987). *Designing the User Interface: Strategies for Effective Human-Computer-Interaction.* Boston, MA: Addison Wesley Longman.

Shneiderman, B. (2000). Universal usability. *Communications of the ACM, 43*(5), 84–91. doi:10.1145/332833.332843.

Shneiderman, B. (2003). *Leonardo's Laptop: Human Needs and the New Computing Technologies.* Cambridge, MA: MIT Press.

Short, J., Williams, E., and Christie, B. (1976). *The Social Psychology of Telecommunications.* London, U.K.: Wiley.

Siibak, A. (2009). Constructing the self through the photo selection—Visual impression management on social networking websites. *Cyberpsychology, 3*(1), Art. 1. Retrieved September 15, 2012, from http://cyberpsychology.eu/view.php?cisloclanku = 2009061501&article = 1

Slimani, P. L. (2011, February 11). Révolution tunisienne: "Facebook m'a tuer". [Tunisian Revolution: "Facebook killing me"]. *Jeune Afrique, 51, 49.*

Smith, S. L. and Mosier, J. N. (1986). *Guidelines for Designing User Interface Software.* (ESD–TR–86–278/MTR 10090). Retrieved from MITRE Corporation website.

Sperry, R. A. and Fernandez, J. D. (2008). Usability testing using physiological analysis. *Journal of Computing Sciences in Colleges, 23*(6), 157–163.

Spool, J. and Schroeder, W. (2001, March 31–April 5). Testing web sites: Five users is nowhere near enough. Paper presented at the *Human Factors in Computing Systems: CHI '01.* Seattle, WA. doi:10.1145/634067.634236.

Stanton, N. A. (2006). Hierarchical task analysis: Developments, applications, and extensions. *Applied Ergonomics, 37*(1), 55–79. doi:10.1016/j.apergo.2005.06.003.

Stanton, N. A. and Stammers, R. B. (2002). Creative (dis)agreement in ergonomics. *Ergonomics, 45*(14), 963–965. doi:10.1080/00140130210166960.

Stanton, N. A. and Young, M. S. (1999). *A Guide to Methodology in Ergonomics: Design for Human Use.* London, U.K.: Taylor & Francis.

Stephanidis, C. (1995). Towards user interfaces for all: Some critical issues. In K. O. Yuichiro Anzai and M. Hirohiko (Eds.), *Advances in Human Factors/Ergonomics* (Vol. 20, pp. 137–142). Amsterdam, the Netherlands: Elsevier. doi:10.1016/s0921-2647(06)80024-9.

Stephanidis, C. (1997). Unified user interface development. *ERCIM News,* (28). Retrieved September 15, 2012, from Ercim.eu website: http://www.ercim.eu/publication/Ercim_News/enw28/stephanidis.html

Stephanidis, C. (2001). User interfaces for all: New perspectives into human-computer inter-action. In C. Stephanidis (Ed.), *User Interfaces for All: Concepts, Methods, and Tools* (pp. 3–17). Mahwah, NJ: Lawrence Erlbaum Associates.

Stephanidis, C. and Emiliani, P. L. (1998, June 23). Design for All in the TIDE ACCESS Project. Paper presented at the *TIDE '98*, Helsinki, Finland. Retrieved September 15, 2012, from http://www.dinf.ne.jp/doc/english/Us_Eu/conf/tide98/164/stephanidis_emiliani.html

Stephanidis, C., Paramythis, A., Sfyrakis, M., Stergiou, A., Maou, N., Leventis, A. et al. (1998). Adaptable and adaptive user interfaces for disabled users in the AVANTI project. In S. Trigila, A. Mullery, M. Campolargo, H. Vanderstraeten, and M. Mampaey (Eds.), *Intelligence in Services and Networks: Technology for Ubiquitous Telecom Services* (Vol. 1430, pp. 153–166). Berlin, Germany: Springer. doi:10.1007/BFb0056962.

Stiegler, B. (1992). Leroi-Gourhan, part maudite de l'anthropologie. *Les Nouvelles de l'Archologie, 48–49*, 23–30.

Still, A. W. (1969). Proactive interference and spontaneous alternation in rats. *Quarterly Journal of Experimental Psychology, 21*(4), 339–345. doi:10.1080/14640746908400229.

Strain, P., Shaikh, A. D., and Boardman, R. (2007, April 30–May 3). Thinking but not seeing: Think-aloud for non-sighted users. Paper presented at the *Human Factors in Computing Systems: CHI '07*. San Jose, CA. doi:10.1145/1240866.1240910.

Streitz, N., Kameas, A., and Mavrommati, I. (2007). Preface. In N. Streitz, A. Kameas, and I. Mavrommati (Eds.), *The Disappearing Computer: Interaction Design, System Infrastructures and Applications for Smart Environments* (pp. iv–x). Berlin, Germany: Springer-Verlag.

Streitz, N. and Nixon, P. (2005). The disappearing computer. *Communications of the ACM, 48*(3), 33–35. doi:10.1145/1047671.1047700.

Subrahmanyam, K. (2007). Adolescent online communication: Old issues, new intensi-ties. *Cyberpsychology: Journal of Psychosocial Research on Cyberspace, 1*(1), Art. 1. Retrieved September 15, 2012, from http://cyberpsychology.eu/view.php?cisloclanku = 2007070701&article = 1

Sutherland, I. E. (1964, June 24–26). Sketch pad a man-machine graphical communication system. Paper presented at the *SHARE Design Automation Workshop: DAC '64*. Atlantic City, NJ. doi:10.1145/800265.810742.

Sutherland, I. E. (2003). Sketchpad: A man-machine graphical communication system. Retrieved September 15, 2012, from http://www.cl.cam.ac.uk/TechReports/

Swain, A. D. and Guttmann, H. E. (1980). Handbook of human reliability analysis with empha-sis on nuclear power plant applications. (NUREG/CR-1278). Retrieved September 15, 2012, from US Nuclear Regulatory Commission website. http://pbadupws.nrc.gov/docs/ML0712/ML071210299.pdf

Tajfel, H. (1978). *Differentiation between Social Groups: Studies in the Social Psychology of Intergroup Relations*. London, U.K.: Academic Press.

Tassé, M. J., Schalock, R. L., and Thompson, J. R. (2008). International implementation of the supports intensity scale. Retrieved September 15, 2012, from http://www.siswebsite.org/galleries/default-file/SISWPInternational.pdf

Termens, M., Ribera, M., Porras, M., Boldú, M., Sulé, A., and Paris, P. (2009 April 20–24). Web content accessibility guidelines: From 1.0 to 2.0. Paper presented at the *18th International Conference on World Wide Web: WWW '09*. Madrid, Spain. doi:10.1145/1526709.1526912.

Tognazzi, B. (2005). First principles of interaction design. Retrieved September 15, 2012, from http://www.asktog.com/basics/firstPrinciples.html

Tonn-Eichstädt, H. (2006, October 23–25). Measuring website usability for visually impaired people —A modified GOMS analysis. Paper presented at the *8th International ACM SIGACCESS Conference on Computers and Accessibility: ASSETS '06*. Portland, OR. doi:10.1145/1168987.1168998.

Tullis, T. and Albert, W. (2008). *Measuring the User Experience: Collecting, Analyzing, and Presenting Usability Metrics (Interactive Technologies)*. San Francisco, CA: Morgan Kaufmann.

Turkle, S. (1995). *Life on the Screen: Identity in the Age of the Internet*. New York: Touchstone.

Turner, C. W., Lewis, J. R., and Nielsen, J. (2006). *Determining Usability Test Sample Size* (Vol. 2, 2nd edn.). Boca Raton, FL: CRC Press.

U.S. Access Board. (2004). *Revised ADA and ABA accessibility guidelines*. Retrieved September 15, 2012, from http://www.access-board.gov/ada-aba/final.pdf

U.S. Congress. (1973). *Individuals with disabilities education Act. Pub. L. 93–112—Sep. 26, 1973*.

U.S. Department of Health and Human Services. (2011). Draft guidance for industry and food and drug administration staff—Applying human factors and usability engineering to optimize medical device design. Retrieved September 15, 2012, from http://www.fda.gov/MedicalDevices/DeviceRegulationandGuidance/GuidanceDocuments/ucm259748.htm

UN Enable. (2006). Some facts about person with disabilities, Retrieved September 15, 2012, from http://www.un.org/disabilities/convention/pdfs/factsheet.pdf

Underwood, B. J. (1957). Interference and forgetting. *Psychological Review, 64*(1), 49–60. doi:10.1037/h0044616.

United Nations (UN). (1975). Declaration on the rights of disabled persons (3447). Retrieved September 15, 2012, from http://www2.ohchr.org/english/law/res3447.htm

United Nations (UN). (1982). World programme of action concerning disabled persons. (A/RES/37/52). Retrieved September 15, 2012, from UN website. http://unstats.un.org/unsd/demographic/sconcerns/disability/A-RES-37-52.htm

United Nations (UN). (1993). Vienna declaration and programme of action. (48/121). Retrieved September 15, 2012, from UN website. http://www.unhchr.ch/huridocda/huridoca.nsf/(symbol)/a.conf.157.23.en

United Nations (UN). (2006). Convention on the rights of persons with disabilities. (A/RES/61/106). New York: UN. Retrieved September 15, 2012, from http://www.un-documents.net/a61r106.htm

United Nations (UN). (2007). World population prospects: The 2006 revision. Retrieved September 15, 2012, from UN website. http://www.un.org/esa/population/publications/wpp2006/English.pdf

United States Congress. (1998). Section 508 of The Rehabilitation Act (Public Law 29 U.S.C. 794d). Retrieved September 15, 2013, from http://www.section508.gov

Urokohara, H., Tanaka, K., Furuta, K., Honda, M., and Kurosu, M. (2000 April 20–24). NEM: "novice expert ratio method" a usability evaluation method to generate a new performance measure. Paper presented at the *Human Factors in Computing Systems: CHI '00*. Hague, the Netherlands. doi:10.1145/633292.633394.

Üstün, T. B., Chatterji, S., Bickenbach, J. E., Kostanjsek, N., and Schneider, M. (2003a). The international classification of functioning, disability and health: A new tool for understanding disability and health. *Disability and Rehabilitation, 25*(11–12), 565–571. doi:10.1080/0963828031000137063.

Üstün, T. B., Chatterji, S., Kostanjsek, N., Rehm, J., Kennedy, C., Epping-Jordan, J. et al. (2010). Developing the World Health Organization disability assessment schedule 2.0. *Bulletin of the World Health Organization*, 1–23. doi:10.2471/BLT.09.067231.

Üstün, T. B., Chatterji, S., Mechbal, A., Murray, C. J. L., and WHS Collaborating groups. (2003b). The World Health Surveys. In C. J. L. Murray and D. B. Evans (Eds.), *Health Systems Performance Assessment: Debates, Methods and Empiricism* (pp. 797–808). Geneva, Switzerland: World Health Organization.

Väänänen-Vainio-Mattila, K., Väätäjä, H., and Vainio, T. (2008). Opportunities and challenges of designing the Service User eXperience (SUX) in Web 2.0. In P. Saariluoma and H. Isomäki (Eds.), *Future Interaction Design II*. London, U.K.: Springer. doi:10.1007/978-1-84800-385-9_6.

Väänänen-Vainio-Mattila, K. and Wäljas, M. (2009, April 4–9). Development of evaluation heuristics for web service user experience. Paper presented at the *Human Factors in Computing Systems: CHI '09.* Boston, MA. doi:10.1145/1520340.1520554.

van den Haak, M. J. and de Jong, M. D. T. (2003, September 21–24). Exploring two methods of usability testing: Concurrent versus retrospective think-aloud protocols. Paper presented at the *IEEE International Professional Communication Conference: IPCC '03.* Orlando, FL. doi:10.1109/IPCC.2003.1245501.

van den Haak, M. J., de Jong, M. D. T., and Jan Schellens, P. (2003). Retrospective vs. concurrent think-aloud protocols: Testing the usability of an online library catalogue. *Behaviour & Information Technology, 22*(5), 339–351. doi:10.1080/0044929031000

Vidulich, M. A. and Tsang, P. S. (1985). Assessing subjective workload assessment: A comparison of SWAT and the NASA-bipolar methods. *Proceedings of the Human Factors and Ergonomics Society Annual Meeting, 29*(1), 71–75. doi:10.1177/154193128502900122.

Vidulich, M. A. and Tsang, P. S. (1986). Techniques of subjective workload assessment: A comparison of SWAT and the NASA-Bipolar methods. *Ergonomics, 29*(11), 1385–1398. doi:10.1080/00140138608967253.

Virzi, R. A. (1990). Streamlining the design process: Running fewer subjects. *Proceedings of the Human Factors and Ergonomics Society Annual Meeting Proceedings, 34,* 291–294. doi:10.1177/154193129003400411.

Virzi, R. A. (1992). Refining the test phase of usability evaluation: How many subjects is enough? *Human Factors, 34*(4), 457–468.

W3C-WAI. (2006). Introduction to web accessibility. Retrieved September 15, 2012, 2011, from http://www.w3.org/WAI/intro/accessibility.php

W3C-WAI. (2008). Web content accessibility guidelines (WCAG) 2.0. Retrieved September 15, 2012, from http://www.w3.org/TR/WCAG20

W3C-WAI. (2012). Accessibility. Retrieved September 15, 2012, from http://www.w3.org/standards/webdesign/accessibility

W3C—World Wide Web Consortium. (2012). W3C. Retrieved September 15, 2012, from http://www.w3.org/

Walther, J. B. (1996). Computer-mediated communication. *Communication Research, 23*(1), 3–43. doi:10.1177/009365096023001001.

Ward, R. D., Marsden, P. H., Cahill, B., and Johnson, C. (2001, September 10–14). Using skin conductivity to detect emotionally significant events in human-computer interaction. Paper presented at the *13th Annual Conference of the Association Francophone d'Interaction Homme-Machine: AFIHM 'oi and 15th Annual Conference of the Human–Computer Interaction Group of the British Computer Society: IHM-HCI '01.* Lille, France.

Ware, C., Purchase, H. C., Colpoys, L., and McGill, M. (2002). Cognitive measurements of graph aesthetics. *Information Visualization, 1*(2), 103–110. doi:10.1057/palgrave.ivs.9500013.

Warschauer, M. (2003). *Technology and Social Inclusion: Rethinking the Digital Divide.* Cambridge, MA: MIT Press.

Wastell, D. G. and Newman, M. (1996). Stress, control and computer system design: A psychophysiological field study. *Behaviour & Information Technology, 15*(3), 183–192. doi:10.1080/014492996120247.

Waterson, S., Landay, J. A., and Matthews, T. (2002, April 20–25). In the lab and out in the wild: Remote web usability testing for mobile devices. Paper presented at the *Human Factors in Computing Systems: CHI '02.* Minneapolis, MN. doi:10.1145/506443.506602.

Waterworth, J. A., Waterworth, E. L., Mantovani, F., and Riva, G. (2010). On feeling (the) present: An evolutionary account of the sense of presence in physical and electronically-mediated environments. *Journal of Consciousness Studies, 17*(1–2), 167–178.

Wegner, D. M. (1986). Transactive memory: A contemporary analysis of the group mind. In B. Mullen and G. R. Goethals (Eds.), *Theories of Group Behavior* (pp. 185–208). New York: Springer-Verlag.

Weiser, E. B. (2001). The functions of internet use and their social and psychological consequences. *Cyberpsychology and Behavior, 4*(6), 723–743. doi:10.1089/109493101753376678.

Weiser, M. and Shertz, J. (1983). Programming problem representation in novice and expert programmers. *International Journal of Man-Machine Studies, 19*(4), 391–398. doi:10.1016/S0020-7373(83)80061-3.

Wellman, H. M. (Ed.). (1990). *The Child's Theory of Mind.* Cambridge, MA: MIT Press.

Wharton, C., Bradford, J., Jeffries, R., and Franzke, M. (1992, May 3–7). Applying cognitive walkthroughs to more complex user interfaces: Experiences, issues, and recommendations. Paper presented at the *SIGCHI Conference on Human Factors in Computing Systems: CHI '92.* Monterey, CA. doi:10.1145/142750.142864.

Wharton, C., Rieman, J., Lewis, C., and Polson, P. G. (1994). The cognitive walkthrough method: A practitioner's guide. In J. Nielsen and R. L. Mack (Eds.), *Usability Inspection Methods* (pp. 105–140). New York: John Wiley & Sons.

Widyanto, L. and McMurran, M. (2004). The psychometric properties of the internet addiction test. *Cyberpsychology and Behavior, 7*(4), 443–450. doi:10.1089/1094931041774578.

Wiederhold, B. K. and Riva, G. (2012). Positive technology supports shift to preventive, integrative health. *Cyberpsychology, Behavior and Social Networking, 15*(2), 67–68. doi:10.1089/cyber.2011.1533.

Wikipedia contributors. (2011). Ecological niche. *The Free Encyclopedia. Wikipedia.* Retrieved September 15, 2012, from http://en.wikipedia.org/wiki/Ecological_niche

Wikipedia contributors. (2012a). History of the Internet. *Wikipedia, The Free Encyclopedia.* Retrieved September 15, 2012, from http://en.wikipedia.org/wiki/History_of_the_Internet

Wikipedia contributors. (2012b). Interference theory. *Wikipedia, The Free Encyclopedia, 2013.* Retrieved September 15, 2012, from http://en.wikipedia.org/w/index.php?title = Interference_theory&oldid = 526399489

Wikipedia contributors. (2012c). Semantic web. *Wikipedia, The Free Encyclopedia.* Retrieved September 15, 2012, from http://en.wikipedia.org/wiki/Semantic_web

Wikipedia contributors. (2012d). Social stigma. *Wikipedia, The Free Encyclopedia.* Retrieved September 15, 2012, from http://en.wikipedia.org/wiki/Social_stigma

Wikipedia contributors. (2012e). Web browsers. *Wikipedia, The Free Encyclopedia.* Retrieved September 15, 2012, from http://en.wikipedia.org/wiki/Web_browser

Wikipedia contributors. (2012f). World Wide Web. *Wikipedia, The Free Encyclopedia.* Retrieved September 15, 2012, from http://en.wikipedia.org/wiki/World_wide_web

Wilson, G. and Sasse, M. A. (2000). Do users always know what's good for them? Utilising physiological responses to assess media quality. In S. McDonald, Y. Waern, and G. Cockton (Eds.), *People and Computers XIV: Usability or Else!* (pp. 327–339). Sunderland, U.K.: Springer.

Winsberg, E. (2003). Simulated experiments: Methodology for a virtual world. *Philosophy of Science, 70*(1), 105. doi:10.1086/367872.

Wohldmann, E. L., Healy, A. F., and Bourne, L. E. (2008). A mental practice superiority effect: Less retroactive interference and more transfer than physical practice. *Journal of Experimental Psychology: Learning, Memory, and Cognition, 34*(4), 823–833. doi:10.1037/0278-7393.34.4.823.

Woolrych, A. and Cockton, G. (2001, September 10–14). Why and when five test users aren't enough. Paper presented at the *Proceedings of IHM-HCI 2001 Conference.* Toulouse, France. http://www.netraker.com/nrinfo/research/FiveUsers.pdf

World Health Organization (WHO). (1980). *International Classification of Impairments, Disabilities, and Handicaps. A Manual of Classification Relating to the Consequences of Disease.* Geneva, Switzerland: WHO.

World Health Organization (WHO). (2001). *ICF: International Classification of Functioning, Disability and Health*. Geneva, Switzerland: WHO.

World Health Organization (WHO). (2002–2004). *World Health Survey*. Retrieved September 15, 2012, from WHO website. http://www.who.int/healthinfo/survey/en/

World Health Organization (WHO). (2008). *The Global Burden of Disease: 2004 Update*. Geneva, Switzerland: WHO.

World Health Organization (WHO). (2011). European report on preventing elder maltreatment. Retrieved September 15, 2012, from http://www.euro.who.int/__data/assets/pdf_file/0010/144676/e95110.pdf

World Health Organization (WHO) and World Bank. (2011). *World Report on Disability*. Geneva, Switzerland: WHO.

Xu, Q., Zhou, F., and Jiao, J. (2011). Affective-cognitive modeling for user experience with modular colored fuzzy petri nets. *Journal of Computing and Information Science in Engineering, 11*(1), 1–10. doi:10.1115/1.3563047.

Yannakakis, G. N. and Hallam, J. (2007). Capturing player enjoyment in computer games. In N. Baba and H. Handa (Eds.), *Advanced Intelligent Paradigms in Computer Games* (Vol. 71, pp. 175–201). London, U.K.: Springer-Verlag.

Young, K. S. (1998). Internet addiction: The emergence of a new clinical disorder. *Cyberpsychology and Behavior, 1*(3), 237–244. doi:10.1089/cpb.1998.1.237.

Zarghooni, S. (2007). A study of self-presentation in light of Facebook. From http://folk.uio.no/sasanz/Mistorie/Annet/Selfpresentation_on_Facebook.pdf

Zhang, P., Carey, J., Te'eni, D., and Tremaine, M. (2005). Integrating human-computer interaction development into the systems development life cycle: A methodology. *Communications of the Association for Information Systems, 15*(1), 512–544. Retrieved September 15, 2012, from http://aisel.aisnet.org/cgi/viewcontent.cgi?article = 3151&context = cais

Zimmerman, D. E., Akerelrea, C. A., Buller, D. B., Hau, B., and Leblanc, M. (2003). Integrating usability testing into the development of a 5 a day nutrition website for at-risk populations in the American Southwest. *Journal of Health Psychology, 8*(1), 119–134. doi:10.1177/1359105303008001448.

Zola, I. K. (1989). Toward the necessary universalizing of a disability policy. *Milbank Quarterly, 67*(Suppl. 2 Pt. 2), 401–428. doi:10.2307/3350151.

Zola, I. K. (1993). Disability statistics, what we count and what it tells us: A personal and political analysis. *Journal of Disability Policy Studies, 4*(2), 9–39. doi:10.1177/104420739300400202.

ZURBlog. (2011). User experience cannot be 'Designed'. Retrieved December 1, 2012, from http://www.zurb.com/article/655/user-experience-cannot-be-designed

Index

Printed and bound by CPI Group (UK) Ltd, Croydon, CR0 4YY

18/10/2024

01776262-0008